.A407
3

THE KILLERS
AND CRIPPLERS

THE KILLERS AND CRIPPLERS

Facts on Major Diseases in the United States Today

•

Compiled by
The National Health Education Committee

David McKay Company, Inc.
New York

Copyright © 1976 by National Health Education Committee
All rights reserved, including the right to reproduce
this book, or parts thereof, in any form, except for
the inclusion of brief quotations in a review.

Library of Congress Catalog Card Number: 74-25725
ISBN: 0-679-50541-5 cloth
0-679-50696-9 paper

MANUFACTURED IN THE UNITED STATES OF AMERICA

Contents

Introduction
What Are the Facts About Allergies and Infectious Diseases?	1
What Is the Prevalence and Cost of Arthritis and Rheumatism?	15
What Are We Doing About Blinding Eye Diseases?	34
What Are the Facts About Cancer?	51
What Are the Facts About Cerebral Palsy?	75
What Are the Facts About Deafness?	93
What Are the Facts About Digestive Diseases?	105
What Are the Facts About Epilepsy?	109
What Are the Facts About Genetic Disease?	120
What Are the Facts About High Blood Pressure?	140
What Are the Facts About Mental Illness?	153
What Are the Facts About Mental Retardation?	175
What Are the Facts About Multiple Sclerosis?	185
What Are the Facts About Muscular Dystrophy?	197
What Are the Facts About Parkinsonism?	208
What Are the Facts About the Population Problem?	214
What Are the Facts About Disabled People in this Country?	230
What Are the Facts About Tuberculosis?	245
Medical Research—Does It Pay Off in Lives and Dollars?	261
Vital Statistics and Other Tables	318

Introduction

The current publication of *The Killers and Cripplers* marks the eleventh edition of this source book of vital statistics on the principal causes of death and disability in the United States. Compiled by Jane E. McDonough, Executive Secretary of the National Health Education Committee, this up-to-date and thoroughly revised book portrays the triumphs and deficits of our national effort against the major killing and crippling diseases. It provides factual background for evaluating the progress and effectiveness of the various health and medical research programs, and it helps to pinpoint the areas of greatest need by identifying those programs in which research has progressed to a stage where more adequate funding could provide the greatest benefit to mankind.

There is no other comparable publication available today. I can strongly recommend this volume as an indispensable source of information to all those working in public health, medical research, and medical reporting.

The National Health Education Committee, which sponsors the book, was organized in 1953 to provide investigative facilities for finding means to provide better health and to reduce the incidence of disabilities and deaths in the United States. Its chairman is Mrs. Albert D. Lasker, and its board includes Howard A. Rusk, M.D.; Jeremiah Stamler, M.D.; Russel V. Lee, M.D.; Frederick J. Stare, M.D.; Mrs. John Gunther; Leonard Goldenson; and William McC. Blair, Jr.

MICHAEL E. DeBAKEY, M.D.

THE KILLERS AND CRIPPLERS

What Are the Facts About Allergies and Infectious Diseases?

I. What Are Infectious Diseases?

1. Infectious diseases occur whenever pathogenic microbes invade the body and disrupt or destroy any of the vital biologic processes. Infectious diseases, therefore, are always linked with microbes. The classic way of showing that a disease is infectious is to demonstrate its transmission from human to human or from animal to human.

II. What Are the Different Types of Infectious Diseases?

1. Infectious diseases are usually defined in terms of the disease-causing microbes. These microbes may be classified under the following headings:
    a. *Bacteria* are one-celled plants. Many of the more serious diseases—diphtheria, scarlet fever, tuberculosis—are caused by bacteria.
    b. *Parasites* are one-celled or multiple-celled. One of the most significant parasitic diseases is malaria. Others are schistosomiasis and filariasis, which are serious medical and socioeconomic problems in many of the developing nations of Asia and Africa.
    c. *Rickettsiae* are microbes that flourish only within cells of susceptible species. *Typhus fever,* a notorious affliction of mankind for more than 4 centuries, is caused by a rickettsial agent.

So is *Rocky Mountain spotted fever*. Rickettsiae are usually carried by arthropods—such as ticks, lice, fleas, and mites—and transmitted to man through bites.

d. *Viruses,* the smallest and simplest of the infectious disease microbes, are cellular parasites like the rickettsiae. Scientists have identified about 300 viruses that infect man; 150 cause respiratory tract infections alone. Viral diseases include smallpox, measles, polio, rabies, rubella (German measles), influenza, and the common cold.

e. *Fungi* are parasitic organisms of simple structure that live in soil, rotting vegetation, and bird excreta. Only a few fungal diseases—such as ringworm and athlete's foot—are contagious from man to man or from animal to man. The more serious fungal diseases are caught by inhaling contaminated material.

f. *Mycoplasmas* are the smallest of free-living organisms capable of reproducing themselves without assistance from other forms of life. They were formerly of most concern to veterinarians. Now mycoplasmas, particularly one called *M. pneumoniae,* have been implicated in human disease.

2. Many medical authorities suspect that repeated *acute respiratory infections* contribute to the development of emphysema and other crippling chronic lung disorders.

3. There is growing evidence from comparative animal studies that *slow-acting viruses or other microbes may cause such chronic disorders as rheumatoid arthritis and degenerative diseases of the nervous system.*

III. What Is the Incidence of Infectious Diseases in the United States?

1. In 1973, there were 228,820,000 episodes of infectious disease.[1]

Infectious and parasitic diseases	40,003,000
Common childhood diseases	5,002,000
Viruses, not otherwise specified	14,300,000
Other infective and parasitic	20,701,000

Respiratory conditions	188,817,000
Upper respiratory conditions (cold, etc.)	100,578,000
Influenza	79,143,000
Other respiratory (including pneumonia, bronchitis)	9,097,000
Total episodes of infectious and parasitic diseases and respiratory conditions	228,820,000

An average acute illness curtailed the patient's normal activities for approximately 5 days, for a total of more than 1 billion days of restricted activity.[1]

2. *Acute respiratory illnesses alone account for over half* of all *reported acute conditions. Viruses* are the infectious agents that cause most acute respiratory illness.[2]

3. But the total incidence of acute respiratory illness is estimated to be much higher because so much of acute respiratory illness is unrecorded. The typical American has 0.9, his under-6 child 1.6 nose, throat and lung infections each year.[1]

IV. How Many Days Do Americans Lose from Work and from School Due to Infectious Diseases?

1. 156,023,000 days were lost from work due to infectious diseases in 1973. *Infectious diseases caused approximately 50% of all days lost from work due to acute illness.*[1]

Infectious and parasitic diseases	20,868,000
Respiratory conditions	
Upper respiratory conditions (common cold)	40,345,000
Influenza	77,199,000
Other respiratory conditions (bronchitis, etc.)	17,611,000
Total days of work lost	156,023,000

The mean income for a full-time year-round worker in 1973 was $9,106, so that the *loss in income* is close to $37.32 per day, or a total of nearly *$6 billion for infectious diseases in 1973.*

2. 147,372,000 days were lost from school due to infectious and parasitic diseases and respiratory conditions in 1973. An

infectious disease accounted for 3 out of every 4 days lost from school due to an acute condition.[1]

3. More than 135,156,000 days were lost from work and another 110,928,000 days were lost from school in 1973 due to acute respiratory illnesses alone.[1]

V. How Many People Die of Infectious Diseases in the United States?

1. 107,612 Americans died of infectious diseases in 1973.[3] This is based on statistics for the underlying cause of death. The figure would be larger if contributory causes were considered.

Among the leading causes of death from infectious diseases were:

Influenza and pneumonia	62,559
Bronchitis	6,452
Kidney infections	6,134
Septicemia (blood poisoning)	4,560
Tuberculosis	3,875

2. Thus, among diseases, infections, as a group, ranked as the Number 4 killer after heart disease, cancer, and stroke.

VI. What Age Groups Are the Principal Victims of Infectious Diseases?

Infectious diseases kill chiefly the very young and very old, but they also take a great toll among people of working age.[3]

VII. What Do These Deaths Mean in Economic Terms?

1. If the 29,189 persons of working age who died of infectious diseases in 1973 had lived just one extra, healthy year, they could perhaps have *earned $265,795,030 in that one year alone.*

2. *The Federal Government could have gained at least $30 million in income tax revenue on those earnings in 1973.*[4]

VIII. How Much Do People Spend on Medical Treatment for Infectious Diseases in the United States?

In 1973, of the total pharmaceutical preparations shipped for human use, the wholesale value of prescription and non-prescription preparations purchased by Americans for respiratory infections alone amounted to *$613.6 million.*[5]

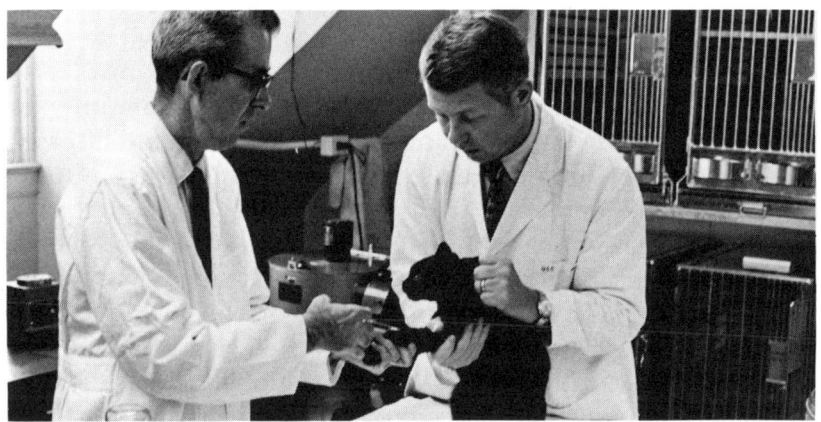

Scientists in the Laboratory of Parasitic Diseases of the National Institute of Allergy & Infectious Diseases take a blood sample from a cat as part of their studies of the role of the cat in the transmission of toxoplasmosis—a widespread parasitic infection which, in a pregnant woman, may severely damage an unborn child. (COURTESY OF NATIONAL INSTITUTES OF HEALTH)

IX. What Are Allergic and Immunologic Disorders?

1. Allergic disorders are the result of the abnormal reaction of some people to certain substances which are harmless to others. The tendency to hypersensitivity (allergy) seems to be inherited: Allergic parents often have allergic children. A person may be allergic to one or to many things. To develop a hypersensitivity, he must first be exposed to the specific substance to which he is sensitive. His body then "fights off" the ordinarily harmless material, very much as normal people resist infectious diseases. This "resistance" by the sensitive individual brings about allergic symptoms.

2. A wide variety of substances can cause allergies in the susceptible person. Substances he breathes in, such as pollens or molds, can cause hay fever or asthma.

The things he eats, including ordinary foods, can cause rashes or even respiratory problems. Some of the most violent reactions may result from drugs which he is given orally or by injections. Tetanus antitoxin (or other preparations containing horse serum), or penicillin, can cause shock and sudden death. So can insect stings.

Contact dermatitis—a skin eruption—is the usual reaction if a person touches a substance to which he is allergic. Cold, heat, light, chemicals and plants, such as poison ivy, can cause skin eruptions.

3. The more scientists learn about the body's immune system, the more they are coming to believe that many diseases, in addition to allergies, are immunologic in nature. Under suspicion are rheumatoid arthritis, systemic lupus erythematosus, Hashimoto's disease (a form of goiter), pernicious anemia, and a number of neurologic diseases—all of which display some characteristics of autoimmunity, or the production of antibodies which attack a person's own tissues. In addition, some rare childhood diseases—agammaglobulinemia, the Wiskott-Aldrich syndrome, and ataxia-telangiectasia—have been identified as ones in which one or more components of the immune response is missing at birth. Immunologic factors in various kinds of cancer are being investigated.

X. How Many People Are Suffering from Allergic Disorders in the United States?

1. *About 35 million Americans*—or about *17% of the total population*—are estimated to *suffer from an allergy at any given time*, according to the National Institute of Allergy and Infectious Diseases. Of this total, 23 million persons suffer from asthma and/or hay fever.[6]

2. Accurate figures on allergic conditions are hard to collect. This difficulty is complicated by the fact that many people suffer from more than one allergic condition. New disorders are being recognized and identified as allergic. Technology continually brings on new materials to which people may become allergic. Notable among these are detergents, cosmetics, plastics, perma-press cloth, and drugs.

XI. What Age Groups Are the Principal Sufferers of Asthma—One of the Most Serious Allergic Disorders?

1. Allergies may start early in childhood and last a lifetime. For example, asthma, one of the most serious allergic disorders, has a prevalence rate of 29.3 per 1,000 population in children under age 6, and 35.8 for persons 65 years of age and older.[7]

XII. How Much Do People Spend on Medical Treatment for Allergies in the United States?

1. Expenses for medical treatment for allergic conditions can only be estimated. It should be kept in mind that allergies may persist over long periods of time. Treatment includes skin tests for specific diagnosis, desensitization injections, steroid therapy, and the use of antihistamines, bronchodilators, sedatives, tranquilizers, and topical preparations. Secondary infections, particularly in patients with respiratory allergies, must be kept under control. Ideally, the severely allergic patient is continually in touch with his physician since his treatment must constantly be reevaluated as new drugs appear or the character of his allergy changes.

2. There are two figures which give some idea of the annual cost of medical treatment for allergic disorders.

   a. It is estimated that the number of patients in this country who are receiving injection therapy to relieve ragweed pollen hay fever is at least 1,000,000.[8] Assuming that this therapy costs each patient approximately $200 a year, the total annual cost would come to *$200,000,000.*

   b. Drug store sales of antihistamines—used largely by allergy sufferers—have a retail value of *more than $53 million.*[9] Separate figures for shipment of other products used in the treatment of allergies are not given. If these figures were available they would probably be enormous, since the Physicians Desk Reference lists pages of ethical drugs under the section on allergies. Some of the types of products in use are sun protectants, special food products, ear drops, eye drops and ointments, nasal sprays, hypoallergenic hair spray, cosmetics, and soaps; also pollen extracts, antihistamines, antipruritics, antitussives and expectorants, local and systemic steroids, bioflavonoids and other antihemorrhagic products; and bronchodilators, topical creams and ointments, as well as narcotics, tranquilizers, and vitamins.

XIII. How Much Is Being Spent for Research in Infectious and Allergic Diseases?

1. Out of an estimated budget of $119,452,000 for fiscal year 1975, the National Institute of Allergy and Infectious Diseases spent approximately *$96,957,000* for research in this area.[6]

2. *Another $8,960,000 was spent for training* in research in infectious diseases and allergies.[6]

3. Other expenditures of the National Institute of Allergy and Infectious Diseases fiscal year 1975 budget include nearly $12 million for institutional and resources support and development, and $1.6 million for program management.[6]

4. Other components of the National Institutes of Health awarded in 1975 over $50 million in grants for research in areas related to immunology and microbiology.[10]

XIV. What Have Been the Major Payoffs of Research in Infectious Diseases?

1. The really big research payoffs in infectious diseases have been the development of numerous vaccines, antibiotics, and sulfa drugs. Many major infectious diseases have been brought under complete control in the United States through the use of these products although the diseases are still rampant in other parts of the world.

    a. *Poliomyelitis,* which until a few years ago killed and crippled thousands of young people every year, has been eliminated as a public health problem in this country by the Salk and Sabin vaccines.

    b. *Measles* vaccine has almost wiped out this dangerous

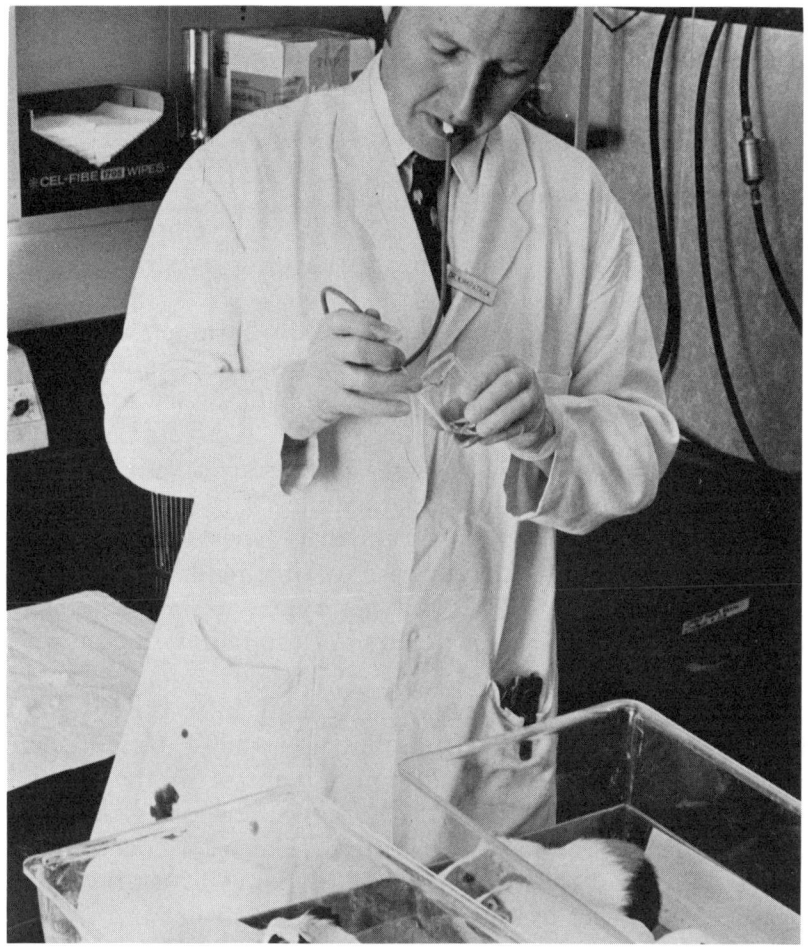

The passive transfer of an allergic reaction is used to study contact dermatitis. In this type of allergy, exposure of the skin to an antigen—the foreign protein in an allergy-causing substance—results in the formation of sensitized lymphocytes (white cells), which circulate in the individual's blood. These cells can be injected into a nonallergic subject and subsequent exposure to the antigen will cause an allergic reaction. As part of a study of contact dermatitis, a scientist in the Laboratory of Clinical Investigations of the National Institute of Allergy & Infectious Diseases paints the antigen (in this case a chemical known as chlorodinitrobenzene) on the skin of passively sensitized guinea pigs. (COURTESY OF NATIONAL INSTITUTES OF HEALTH)

disease of childhood. Its use has resulted in a sharp decrease in incidence of the disease, from 4 million in 1963 to 26,690 cases in 1973. From 1963 to 1968 alone, immunization efforts are estimated to have *saved the nation about $278 million in direct costs for medical care and another $253 million in indirect costs, or loss of productivity.*[11]

   c. *Smallpox, diphtheria, whooping cough, and tetanus vaccines* have been so effective that Americans now take freedom from these diseases for granted.

   d. A live *mumps* virus vaccine has been developed which is of particular value in children approaching puberty, adolescents, and adults.

   e. A *rubella* (German measles) vaccine became available in 1969 and is being used on a national basis. This should drastically reduce the number of malformed babies born to women acquiring this disease in early pregnancy. It is estimated that 20,000 infants in the United States suffered congenital defects as a result of the 1964 rubella epidemic.[11]

   f. Oral vaccines against Adenovirus types 4 and 7—common causes of respiratory disease among military recruits—have been developed. Both vaccines appear to be 95% effective, thus saving millions of dollars in hospitalization costs and training time.

2. Following the discovery of streptomycin in the 40's and other effective anti-TB drugs in the 1950's this former scourge began to be brought under control in the United States. In the period 1965-1973, active new cases reported have declined from 45,647 to 31,015. The most encouraging aspect of control efforts is use of TB drugs as a preventive measure. With the use of these drugs, which began in 1946, the TB death rate has declined 95%.[11]

3. Advances have been made in the prevention and treatment of other diseases:[12]

   a. Methods have been developed that show promise for synthesizing a whole new family of antibiotics tailor-made to combat bacterial infections.

   b. An experimental drug, rifampicin, has been found effective against viruses in the test tube and, when administered to carriers of meningococcal meningitis, appears to eliminate the bacteria in most cases.

   c. A vaccine against Group C meningococcal meningitis has been licensed for epidemic use in the U.S. A group A meningococcal vaccine has also been developed and is undergoing field trials in foreign countries where epidemics of the disease have occurred.

d. A new drug, disodium cromoglycate, has helped open up a new approach to treatment of severe asthma. In some patients, this drug produces clinical improvement and reduces dependence on costicosteroid drugs.

e. A derivative of penicillin—called carbenicillin—has been shown effective in treating *meningitis* and bacterial infections of the urinary tract and burns, when due to pseudomonas, proteus, and enterobacteria.

f. Significant progress has been made towards the prevention of hepatitis. The Dane particle has been confirmed as the virus responsible for serum hepatitis (hepatitis B) and a prototype vaccine—which has proved effective in chimpanzee tests—has been developed. The virus which causes infectious hepatitis, or hepatitis A, has been visualized. This discovery should accelerate the development of a vaccine against this form of the disease.

g. Identification of the two chemicals on the surface of the influenza virus responsible for its shifty nature has opened new areas for vaccine research on this agent. A vaccine directed against one of these chemical antigens has proven effective in preventing illness, inducing resistance to that virus and antigenically similar ones, and may also provide a more potent, longer-lasting immunity.

XV. What Are Recent Research Payoffs Against Tropical Diseases?

1. Cooperative efforts by U.S. and Asian scientists have laid the groundwork for *development of an effective vaccine against cholera*. A simple therapeutic regimen has also been worked out which is already resulting in significant improvement in treating patients in rural areas.[13]

2. Research on *filariasis and schistosomiasis*—two major parasitic diseases of man—has increased scientific understanding of the immunological factors involved in the development of

schistosomiasis and of the roles played by vectors in the spread of both these diseases.[13]

XVI. What Are the Recent Research Payoffs in Immunology?

1. Studies in immunology are essential to progress in the areas of both allergic and infectious diseases and much is being accomplished.

2. *The key to the problem of graft rejection in organ transplantation lies in understanding the immune system and learning how to control its undesirable effects.*

Scientists have developed tissue typing techniques—analogous to the red blood cell matching used in transfusions—which increase the likelihood of successful organ transplants.

Better "matching" of organ donor and recipient has resulted in a dramatic increase in the use of transplants as treatment for end-stage kidney disease. Figures from the American Cancer Society/National Institutes of Health Organ Transplant Registry show that in 1972, kidneys obtained from brothers or sisters had a 1-year survival rate of 80%, and a 2-year rate of 74%. Kidneys from cadaver donors had a 1-year survival rate of 51% and a 2-year rate of 43%.[12]

XVII. What Are the Principal Needs in the Fight Against Allergy and Infectious Diseases?

1. More research workers need to be trained. New knowledge and new methods create a need for trained people capable of developing and enlarging this knowledge. The need is particularly acute in the fields of allergy and immunology.

2. *New vaccines are needed.* A vaccine against hepatitis A is needed; and vaccines are still needed against parainfluenza and respiratory syncytial viruses, which kill about 5,000 children a year.

3. Research on *drug resistance* is sorely needed. Studies on the physiology, biochemistry, and genetics of bacteria need to

be stepped up. New drugs are needed to take the place of those to which resistance is growing, and for use in conditions for which there is no effective drug at present.

4. Few effective drugs or methods of treatment for many of the *parasitic and systemic fungal infections* exist, and too little known about many of these diseases. Some of them occur in the United States; others are a threat to U.S. military and civilian personnel serving overseas.

5. Basic research in virology is opening up completely new areas of knowledge and has the potential for answering many unanswered questions in medicine and in biology itself. *Antiviral substances* are needed and progress is being made, but much remains to be done.

6. Basic research for a better understanding of the *immune response* and its role in allergic disorders and organ transplantation is of prime importance.

7. We need stepped-up research on the role of *microbial agents* in *chronic disorders,* such as emphysema, rheumatoid arthritis, and degenerative disorders of the respiratory and nervous systems.

Comparative studies with animals have shown that viruses, for example, can cause chronic degenerative nervous system disorders such as scrapie in sheep. Such important leads need to be followed up.

8. Increased knowledge of the basic biology of the organisms causing *venereal diseases* is needed and vaccines or other methods of control developed if the present epidemic of these diseases is to be halted through vaccines.

Notes

1. Data from the National Health Survey—Series 10, No. 95, Current Estimates, from the Health Interview Survey, United States, 1973. U.S. Dept. of Health, Education, and Welfare, Public Health Service, Health Services and Mental Health Administration.
2. Conference on Newer Respiratory Disease Viruses, U.S. Public Health Service, 1962.

3. Monthly Vital Statistics Report, Annual Summary for the United States, 1973. National Center for Health Statistics, Rockville, Md. 20852.
4. Computations based on data from Statistical Abstract of the United States, 1973, p. 395.
5. From Current Industrial Reports, Pharmaceutical Preparations, Except Biologicals, 1973.
6. Figures furnished by the National Institute of Allergy and Infectious Diseases, National Institutes of Health, Bethesda, Md. May, 1975.
7. Data from the National Health Survey—Series 10, No. 84, Prevalence of Selected Chronic Respiratory Conditions, United States, 1970. U.S. Dept. of HEW, PHS, Health Resources Administration.
8. From a report by the Allergy Foundation of America, New York, 1971.
9. 1974 Drug Topics Marketing Guide. Litton Publications, 550 Kinderkamack Rd., Oradell, N. J.
10. From a report prepared in the Office of Research, Division of Research Grants, National Institutes of Health.
11. From "Contributions of the Biological Sciences to Human Welfare," Federation Proceedings, Vol. 31, 1972.
12. Opening Statements by the Director of the National Institute of Allergy and Infectious Diseases, appearing before Congressional Appropriations Committees, 1975.
13. From "The First Five Years, 1965-1970, The United States-Japan Cooperative Medical Science Program," Geographic Medicine Branch, National Institute of Allergy and Infectious Diseases, National Institutes of Health, Bethesda, Md. 20014.

What Are the Prevalence and Cost of Arthritis and Rheumatism?

What Is Being Done for People with These Diseases?

I. How Many People in the United States Have Arthritis and Rheumatism?

1. About *20.2 million people* in the United States today (1 out of every 10 Americans) are afflicted with arthritis severe enough to require medical care.[1]

   a. No other disorder causes more prolonged misery to a greater number of people in the United States than do the arthritic and rheumatic diseases.

2. *Arthritis and rheumatism are second only to heart diseases* as the most widespread *chronic illness* in the United States today.[2]

   a. The leading causes of activity limitation in the United States today are:

   > Heart conditions—16.4%
   > Arthritis and rheumatism—14.0%

   b. Arthritis and rheumatism ranked second among the chronic conditions that prevented people from carrying on their major activity (work, keeping house, school).[2] Of those people unable to carry on their major activity, 22 percent reported heart conditions as the cause and 15.1 percent reported arthritis and rheumatism as the cause.[2]

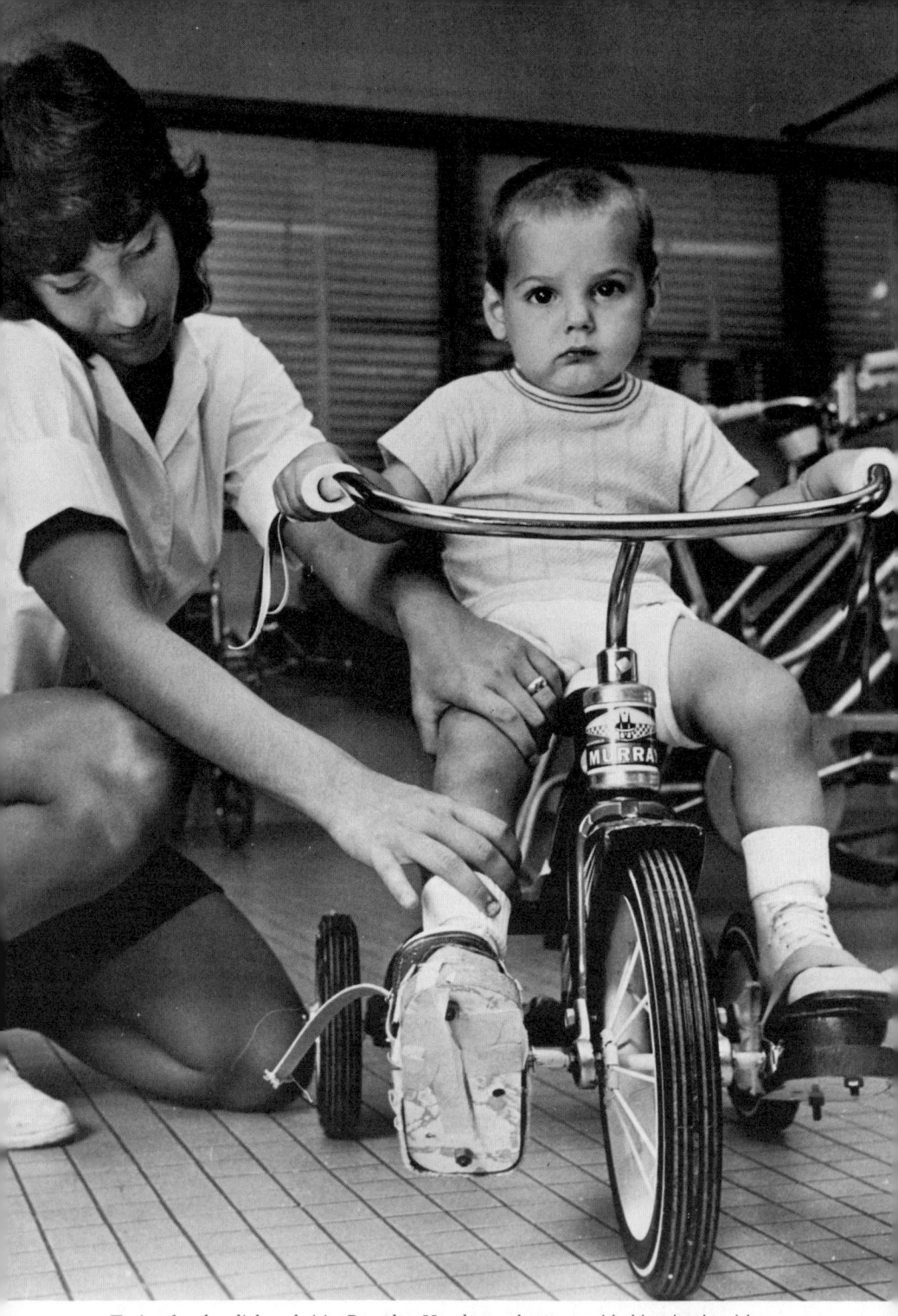

Trying hard to lick arthritis, Douglas Henderson learns to ride his tricycle with some help from a physical therapist. Contrary to popular belief, arthritis isn't just a disease for older adults; it also strikes children like Douglas. (COURTESY OF THE ARTHRITIS FOUNDATION, NEW YORK)

3. An estimated 3.5 million arthritis victims are disabled—limited in their usual activities—at any one time.[2]
   a. Of these, *321,000 are under 45 years of age.*[2]
   b. 857,000 or 26.8 percent are unable to carry on their major activity (work, keeping house, school) because of arthritis and rheumatism.[2]

4. Arthritis and rheumatism cause about *238 million days of restricted activity* annually and 14.2 million days lost from work (regular job) annually.[1]

II. What Are the Major Forms of Arthritis and Rheumatism?

Arthritis (which literally means inflammation of a joint) is an umbrella term covering more than 80 forms of rheumatic disease that attack the joints and/or other connective tissues of the body. Some are very common; some are very rare.[19]

The three major forms (in terms of prevalence and morbidity) are:[19]

>Rheumatoid arthritis
>Osteoarthritis
>Gout

Other diseases associated with arthritis that are common and serious enough to be of concern include:[19]

>Rheumatic fever
>Ankylosing spondylitis
>Scleroderma
>Systemic lupus erythematosus

III. How Many People Have Rheumatoid Arthritis?

Rheumatoid arthritis affects 3.2 percent of adults aged 18 through 79 years, or about *5 million people* in the United States

ARTHRITIS AND RHEUMATISM ARE SECOND ONLY TO HEART DISEASE AS CAUSE OF ACTIVITY LIMITATION
1969-70
(Percent of Limited Persons)

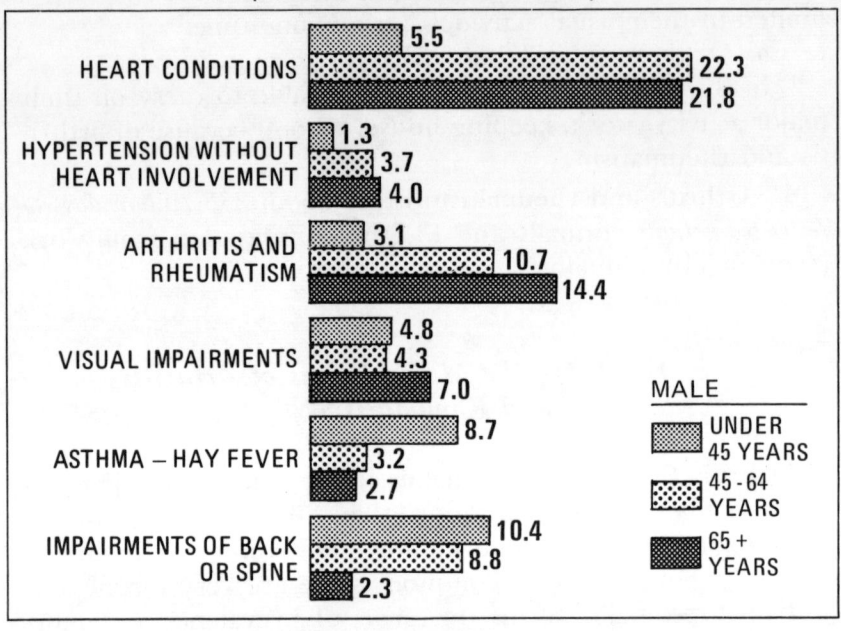

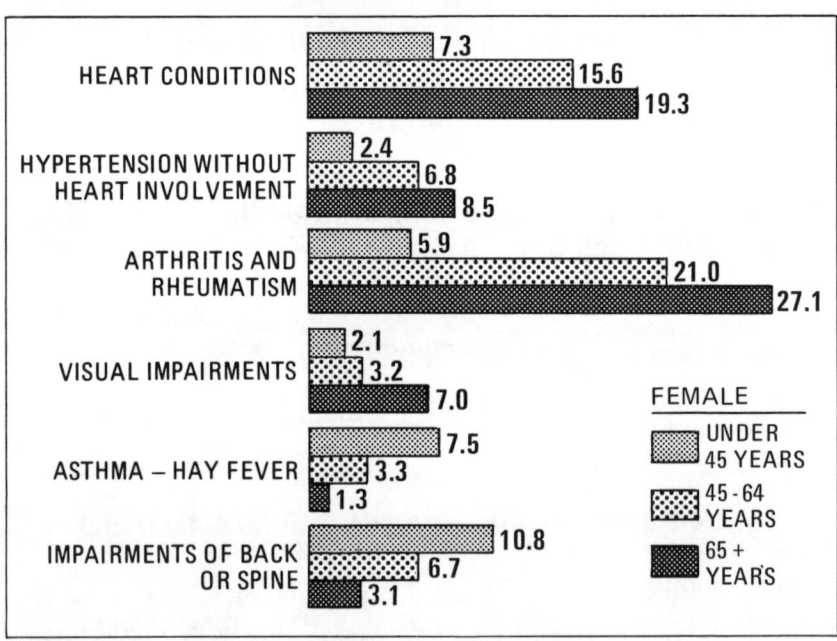

Percent of persons with activity limitation who reported selected chronic conditions as a cause of their limitation, by sex and age. (2)

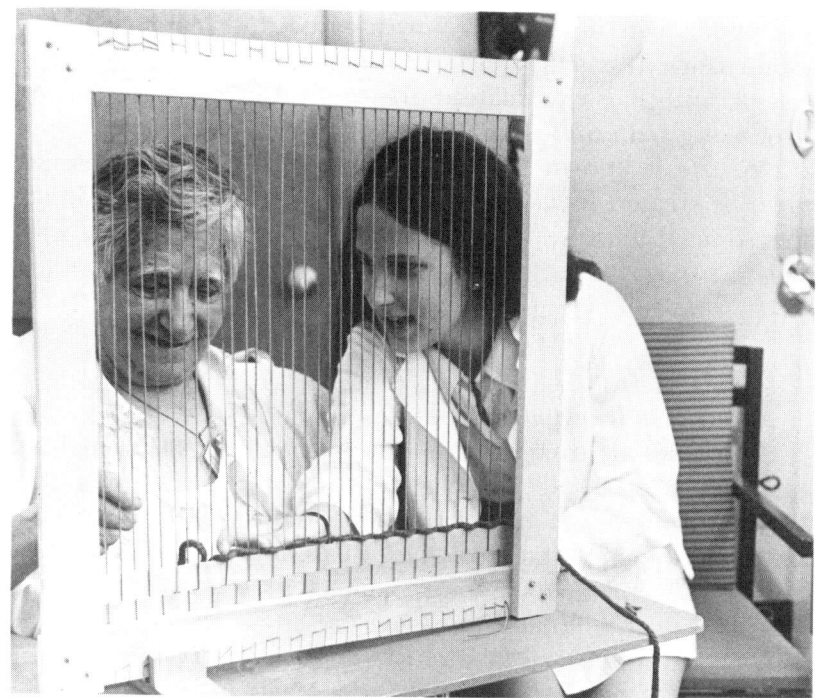

Arthritis knows no generation gap. Debbie Mikels, who has suffered from the childhood form of the disease, helps Mrs. Marie C. Picone, another arthritis patient, to regain and retain use of her arthritic hands. (COURTESY OF THE ARTHRITIS FOUNDATION, NEW YORK)

today, and is the most devastating and crippling form of arthritis.[3]

A majority of its victims are young and middle-aged adults in their most productive years, between 20 and 45 years of age, although it can begin both earlier and later.[3]

It is a chronic inflammatory connective tissue disease that leads to permanent joint deformities and other complications producing disability and chronic invalidism.[19]

The primary cause is still unknown. There is no cure, though it is often possible to control the disease or ameliorate its manifestations.[19]

IV. How Many People Have Osteoarthritis?

About *10 million Americans* have osteoarthritis severe enough to cause pain and require medical care.[4]

Osteoarthritis is associated with aging and degeneration of joint tissues. It usually develops more slowly and is milder and less painful than rheumatoid arthritis, although it can end up producing pain and disability in some victims.[19]

No cure is known for osteoarthritis. This form of arthritis must be treated by controlling symptoms, relieving strains on the affected joints, and by surgery.[19]

V. How Many People Suffer from Gout?

About *a million Americans* suffer from gout.[1]

Gout is an arthritic disease that most often affects the joints of the feet, especially the big toe.[5]

A susceptibility to gout is probably inherited, and most of its victims are men. Attacks of the disease last for days or weeks, and usually produce intense pain. Gout is related to excess uric acid in the blood and tissues.[5]

The disease can now be very effectively controlled by drugs and treatment that reduce the uric acid levels in the body.[5] (See Question IX, 3.)

VI. What Is the Economic Loss to the Country from Arthritis and Rheumatism?

1. Arthritis and rheumatism are conservatively estimated to cost the nation $9,200,000,000 annually.[6] Of this amount:

    a. *$3.5 billion is lost in wages and salaries* by persons unable to work because of their ailment.[6]

    b. *$3.8 billion represents annual medical care costs.*[6]

VII. How Much Does the Veterans Administration Pay in Compensation or Pension Payments to Veterans Because of Arthritis and Rheumatic Diseases?

1. As of 1973, there were 324,717 veterans receiving compensation or pension payments whose major disability was clas-

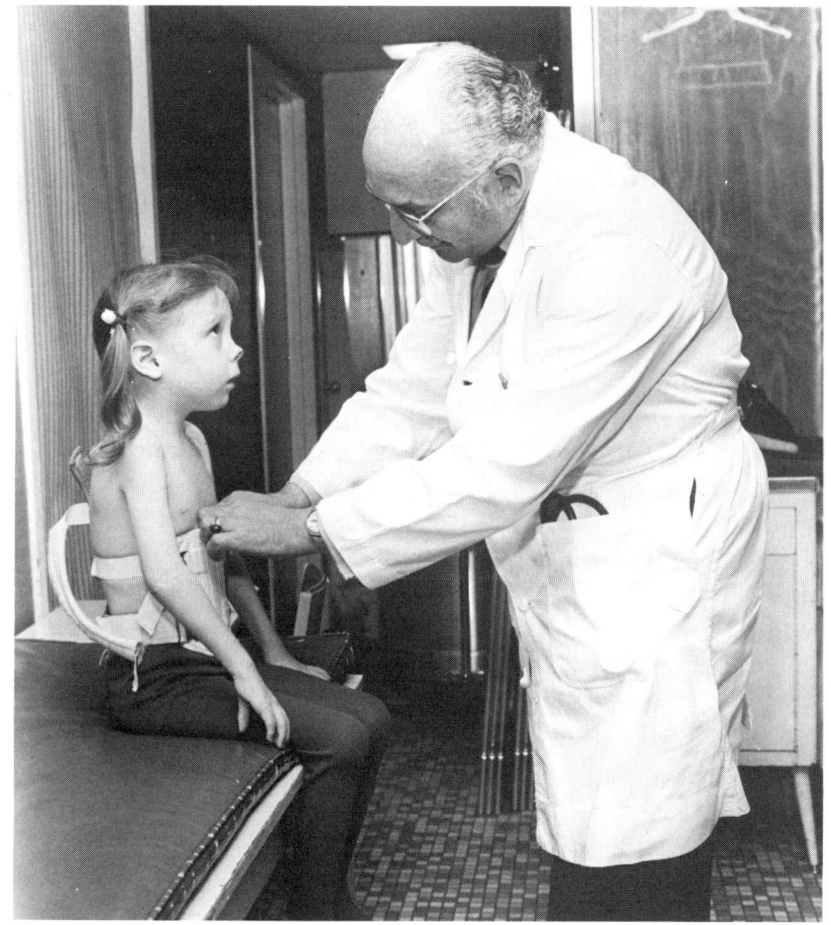

This young victim of juvenile rheumatoid arthritis has her back brace adjusted by Dr. Burton J. Grossman, medical director of LaRabida Children's Hospital in Chicago. Dr. Grossman is one of a handful of physicians who are pediatric rheumatologists, or specialists in caring for children with arthritis. (COURTESY OF THE ARTHRITIS FOUNDATION, NEW YORK)

sified as arthritis or rheumatic disease. The estimated annual value of these payments was $394,428,972.[7]

VIII. How Much Does the Federal Government Lose in Income and Excise Taxes?

In one year alone, the Federal Government loses *more than $773 million* in income and excise taxes on the wages and salaries lost by persons unable to work because of arthritis and rheumatism.[6]

IX. What Methods of Treatment Are Presently in Use for Arthritis and Other Rheumatic Diseases?

1. Rheumatoid arthritis[8]

   a. Lacking a cure for rheumatoid arthritis and since it is a systemic disease, measures of proved value, for the most part, are directed toward reducing inflammation, preventing disability, and controlling pain. Treatment includes rest and specific exercises, drugs, physical therapy and rehabilitation, and sometimes surgery.

   b. Measures for the treatment of rheumatoid arthritis on which there is fairly uniform agreement but not unanimity include:[8]

   i. *Salicylates:* The salicylates, of which *aspirin* is the most common, are perhaps the drugs that over the years have been most widely used in the treatment of rheumatoid arthritis. *Aspirin,* in adequate dosage, has proved to be one of the *most effective* and *least dangerous* of any drug in relieving the symptoms of the disease. Aspirin not only eases aches and pains in the joints, but research indicates that in rheumatoid arthritis the drug probably lessens the inflammatory process that is the basis of the disease.

   Aspirin is available in various forms that permit the use of the drug in persons who are unable to tolerate it because of gastrointestinal distress.

   ii. *Gold salts:* Injections of gold have been effectively used in the treatment of rheumatoid arthritis for at least a quarter of a century. The mode of action of gold on the rheumatoid process is not known. However, experience has shown that many persons given gold undergo a beneficial response.

Not only does gold restrict the disease activity, but it also suppresses many of the inflammatory changes caused by the rheumatoid process. Not all arthritics will benefit from the use of gold and about one-third of them will suffer toxic and undesirable side reactions from it.

iii. *Phenylbutazone:* This drug is a synthetic chemical compound and not a steroid or a hormone. It is an anti-inflammatory agent and alleviates pain in many types of arthritis, especially in spondylitis and gout. In the early and acute stages of rheumatoid arthritis, the drug brings about a decrease in joint swelling and muscle stiffness.

As with gold and the steroids, phenylbutazone cannot be taken by all arthritics; not all will benefit from it and a good many will experience undesirable side reactions.

iv. *Antimalarial* drugs: Certain compounds such as chloroquine, which have been developed against malaria, once widely used in the treatment of rheumatoid arthritis and systemic lupus erythematosus, are now seldom prescribed because of possible systemic toxic effects, including blindness. However, an occasional patient may benefit from it.

v. *Indomethacin:* This is a relatively new anti-inflammatory drug, not related to cortisone or aspirin, which may relieve certain symptoms associated with rheumatoid arthritis. Experience confirms that its greatest usefulness is in spondylitis, gout, and oesteoarthritis.

vi. *Steroid hormones:* Cortisone and related steroid drugs are a special problem. They can bring about sensational reduction of pain and inflammation in a matter of hours, but they have been found to have serious side effects, sometimes worse than the rheumatoid disease. Also, they do not stop the disease process; they merely hide the fact that joint damage is still going on. Thus, although they are useful in special situations, they are being prescribed less often by arthritis specialists today in the routine treatment of rheumatoid arthritis.

vii. *Cyclophosphamide,* a new anti-inflammatory agent, has shown great promise in recent studies. But under Federal Food and Drug Administration regulations, it may be used for arthritis only under investigatory conditions. In any case, this drug is extremely toxic and should be given only in severe, intractable cases.[9]

2. Osteoarthritis[19]

a. No specific therapy is known for the treatment of degenerative joint disease. Treatment is symptomatic and includes rest for the involved joints, physical therapy, weight reduction, drugs, and, in some cases, reconstructive surgery to correct badly deformed joints or other mechanical disturbances.

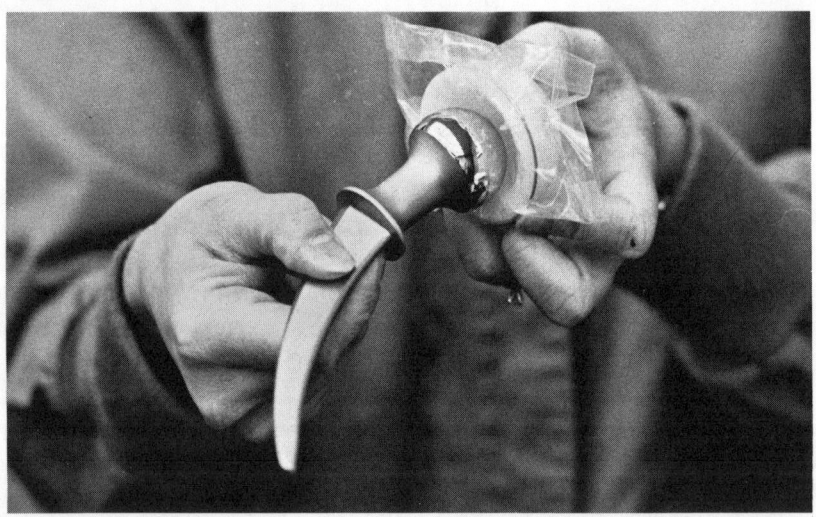

One of the greatest recent advances in arthritis treatment has been the development of new procedures for "total hip replacement." The artificial hip joint consists of a lower half—to be cemented into the femur—made of vitallium, with a polished ball-like top. The upper half is a cup made of polyethylene that functions as a socket and is cemented into the pelvic bone. (COURTESY OF THE ARTHRITIS FOUNDATION, NEW YORK)

An operation, developed by Dr. John Charnley of Lancaster, England, and now widely used by leading orthopedic surgeons in the United States, involves complete reconstruction of the hip joint to relieve arthritis of the hip. This operation is successful in the majority of the cases and represents one of the greatest recent advances in arthritis treatment.[10]

Cortisone-like drugs are rarely used in osteoarthritis except in instances where they are injected into joint spaces. Aspirin, phenylbutazone, indomethacin, and perhaps other drugs can be helpful.

3. Gout[5]

The acute, painful attacks of gout can be controlled quite well with several drugs now available, particularly colchicine, phenylbutazone, and indomethacin. Also, allopurinol, probenecid, and sulfinpyrazone now can be prescribed in the long-term treatment to prevent the excessive accumulation of uric acid. Early treatment is important. If the gouty patient closely follows his treatment regimen, he can lead a virtually normal life free of the pain and complications of this form of arthritis.

4. Rheumatic fever[19]

Rheumatic fever is an acute systemic disease accompanied by fever and painful joints. It frequently damages the heart. Anyone of any age can be attacked by rheumatic fever, which nearly always follows a streptococcus infection, although it is most frequently observed between the ages of 5 and 15.

Those who have had one rheumatic fever attack may be susceptible to others and frequently contract it again.

Flare-ups of rheumatic fever can be prevented, however, by proper use of antibiotics (especially penicillin) to prevent the streptococcus infection. The avoidance or prevention of streptococcal infection by the systematic use of penicillin or a similar antibiotic will nearly always prevent attacks of rheumatic fever.

The treatment for acute attacks of arthritis associated with rheumatic fever consists of rest, anti-inflammatory drugs such as aspirin, and sometimes cortisone-like compounds.

X. What Are Some of the Current Research Leads Being Pursued Against Arthritis? [19]

1. The key to the problem of rheumatoid arthritis is inflammation, a process that, once started, tends to be self-perpetuating. It is inflammation that causes the pain, heat, swelling, and eventually the damage to joint tissues and rheumatoid arthritis. The focus of current research, therefore, is on decoding the steps in the chain-reaction inflammatory process—and in attempting to develop new drugs to block or interrupt the process.

The ideal agent would suppress inflammation as effectively as the steroids do but without causing serious side effects. There is particular interest in investigations of immuno-suppressive agents because of promising studies with cyclophosphamide and other agents.[11]

2. The primary cause of rheumatoid arthritis is still unknown. Two leading theories, supported by considerable evidence, suggests that an obscure process involving triggering action by a latent virus, or an autoimmune reaction (characterized by manufacture by the body of antibodies that attack its own tissues) may be involved, or possibly a combination of both processes.[11] More research has centered on a possible infectious cause for rheumatoid arthritis during the past 5 years than during the previous 20, but while specific types of arthritis are known to be due to invasion of joints by certain microorganisms, no microbial or viral agent has yet been positively identified as a cause of rheumatoid arthritis.[11]

XI. Are Some People Affected More Than Others by Arthritis and Rheumatism?

1. Persons who work outdoors as manual laborers appear to suffer more from rheumatic diseases than those in indoor sedentary occupations.[19]

2. Three times more women than men suffer from severe arthritis and rheumatism.[19]

XII. How Many Physicians Specialize in the Rheumatic Diseases?

1. There are approximately 2,300 members of the American Rheumatism Association, a professional society of physicians interested in treatment of and research in arthritis and rheumatic diseases. The Association is a section of The Arthritis Foundation.
2. Only 78 of the nation's 114 medical schools offer a full program of courses in rheumatology.[12]

XIII. What Facilities Are Available for Treatment of Arthritis and Rheumatism?

1. A large "delivery gap" exists between the help that can be given to arthritis victims and what they actually receive. An adequate, comprehensive system has yet to be developed. Arthritis is the nation's number one crippler, but its victims are short-changed by a medical system that is oriented to treating acute rather than chronic disease.[13]
2. The Arthritis Foundation has supported pilot programs that have clearly demonstrated the value and effectiveness of comprehensive care for arthritis victims. However, the foundation lacks the funds to provide such treatment for every arthritis sufferer and has sought Federal action to bring these programs into existence throughout the country by the establishment of a nationwide network of arthritis centers and satellite clinics.
3. The Arthritis Foundation in its 1968 Annual Report indicated that there were about *50 first-rate arthritis research-training-care centers in the United States and more than 300 clinics.*

XIV. Are These Facilities Adequate?

1. No. The need for additional clinics, improved out-patient facilities, and trained personnel to treat arthritis is urgent.[13]

2. *Facilities are needed to aid in research on the rehabilitation and restoration to active life of bed-ridden arthritics.*[13]

XV. *What Are the Main National Organizations Concerned with Arthritis Research?*

The two major sources of support for research in arthritis are:

1. *The Arthritis Foundation,* the leading national voluntary health agency devoted to this area.
2. *The National Institute of Arthritis, Metabolic and Digestive Diseases* of the National Institutes of Health, U.S. Department of Health, Education, and Welfare, the leading government agency working in this area.

XVI. *What Are We Spending for Research on Arthritis?*

1. The most recent estimated annual allocations for arthritis research and closely related basic studies total $21 million distributed as follows:

a. *The National Institute of Arthritis, Metabolism and Digestive Diseases,* U.S. Public Health Service, estimated for fiscal 1975 (out of a total appropriation of $173 million).[18]	$16,273,000
b. *Veterans Administration,* Department of Medicine and Surgery, estimated fiscal 1975.[14]	$ 3,377,000
c. *The Arthritis Foundation*—for research in universities, hospitals, and other institutions in 1973[15] (national office only).	$ 1,359,005
Total	$21,009,005

XVII. How Does This Compare with Other National Expenditures?

1. In *contrast* with the $21 million currently being spent for arthritis research, the people of the United States in 1972 spent approximately:

$17 billion for alcoholic beverages.[16]
$13 billion for tobacco products and smokers' accessories.[16]
$303 million for toilet water and cologne.[16]
$249 million for hair coloring preparations.[16]
$66 million for arthritic and rheumatic pain relievers.[16]

2. The current *Federal* allocation for research on rheumatic disease, *the number one crippler,* is about 6 percent of the $289 million budget authority in fiscal 1973 of the Animal and Plant Health Inspection Service of the U.S. Department of Agriculture.[17]

XVIII. How Much Does the Arthritis Foundation Raise Annually Nationwide and How Are These Funds Spent?

According to the 1973 annual report of the Arthritis Foundation, the American people contributed $10,718,000 to the foundation during that year.

Expenditures for the fiscal year ended December 21, 1972, were as follows:

	Amount	% of Total
Patient and community services	$1,906,900	19.8%
Research	2,262,762	23.4%
Management and general	1,233,612	12.8%
Fund-raising	1,488,164	15.4%
Public health education	1,586,677	16.4%
Professional education and training	1,176,630	12.2%
	$9,654,745	100.0%

XIX. What Can Be Done About the Problem of Arthritis and Rheumatism?

1. The public and all agencies in this field should support and cooperate with The Arthritis Foundation, the major national voluntary agency working specifically in this area.
2. Congress should triple or quadruple the funds for research in arthritis so that a vigorous and direct attack upon the rheumatic diseases can go on without interruption.
3. The problem is centered mainly in the nation's medical schools, which have *inadequate personnel, funds, and facilities* to meet the needs of continued clinical and basic research in the rheumatic diseases.

    a. *Federal funds should be provided for the construction of laboratories and other research facilities* needed to make possible the greater study of these diseases.

    b. Federal funds must be increased to make possible more grants-in-aid to non-federal institutions, *to provide for the purchase of equipment and the payment of stipends to investigators and their staffs,* and to finance the laboratories of the National Institute of Arthritis, Metabolism and Digestive Diseases.

4. A major problem is the need for the *training of more physicians* in the diagnosis and treatment of arthritis and rheumatism.

    a. *Congress should make available* to the National Institute of Arthritis, Metabolism and Digestive Diseases *additional funds for training* so that young physicians may be provided the opportunity for an academic research career in rheumatology. In fiscal 1973, the National Institute of Arthritis, Metabolism and Digestive Diseases spent an estimated $1,128,000 in training grants for arthritis and the rheumatic diseases, which is inadequate.[18]

5. The total of $21 million currently being spent by major sources for arthritis research is inadequate to solve the arthritis problem that afflicts over 20 million Americans. These diseases cause suffering and severe economic loss for which the only hope is more intensive medical research and training.

Notes

1. National Health Interview of 1969. Unpublished data. National Center for Health Statistics. Rockville, Md.
2. Chronic Conditions Causing Activity Limitation, U.S. 1969-1970. U.S. Department of Health, Education and Welfare, Washington, D. C.
3. Rheumatoid Arthritis in Adults, U.S.—1960-1962, Series 11, No. 17, 1966. U.S. Department of Health, Education and Welfare. Washington, D. C.
4. Prevalence of Osteoarthritis in Adults—U.S. 1960-1962, Series 11, No. 15, 1966. U.S. Department of Health, Education and Welfare.
5. Primer on The Rheumatic Diseases—7th Edition, The Arthritis Foundation, New York, N. Y. 1973.
6. Unpublished data, compiled by The Arthritis Foundation, 1973.
7. Unpublished data from Veterans Administration files, Veterans Administration central office, Washington, D.C. Personal communication to The Arthritis Foundation from Mr. Scott Mason.
8. Information on current therapies for rheumatoid arthritis from "Today's Facts About Arthritis," The Arthritis Foundation, New York, N.Y.
9. Cooperating clinics of the American Rheumatism Association. A Controlled Trial of Cyclophosphamide in Rheumatoid Arthritis. New England Journal Medicine 283: 883, 1970.
10. Rosenburg E.F., et al, Total Hip Placement in England. Journal of the American Medical Association 212: 611, 1970.
11. Johnson J.S., et al, Rheumatoid Arthritis 1970-1972. Annals of Internal Medicine 78: 937, 1973.
12. Rheumatology Manpower Study. The Arthritis Foundation, N.Y., N.Y. 1973.
13. 1968 and 1969 Annual Reports of The Arthritis Foundation, New York, N.Y.
14. Veterans Administration, Department of Medicine and Surgery, Washington, D.C., personal communication dated April 16, 1975 from Lawrence B. Hobson, M.D., Deputy Assistant Chief Medical Director for Research and Development.
15. 1973 Annual Report of The Arthritis Foundation, New York, N. Y.

16. *1973 Marketing Guide* published by *Drug Topics,* Medical Economics Company, Oradell, N. J.
17. Budget of the United States Government, 1974.
18. Information from the National Institute of Arthritis, Metabolism and Digestive Diseases, National Institutes of Health, Bethesda, Md.
19. Information from The Arthritis Foundation, New York, 1973.

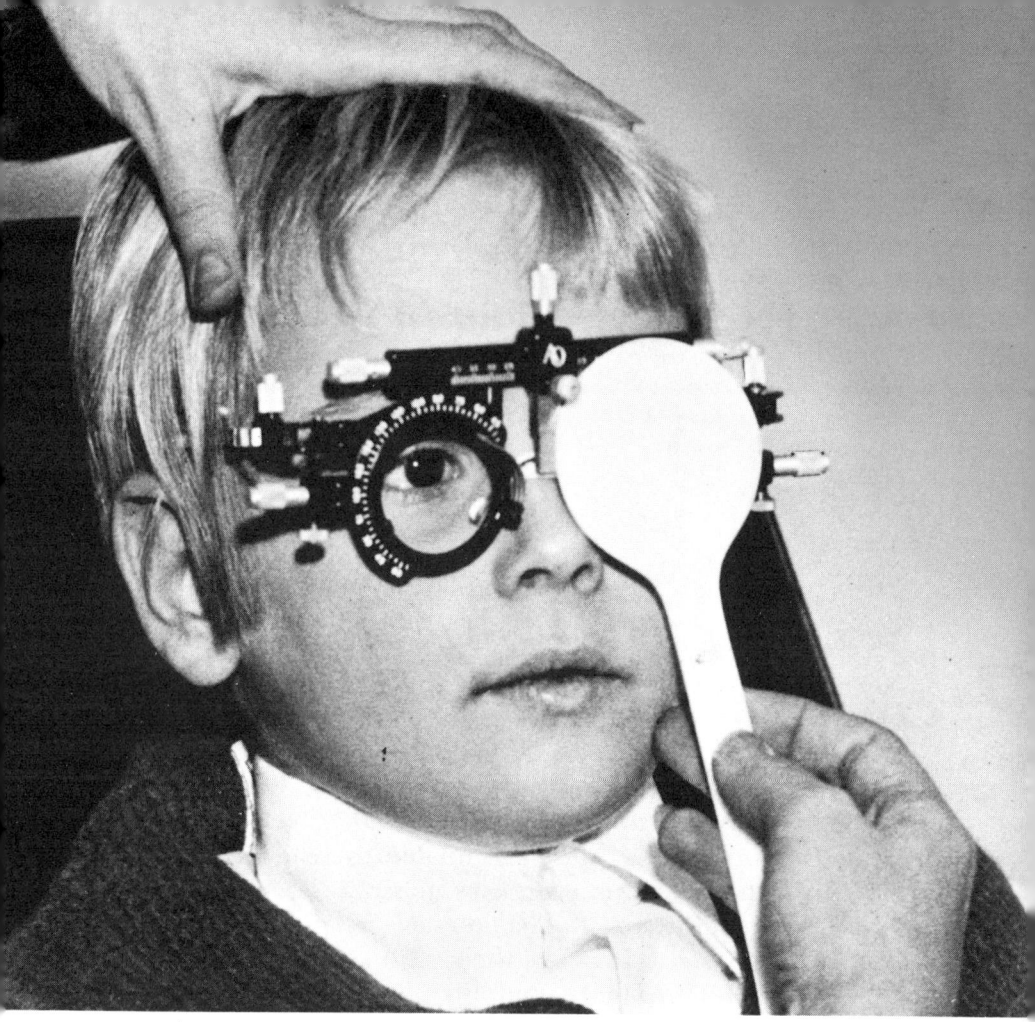
(COURTESY OF RESEARCH TO PREVENT BLINDNESS, INC., NEW YORK)

What Are We Doing About Blinding Eye Diseases?

I. How Many People in the United States Are Blind or Visually Impaired?

1. An estimated *9,596,000* people in the United States have some degree of *visual impairment.*[1]

    a. Of these, approximately *1,306,000* have such *severe visual impairment* that they are unable to read ordinary newsprint with either eye, even with glasses.[1]

    b. In addition, *94,000,000 people in this country wear glasses or contact lenses* to improve their vision.[1]

2. At least 475,000 people in the United States are *legally blind.*[3] (Their measured visual acuity is 20/200 or worse in the better eye [a measurement of 20/20 is considered normal], or their visual field measurement is 20 degrees or less at its widest point.)

3. An estimated 44,350 people in this country *become blind each year.*[3]

4. Visual impairments rank:

    - Third among diseases that restrict Americans from leading productive lives[4]
    - Sixth in number of hospital discharges[4]
    - Tenth in number of hospital days[4]
    - Twelfth as a cause of bed disability[4]

II. What Are the Main Causes of Blindness?

Retinal diseases, glaucoma, and cataract together account for more blindness in this country than all other visual disorders combined.[5]

1. Retinal diseases

   a. Conditions affecting the retina—the light-sensitive tissue at the back of the eye—are the leading causes of blindness in the United States, accounting for 25 percent of all blindness in the country.[5]

   b. An estimated 145,000 people have retinal detachment.[1]

   c. A minimum of 76,500 people are blind from retinal diseases, and this does not include the thousands of individuals who suffer disability from these diseases but are not legally blind.[5]

   d. In 1972, an estimated 8,800 people became blind from retinal diseases, making it the leading cause of new blindness (29.7 percent) for the year.[5]

   e. Of the total number of people blind from retinal diseases, 22,000 cases are attributable to prenatal causes and 14,400 to complications of diabetes.[5]

   f. In 1972 senile retinal degeneration alone accounted for 12.6 percent of all new blindness, and diabetic retinopathy (a progressive disorder in the blood vessels of the retina stemming from diabetes) was responsible for 11.1 percent.[5]

2. Glaucoma

   a. Nearly 797,000 have glaucoma. Of these, 470,000 are 65 years of age and older, 268,000 are 45 to 64 years of age, and 52,000 are 17 to 44 years of age.[1] Glaucoma has claimed the sight of more than 34,000 Americans now living and accounts for *11 percent of all blindness* in the United States.[5]

   b. In glaucoma, visual function is lost because of damage to the optic nerve associated with an increase in intraocular pressure. Vision lost from glaucoma cannot be restored.[6]

c. There are three basic kinds of glaucoma. In *closed-angle glaucoma* there is a gross structural defect which causes a narrowing of the angle between the iris (the colored, circular membrane that controls the pupil) and the back of the cornea (the transparent membrane that covers the front of the eye). This can lead to an acute attack of glaucoma which is very painful and may cause permanent blindness unless there is prompt medical attention.[6]

d. *Secondary glaucoma* results from a preexisting, generalized eye disease such as inflammation, tumor, vascular disorder, or diabetes. This kind of glaucoma is most difficult to treat.[6]

e. The most common form of glaucoma, called *open-angle or chronic glaucoma,* is insidious. Although there is no apparent defect that blocks the outflow of fluid from the eye, a blockage does occur somewhere in the outflow channels. This form of the disease is usually painless and, because it slowly restricts peripheral vision, may develop unnoticed by the patient. The person with this disease may seek medical attention only when the condition is far advanced and a considerable amount of irreparable damage has occurred. Once diagnosed, chronic glaucoma can usually be arrested and controlled by medication, but the vision already lost cannot at present be restored. In some cases surgery may be necessary eventually to provide a new outflow channel.[6]

f. It is estimated that *in 1972 alone, 3,100 people lost their sight* because of *glaucoma.*[5]

3. Cataract

A cataract is a cloudiness in the lens of the eye that interferes with vision.

a. Approximately 3,013,000 individuals suffer from cataract.[1] Of these, 2,212,000 are 65 years of age and older; 565,000 are 45 to 64 years of age; and 197,000 are 17 to 44 years old.[1] More than 40,000 people are *blind* because of cataract and more than 4,400 people lost their sight in 1972 alone because of cataract.[5]

b. Cataracts are most common among the elderly; senile

Leading Causes of Blindness in United States Today[5]

Disease	Estimated Number of Blind People in U.S.	Percentage of Total Cases of Legal Blindness
Retinal diseases	76,500	25.0
Cataract	40,000	13.2
Glaucoma	34,000	11.0
Optic nerve disorders	28,000	9.2
Uveitis	16,000	5.1
Cornea or sclera disease	14,000	4.7
Myopia	9,000	3.0
Retrolental fibroplasia	8,000	2.5
Multiple afflictions	13,000	4.4
Unknown causes	34,000	11.1
Multiple causes	33,000	10.8

New Cases of Blindness in 1972[5]

Disease	Minimum Number Newly Blind People	Percentage of New Cases of Legal Blindness
Retinal disease	8,800	29.7
Cataract	4,400	14.6
Glaucoma	3,100	10.2
Optic nerve disorders	1,900	6.6
Uveitis	800	3.0
Cornea or sclera disease*	800	2.6
Myopia	600	2.2
Retrolental fibroplasia	200	1.0
Multiple afflictions	2,700	9.4
Other	2,500	8.3
Unknown causes	3,800	12.4

These figures do not include the number of people who became visually impaired—no matter how severely—but were not considered *legally* blind.

*Difference in percentage due to rounding of figures to nearest hundred.

cataract alone accounted for 8.5 percent of all new blindness in 1972. However, cataracts can also result from congenital factors, injury, or in association with other eye diseases.[6]

c. Tragically, blindness caused by cataracts is usually needless, unless there are other complications in the eye or general health reasons that preclude surgery. Cataract extraction is one of the most successful operations performed today. From 90 to 95 percent of patients enjoy a restoration of useful vision.[6]

d. In 1968 alone, more than 200,000 people regained their sight through cataract surgery.[7]

III. Is Age a Factor in Blindness and Visual Impairment? Yes

1. There is a high prevalence of visual impairment among the elderly, as shown in National Center for Health Statistics data for the three leading causes of visual impairment.[1]

Disease	Total Number Visually Impaired	Number Visually Impaired Age 65+	Percent of Total Visually Impaired Age 65+
Cataract	3,013,000	2,212,000	73.4
Glaucoma	797,000	470,000	59.0
Retinal detachment	145,000	66,000	45.5

2. Yet, despite the fact that the highest rates of blindness occur among the elderly, there are at least 32,000 blind persons under age 20.[2]

Disease	Percentage of Legal Blindness Under Age 20	Number
Prenatal influences	57.3	18,300
Infectious disease	8.0	2,600
Injury or poisoning	5.8	1,800
Neoplasm	4.1	1,300
All others	24.8	8,000

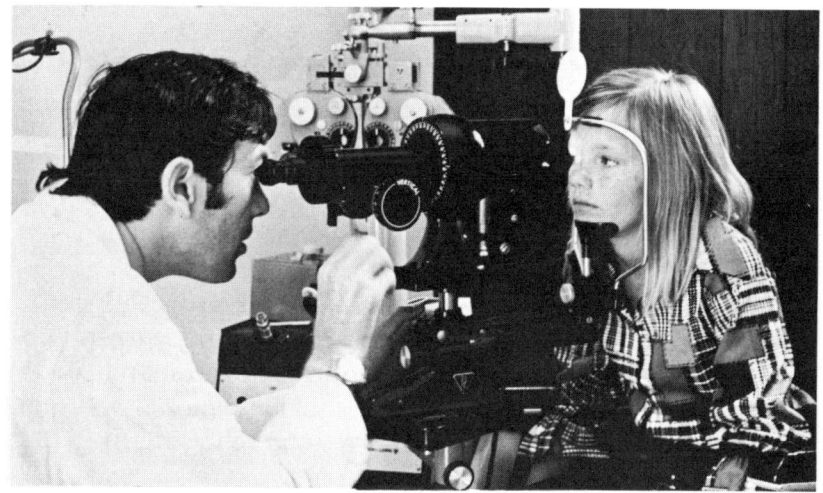
(COURTESY OF RESEARCH TO PREVENT BLINDNESS, INC., NEW YORK)

IV. What Is the Economic Cost of Blindness?

1. *Annual income lost* due to blindness ranges from *$600 million to $1 billion.*[9]

2. A minimum of *$140 million is lost in Federal taxes each year* due to blindness.[9]

3. The *cost of blindness to public welfare agencies is $468,567,000* annually. Of this, the Federal Government spends $267,724,000; state governments spend $131,254,000, and private agencies spend $69,589,000.[11]

4. The average cost of supporting *one* blind person is *more than $2100 per year.*[9]

5. The estimated cost of supporting *all* blind persons in this country is *$500 million.*[9]

V. How Much Money Is Available to Support Research for Improved Prevention, Diagnosis, and Treatment of Visual Impairment and Blinding Eye Diseases?

Approximately $45,842,209 is currently being spent by the major agencies listed for medical research in the cause, treatment, and prevention of eye diseases, as follows:

1. Government funds—$44,785,000

a. Fiscal 1975 appropriations to the National Eye Institute of the National Institutes of Health totaled *$44,133,000* to support programs to improve prevention, diagnosis, and treatment of visual disorders.[6]

b. The *Veterans Administration* spent during fiscal 1975 an estimated $652,000 for ophthalmic research.[12]

2. Nongovernment funds—$1,057,209 (for sources listed)

No reliable estimates are available on amounts currently being spent from nongovernment sources for research in the blinding eye diseases. However, the major national voluntary agencies working in this area reported the following in 1973:[8]

PUBLIC SUPPORT AND OTHER FUNDING

		Funds Raised for Research
Research to Prevent Blindness Committee	$ 751,549	$ 591,927
National Council to Combat Blindness	431,866	316,769
National Society for the Prevention of Blindness	2,473,379	148,513
Total	$3,656,794	$1,057,209

VI. How Does This Compare with What We Spend on Other Things?

1. In contrast with the estimated total of approximately $45.8 million which is available from major public and private sources listed for research in blindness and eye diseases, the American people spent in 1972 approximately:[10]

- $300,230,000 for lipsticks
- $280,840,000 for sunglasses (no corrective lenses)
- $194,100,000 for eye makeup

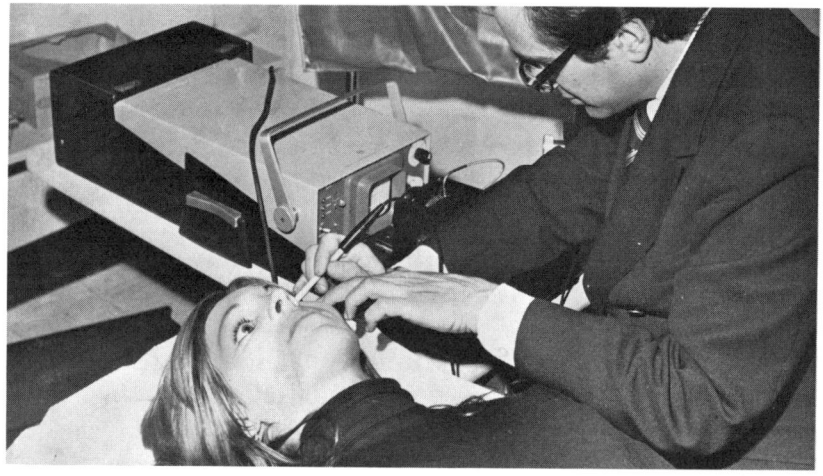

Ultrasound waves, painlessly penetrating the eye, record hidden structural changes due to disease and permit precise localization of tumors and foreign bodies lodged within the eye. (COURTESY OF RESEARCH TO PREVENT BLINDNESS, INC., NEW YORK)

VII. Has Medical Research in Eye Diseases Paid Off? Yes!

1. *Cataract surgery is now safer* and its outcome more satisfactory because of advancements in suture techniques, improved instrumentation, operation under microscopic control, and other technical improvements.[6]

    a. An enzyme is now being used by some ophthalmic surgeons to weaken the ligaments holding the cataract in place. The cataract is then easily removed by grasping it with special forceps or a suction cup.[6]

    b. Another technique recently developed employs a very cold probe. In this technique, cryoextraction, the lens is frozen and the probe adheres to it. This produces a firm connection, and the cataract can be lifted easily from the eye.[6]

    c. Ultrasound is also being used for cataract extraction. In this method, called phacoemulsification, a hollow needle is attached to an ultrasound unit and inserted into the lens. The sound vibrations break up the cataract so it can be drawn out by suction through the hollow needle. This technique involves a smaller incision in the white of the eye than conventional cataract extraction. The period of hospitalization may be shorter. Clinical evaluation of this technique is still under way.[6]

2. Through research, *new and improved drugs* have been developed to control the high intraocular pressure associated with *glaucoma*. Glaucoma develops when the intraocular pressure is high enough to damage the optic nerve and cause visual loss. With the use of these drugs, most glaucoma patients can expect to retain useful vision throughout their lives.[6]

3. A few years ago it was found that some cases of *herpes simplex keratitis can be cured by idoxuridine (IDU),* the first drug shown to be effective against any virus. The mechanisms by which antiviral drugs accomplish their task are now better understood, but research is continuing in an effort to broaden the use of antiviral drugs.[6]

4. The *hydrophilic or soft contact lens* is proving to be helpful for those people who have difficulty adjusting to the hard contact lens and is proving to be useful in treating corneal diseases. It has already been shown that the soft lenses may reduce the pain frequently associated with corneal disease. Studies are being conducted to determine whether the soft lens can also be effective in aiding the healing of certain corneal diseases.[6]

5. Progress has been achieved in treating *uveitis* through the use of antibiotics, antitumor drugs, steroids, electron microscopic studies, and other measures.[6]

6. The *Optacon,* a device that enables a blind person to read the same printed material any sighted person would use, has been developed. The user of the Optacon senses the outline of a regular letter conveyed through the raising and lowering of an array of tiny rods that fit onto a single finger. The entire system weighs only eight pounds and can be easily transported.[6]

7. A more complex vision substitution device uses the images captured by a television camera to activate a series of stimulators arranged on a grid and positioned over the skin of the abdomen. A sightless person, with training and practice, can learn to translate these impulses automatically into crude spatial images within his brain. Both the Optacon and this

system were developed with grant support from the National Eye Institute and other Federal agencies.[6]

8. *A new diagnostic technique, fluorescent angiography,* has made possible advancements in understanding *retinal diseases.* The technique involves the injection of a fluorescent dye into the arm. This dye circulates in the bloodstream and permits the direct viewing of the blood flow within the vessels of the retina and choroid, the tissue underlying the retina that is responsible for its nourishment. Fluorescent angiography improves the ability of doctors to distinguish among various kinds of diseases of the eye and to pinpoint the site of any leakage or blocking of blood flow in the retina or choroid. Research indicates that the techniques will also improve the physician's ability to detect malignant melanoma, a cancer in the eye that causes severe visual loss and endangers life.[6]

9. *Cryosurgery,* a technique used for cataract extraction, is now being employed in the treatment of *retinal detachment,* a separation of the inner layer of the retina from its outer layer. The extreme cold produces adhesions between the two layers and can be used in those cases where photocoagulation (intense heat) cannot be used because it is difficult to see clearly the area to be treated. The two procedures complement each other.[6]

10. *Microsurgery* permits meticulous and precise placement of stitches during corneal transplantation so that a more nearly perfect placement of the graft in its recipient can be achieved. This minimizes the risk of scar tissue formation and subsequent growth of unwanted blood vessels. Microsurgery also allows the use of finer sutures which are less irritating to the eye.[6]

11. *New methods of freezing and dehydrating corneas* for long-range storage have also resulted in improved corneal transplants.[6]

12. *Computer technology* is being applied to the ERG (electroretinography, which is an electrical recording of the retina's response to light) in an effort to increase its usefulness in specific clinical diagnostic situations. Research is continuing in an effort to improve this technology and the range of its usefulness.[6]

13. Great advances have been made in the development of

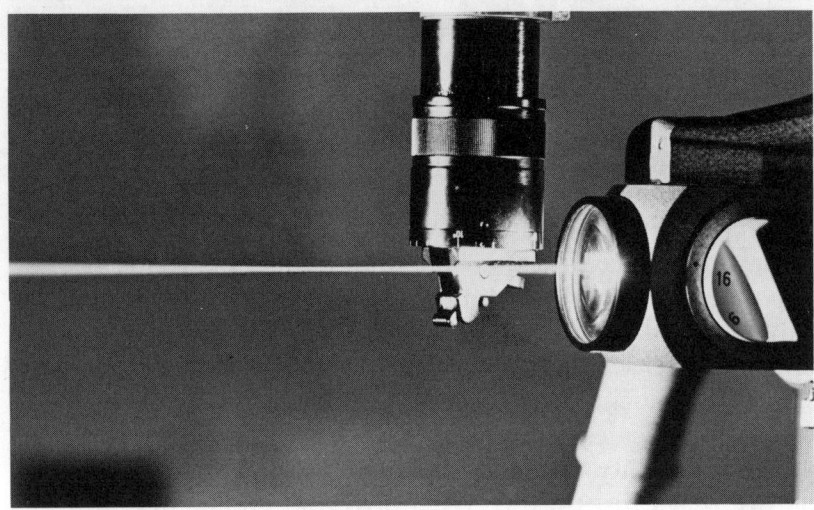

The laser beam, already an important tool of the ophthalmic surgeon, is under continuous development by ophthalmic scientists seeking new uses for its intense power. (COURTESY OF RESEARCH TO PREVENT BLINDNESS, INC., NEW YORK)

optical devices for patients with low levels of visual acuity. These devices include telescopic spectacles and a host of visual aids for the magnification of visual material both for direct observation and by projection.[6]

14. The cause of retrolental fibroplasia (RLF), formerly a major cause of blindness among infants, is now known and preventive measures have been developed. Research supported by the National Institutes of Health, the National Foundation for Eye Research, and the National Society for the Prevention of Blindness established the cause of RLF as the excessive exposure of premature babies to high oxygen concentration. As a result, the number of new cases per year of RLF has been substantially reduced.[6]

VIII. What Are Some of the Current Research Leads Being Pursued by the National Eye Institute?

1. Glaucoma research

The institute conducts and supports a number of *glaucoma research* studies. These are concerned with understanding the mechanism of pressure control within the normal eye, the effect of drugs on the normal flow of fluid through the eye in glaucoma, development of new surgical techniques, and laboratory and epidemiological studies of the eye related to glaucoma. The institute is also supporting the development of new drugs to treat glaucoma patients and the development of an instrument for estimating the rate of blood flow through the back of the eye to be used in understanding the relationship between elevated pressure and the flow of blood to the optic nerve.[6]

a. Recent findings in glaucoma research indicate the possibility of detecting early damage from this disease by identifying changes in the retina at the back of the eye through simple photography. Ophthalmologists must now rely on measurements of intraocular pressure and complicated visual field testing to diagnose glaucoma. These procedures are not completely satisfactory for detecting glaucoma before significant damage has been done.[6]

b. New experimental methods for treating glaucoma, which appeared within the last year, are being further studied. A drug (6-hydroxydopamine or 6HD) which enhances the pressure lowering effects of presently used glaucoma drugs is now being tested clinically with early promising results.[6]

c. Two new techniques for better delivery of drugs used to treat glaucoma have been developed. These are the soft contact lens, which was originally developed as an alternative to the conventional hard lens, and the Ocusert, which is a miniaturized drug dispenser that is placed under the lower lid of the eye. These techniques may make present glaucoma drugs more effective and may make it possible to administer the drugs as infrequently as four times a year. This would make therapy more efficient and easier for the patient. The soft contact lens is already in use, and the Ocusert is expected to be available shortly.[6]

2. Cataract research

a. A researcher who is now at the National Eye Institute was recently able to block the formation of sugar cataracts in rats for the first time. This type of cataract is responsible for blinding babies who suffer from galactosemia, a rare hereditary disorder causing poor weight gain and malnutrition. His studies indicate that a common mechanism is responsible for both cataracts associated with galactosemia and those occurring in conjunction with diabetes. The studies have a direct bearing on the formation of cataracts in humans with diabetes and galactosemia. They are also relevant to understanding the more subtle mechanisms involved in the cause of some congenital cataracts, occurring at or soon after birth.[6]

b. Recent progress has been made, some of it in the National Eye Institute's Laboratory of Vision Research, in understanding how the lens protein clumps together in the type of cataract commonly associated with aging people, the so-called senile cataract. This research has suggested a working hypothesis about how the lens becomes opaque which may open the possibility of either preventing or slowing the development of this type of cataract.[6]

3. Retinal diseases

a. Studies supported and conducted by the institute focus on understanding the mechanism of the retina's response to light and the initial processing of information that is transmitted to the visual centers of the brain, as well as developing animal models of various retinal diseases. Forms of surgery and photocoagulation, a therapy employing an intense beam of light which is directed into the eye, are being evaluated.[6]

b. The institute is supporting a cooperative, nationwide study involving 16 research centers to evaluate forms of treatment of diabetic retinopathy, a progressive disorder in the blood vessels of the retina stemming from diabetes. The purpose of the study is to evaluate the efficacy of photocoagulation treatment of diabetic retinopathy. Photocoagulation is used to coagulate or "weld" the leaking blood vessels associated with the disease. Although photocoagulation treatment is fairly common, this is the first large-scale controlled study designed to determine just how effective and safe the treatment really is.[6]

c. Researchers supported by the institute are studying the

growth of photoreceptor cells in the retina to understand how these light-sensitive cells normally renew themselves. A breakdown in the normal renewal of rod cells may be a basis for inherited degenerative disorders such as retinitis pigmentosa.[6]

4. Corneal disease

a. The development and testing of soft contact lenses for treating these conditions is continuing because they appear to aid corneal healing and reduce pain. Methods for storing corneal tissue to be used in transplants are being improved by refining cryopreservation (extreme cold) techniques. Antiviral drugs and artificial tears are being developed and tested clinically.[6]

b. As part of this corneal research effort, a study is being conducted by the National Eye Institute to learn whether the success rate of corneal transplantation can be improved by the antigenic matching of donors and recipients. In many kinds of corneal disease where transplants are used, tissue matching is not critical. The normal cornea does not have a blood supply, and this is also true in certain disease states. However, in some conditions, blood vessels infiltrate the cornea and thereby circulating antibodies are introduced. When this occurs a rejection of transplanted tissue may result. If investigations indicate that antigenic matching is helpful in these complicated cases, it may be possible to extend the benefits of corneal transplantation to many victims of corneal disease who were previously poor candidates for this procedure.[6]

5. Population studies

An epidemiologic research study aimed at identifying risk factors for the four leading causes of adult blindness in the United States—senile cataract, senile macular degeneration, chronic simple glaucoma, and diabetic retinopathy—is being supported by the National Eye Institute. This study, which is being conducted in Framingham, Massachusetts, involves the same population that has been part of the Framingham Heart Study (conducted by the National Heart and Lung Institute, also a component of the National Institutes of Health) since 1950. This investigation will measure the prevalence of these

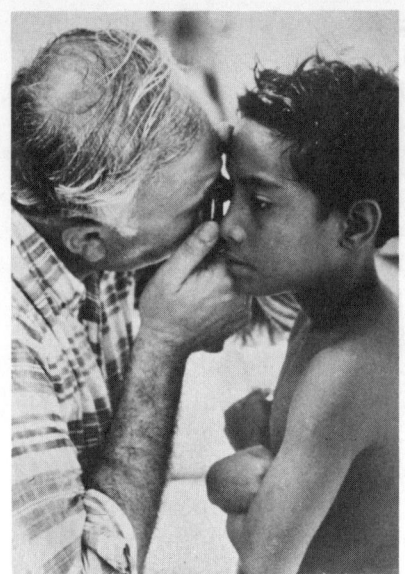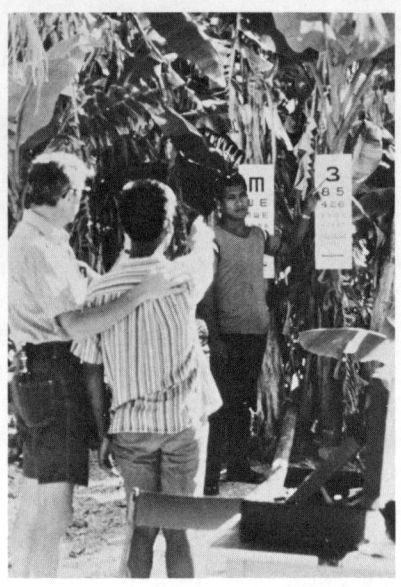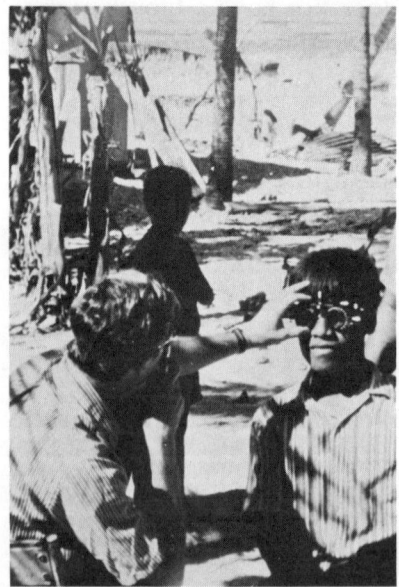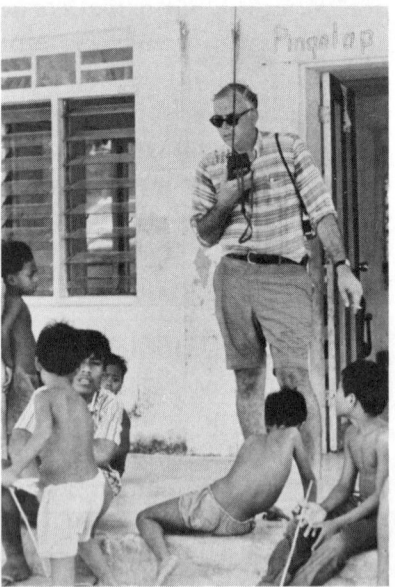

Widespread blindness on a remote Pacific atoll provided clues to a genetic eye disease for an expedition sponsored by Research to Prevent Blindness, Inc., which restored sight to many inhabitants. (COURTESY OF RESEARCH TO PREVENT BLINDNESS, INC., NEW YORK)

conditions in the study population and make use of all the earlier information collected by the National Heart and Lung Institute during the heart study to discover whether factors such as cigarette smoking, diet, blood pressure, and so forth are related to these eye disorders.[6]

IX. What Is Needed in the Fight Against Blindness and the Eye Diseases?

1. More funds are needed by the National Eye Institute to support greater research efforts to find answers to the blinding eye diseases, as well as increased funds for personnel and training and the construction of research facilities and centers.

2. Increased support of medical research and training is needed by Research to Prevent Blindness, Inc., and other voluntary agencies concerned with blindness and eye diseases.

Notes

1. National Center for Health Statistics, unpublished data based on household interviews of the 1971 civilian, noninstitutional population of 202,360,000, 1971.
2. H. A. Kahn and H. B. Moorhead, *Statistics on Blindness* in the Model Reporting Area, 1969-70. D.H.E.W. Publications no. (NIH) 73-427, National Eye Institute, National Institutes of Health, Department of Health, Education and Welfare, Washington, D.C., U.S. Government Printing Office, 1973.
3. Elizabeth Macfarlane Hatfield, M.P.H., "Estimates of Blindness in the United States," *The Sight-Saving Review* 32, no. 2 (Summer, 1973).
4. "Bed Disability, Limitation of Activity, Hospital Discharges, Hospital Days, and Deaths by Selected Conditions, U.S., 1971," unpublished data from the National Center for Health Statistics.
5. Application of the 1970 rate of legal blindness in the Model Reporting Area (14 states) to December 1972 estimate of U.S. resident population of 208,966,000 (Series P-25, no. 495, January 1973, U.S. Bureau of the Census).

6. Information obtained from the National Eye Institute, National Institutes of Health, Bethesda, Md. 20014, 1973.
7. Monthly Vital Statistics Report, Hospital Discharge Survey Data from the National Center for Health Statistics, U.S. Department of Health, Education, and Welfare, National Center for Health Statistics, Pub. no. (HSM) 72-1133, vol. 21, no. 3, supplement (2), 1972, p. 6. This data is included under "operations—lens."
8. Annual reports of the agencies listed.
9. Kenneth Trouern-Trend, *Blindness in the United States*, final summary report, Contract No. PA-43-67-1463 to the National Institute of Neurological Diseases and Blindness (Hartford, Conn.: Travelers Research Center, Inc., 1968), p. 77.
10. *1973 Marketing Guide*—published by *Drug Topics*, Medical Economics Company, Oradell, N. J.
11. *Blindness and Services to the Blind in the United States* (Cambridge, Mass.: OSTI Press, 1971), p. 34, table 1-7.
12. Lawrence B. Hobson, M.D., Deputy Assistant Chief Medical Director, Department of Medicine and Surgery, Veterans Administration, Washington, D.C., in personal communication dated April 16, 1975.

What Are the Facts About Cancer?

I. How Many People Die of Cancer in the United States?

1. The *number two killer* of our people is cancer.[1]
2. In 1973 353,440 Americans died of cancer[1] or about *one out of every 5.6 deaths.*
   a. This means that *cancer killed over 18 percent* of the 1,977,000 Americans who died in 1973.[1]
3. It is estimated that *53 million people now alive* in this country will eventually have cancer, and *35 million people will die from it,* unless new methods of prevention, treatment, or cures are found.[2]
4. Cancer kills one man, woman, or child every two minutes in the United States.
5. More than half (57 percent) of all cancer deaths are in people over 65 years of age.[1]

II. What Is the Economic Loss from Cancer?

Based on 1968 estimates on the economic costs of cancer, it is estimated the costs in 1972 totaled *$20 billion.* This includes direct and indirect costs of morbidity and mortality costs.[5]

III. How Many People Are Suffering from Cancer in the United States?

1. More than one million people were *under medical care* for cancer in 1975.[2]

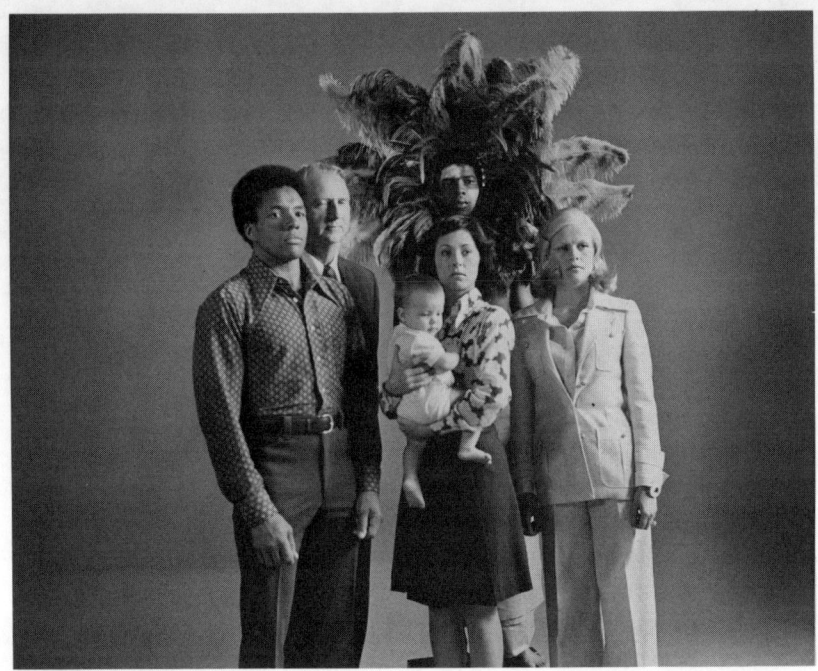

Actors appearing in "Faces," a 30-second TV spot sponsored by the American Cancer Society, which posed questions about cancer to which epidemiologists are seeking answers: Why do Japanese men have a higher incidence of stomach cancer than do American men? Why do the Massai in Africa have a low incidence of colon cancer, which is high in incidence in America? (COURTESY OF AMERICAN CANCER SOCIETY, INC., NEW YORK)

2. About *one out of every four* people now alive in the United States will have cancer *at some time in his life unless new preventive measures are found.*[2] This means that if cancer illness rates are not cut:

    a. Approximately *53 million people now alive* in the United States *will have some form of cancer during their lifetime.*[2]

    b. Approximately *35 million of these cancer victims will die* from cancer unless preventive new treatments or cures are found.

3. On the average, cancer will strike about *two out of every three American families.*[2]

4. Among women, cancer far exceeds any other disease as a cause of "working years lost"; among men, it is third after accidents and heart disease.[2]

Estimated Cancer Deaths and New Cases by Sex for All Sites—1974

	Estimated New Cases		
Site	Total	Male	Female
All Sites	655,000*	326,000*	329,000*
Buccal Cavity and Pharynx (Oral)	23,700	16,700	7,000
Lip	3,700	3,300	400
Tongue	4,800	3,400	1,400
Salivary gland / Floor of mouth / Other and unspecified mouth	8,500	5,100	3,400
Pharynx	6,700	4,900	1,800
Digestive Organs	166,900	86,800	80,100
Esophagus	7,400	5,500	1,900
Stomach	23,100	14,000	9,100
Small intestine	2,200	1,200	1,000
Large intestine (colon-rectum)	68,000	31,000	37,000
rectum	31,000	17,000	14,000
Liver	11,400	5,600	5,800
Pancreas	20,300	11,000	9,300
Other and unspecified digestive	3,500	1,500	2,000
Respiratory System	95,200	77,000	18,200
Larynx	9,500	8,300	1,200
Lung	83,000	67,000	16,000
Other and unspecified respiratory	2,700	1,700	1,000
Bone, Tissue and Skin	14,700	7,300	7,400
Bone	2,000	1,100	900
Connective tissue	4,500	2,400	2,100
Skin (melanoma)	8,200*	3,800*	4,400*
Breast	89,700	700	89,000
Genital Organs	125,800	58,100	67,700
Cervix, invasive } uterus	19,000*	—	19,000*
Corpus uteri	27,000	—	27,000
Ovary	17,000	—	17,000
Other female genital	4,700	—	4,700
Prostate	54,000	54,000	—
Other male genital	4,100	4,100	—
Urinary Organs	42,900	30,000	12,900
Bladder	28,400	21,000	7,400
Kidney and other urinary	14,500	9,000	5,500
Eye	1,700	800	900
Brain and central nervous system	10,700	5,900	4,800

	Estimated New Cases		
Site	Total	Male	Female
Endocrine Glands	8,900	2,600	6,300
Thyroid	7,800	2,100	5,700
Other endocrine	1,100	500	600
Leukemia	21,200	12,000	9,200
Lymphomas	27,600	15,100	12,500
Lymphosarcoma and reticulosarcoma	9,900	5,400	4,500
Hodgkin's disease	6,900	4,100	2,800
Multiple myeloma	7,500	3,800	3,700
Other lymphomas	3,300	1,800	1,500
All other and unspecified sites	26,000	13,000	13,000

SOURCE: *Ca—A Cancer Journal for Clinicians,* published by the American Cancer Society, vol. 24, no. 1 (January–February 1974).

Incidence estimates are based on rates from National Cancer Institute, Third National Cancer Survey.

*Carcinoma in situ of the uterine cervix and superficial skin cancers not included in totals.

ESTIMATED CANCER DEATHS AND NEW CASES BY SEX FOR ALL SITES—1974

	Estimated Deaths		
Site	Total	Male	Female
All Sites	355,000	193,000	162,000
Buccal Cavity and Pharynx (Oral)	7,900	5,700	2,200
Lip	225	200	25
Tongue	1,800	1,300	500
Salivary gland	650	400	250
Floor of mouth	525	400	125
Other and unspecified mouth	1,250	800	450
Pharynx	3,450	2,600	850
Digestive Organs	100,100	53,100	47,000
Esophagus	6,300	4,600	1,700
Stomach	14,300	8,400	5,900
Small intestine	650	300	350
Large intestine (colon-	37,300	17,300	20,000
rectum)	10,700	6,000	4,700
Liver	9,800	4,800	5,000
Pancreas	19,400	10,900	8,500
Other and unspecified digestive	1,650	800	850
Respiratory System	79,900	63,500	16,400
Larynx	3,200	2,800	400
Lung	75,400	59,900	15,500
Other and unspecified respiratory	1,300	800	500

	Estimated New Cases		
Site	Total	Male	Female
Bone, Tissue and Skin	8,700	5,000	3,700
Bone	1,900	1,100	800
Connective tissue	1,700	900	800
Skin (melanoma)	5,100	3,000	2,100
Breast	32,750	250	32,500
Genital Organs	41,800	19,000	22,800
Cervix, invasive } uterus	7,800	—	7,800
Corpus uteri	3,400	—	3,400
Ovary	10,700	—	10,700
Other female genital	900	—	900
Prostate	18,000	18,000	—
Other male genital	1,000	1,000	—
Urinary Organs	16,200	10,700	5,500
Bladder	9,200	6,300	2,900
Kidney and other urinary	7,000	4,400	2,600
Eye	350	150	200
Brain and central nervous system	8,100	4,700	3,400
Endocrine Glands	1,650	650	1,000
Thyroid	1,150	350	800
Other Endocrine	500	300	200
Leukemia	15,300	8,600	6,700
Lymphomas	20,400	11,200	9,200
Lymphosarcoma and heticulosarcoma	7,700	4,100	3,600
Hodgkin's Disease	3,700	2,200	1,500
Multiple Myeloma	4,600	2,400	2,200
Other Lymphomas	4,400	2,500	1,900
All other and unspecified sites	21,850	10,450	11,400

IV. Do More Men Die from Cancer Than Women?

Yes.

1. The 1973 cancer death rate among men was *26 percent higher* than the female cancer death rate. (These are crude death rates.[1])

 a. Of 351,055 cancer deaths in 1973, male deaths totaled 191,320, and female deaths, 159,735.[1]

2. Lung cancer is the leading cause of male cancer deaths—the rate being 18 times greater than 40 years ago.[2]

 a. An estimated 63,500 men (and 17,600 women) died from lung cancer in 1975.[2]

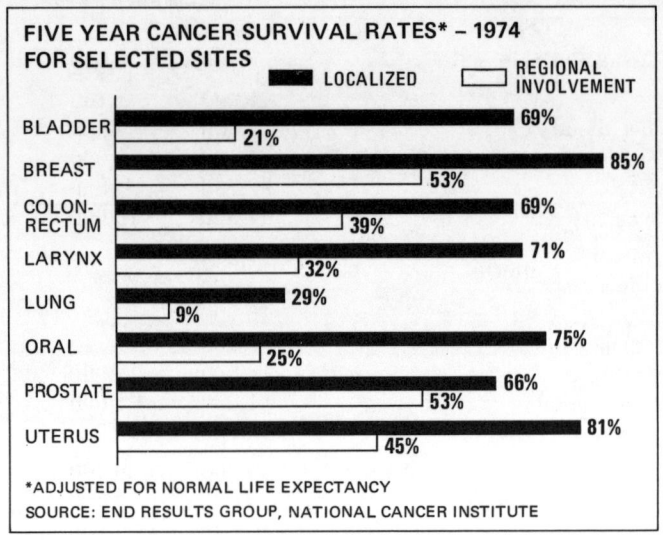

V. How Much Does Cancer Cost the Veterans Administration?

1. It is estimated that the *total annual cost of cancer to the Veterans Administration* is approximately *$208 million.*
   a. *Hospital treatment* accounts for an estimated *$158 million* of this total.[8]
   b. In fiscal year 1972, 26,227 veterans were receiving *compensation or pension payments* where the only or major disability was diagnosed as a malignancy. The approximate annual value of these awards was *$50,822,000.*[9]

VI. What Are the Chances Today of Recovery from Cancer?

1. About 665,000 new cancer cases were diagnosed for the first time in 1975.[2]
One cancer patient in three is now being saved, so about 221,000 of these Americans will be saved from cancer this year. A few years ago only 1 in 4 was saved; this is a *gain in lives saved of 55,000* patients each year.[2]

CANCER INCIDENCE BY SITE AND SEX* — 1974

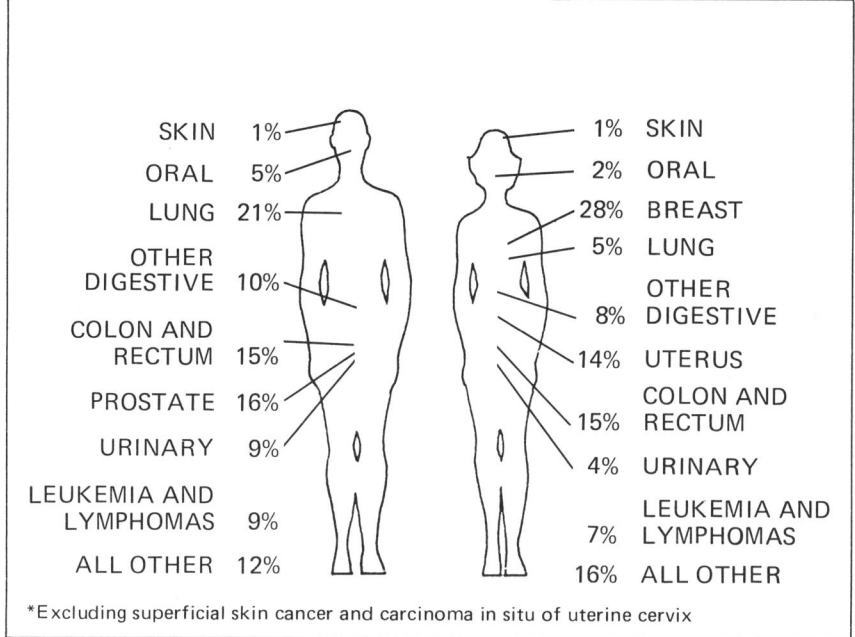

*Excluding superficial skin cancer and carcinoma in situ of uterine cervix

CANCER DEATHS BY SITE AND SEX* — 1974

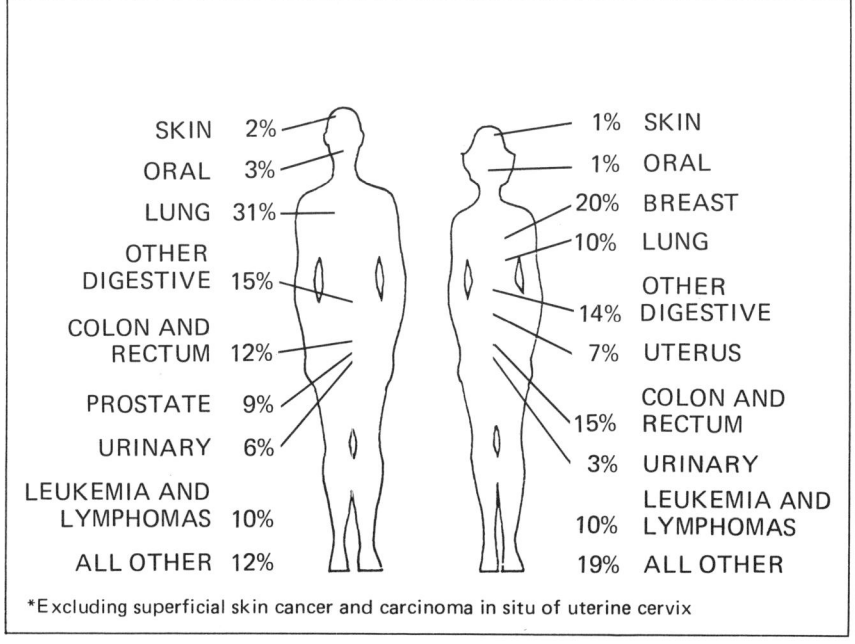

*Excluding superficial skin cancer and carcinoma in situ of uterine cervix

FROM: Ca — A Cancer Journal For Clinicians
January - February, 1974; Vol. 24, No. 1
Published by the American Cancer Society, New York

2. Of every 6 persons who get cancer today, 2 will be saved and 4 will die. Of the 4 who die, *one could have been saved* had proper treatment and early diagnosis been received in time. Thus, half of those who get cancer could be saved with present knowledge.[2]

VII. How Much Money Is Available for Research to Find New Treatments and Cures for Cancer from the Federal Government and Leading Voluntary Agencies?

1. Approximately *$892 million* for fiscal 1974, as follows:[7]

1. National Cancer Institute	$581,114,000
2. Other Federal Agencies	79,000,000
3. State & Local Governments	84,000,000
4. Voluntary agencies	92,000,000
5. Industry	16,000,000
6. Private Institutions	40,000,000
	$892,144,000

2. This means that we are spending about $2,500 per cancer death annually, or *$890* per case under treatment; but only *$16 per American now alive* who will have cancer unless cures or preventive measures are found.

3. In *contrast* to the *$892* million available from the major public and private sources for cancer research:

   a. The people of the United States spent in 1972 approximately:[10]

   $1.3 billion for greeting cards
   $1.3 billion for boxed candy
   $496 million for chewing gum

VIII. How Much Money Has the American Cancer Society Raised for Lay and Professional Education as Well as Service to Cancer Patients, Excluding Research?

1. Out of a total of $86,851,505 raised in 1973 in contributions and legacies, the American Cancer Society and all its state and local divisions allocated 46.3 percent—$37,541,106— for these purposes in 1973, over and above the amount raised

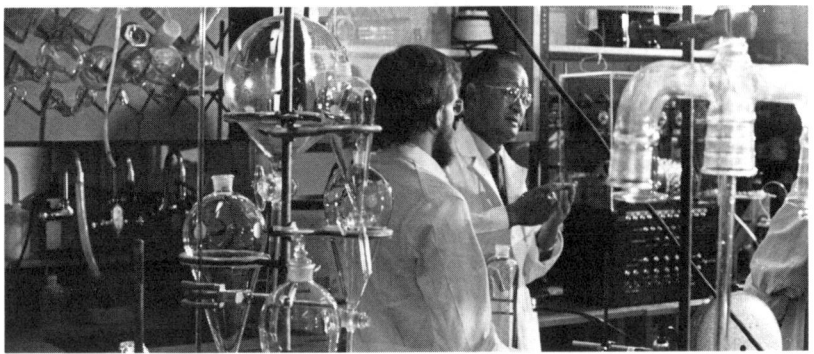

In synthesizing Human Growth Hormone (HGH), Dr. Choh Hao Li, director of the Hormone Research Laboratory, University of California, San Francisco (right in photo), has opened a new area of potential advancement in the battle against cancer. (COURTESY OF AMERICAN CANCER SOCIETY, INC., NEW YORK)

for research.[3] This does not include fund-raising or administration costs.

    a. This is in contrast to $832,862, the total raised nationally by the Cancer Society in 1944, and $372,057.17 in 1943 when the society allocated no funds for research whatever.[11]

  2. The American Cancer Society spent $21,711,897 for *research* in the same year (1973).[3]

IX. Is Cancer Primarily a Disease of Old Age?

1. *No.* Of 351,055 deaths in 1973 from cancer and other malignant tumors:[1]

    a. 149,089 or *42.5 percent were under 65 years old,* and 57.5 percent were over 65.

    b. 23,175 or about 6.6 percent were under 45 years old.

    c. 5,991 or about 2 percent were under 25 years old.

X. How Many Children Does Cancer Kill?

1. In the United States, cancer today *kills more children from 1 to 15 years of age than any other disease.*[1]

    a. In 1973, 2,961 children from 1 to 15 years of age died from cancer; about 43 percent died from leukemia (1,286).[1]

XI. What Are the Major Research Payoffs and Developments in the Treatment of Cancer?

1. *Chemotherapy* is now the key factor responsible for long-term survival in a number of types of widespread cancer occurring largely in children, adolescents, and young adults.[6]

Cancers Highly Responsive to Chemotherapy[6]
1. Choriocarcinoma
2. Retinoblastoma
3. Wilms' tumor (tumor of the kidney in children)
4. Hodgkin's disease
5. Acute lymphocytic leukemia
6. Lymphosarcoma
7. Mycosis fungoides
8. Embryonal testicular cancer
9. Ewing's sarcoma
10. Rhabdomyosarcoma
11. Burkitt's tumor

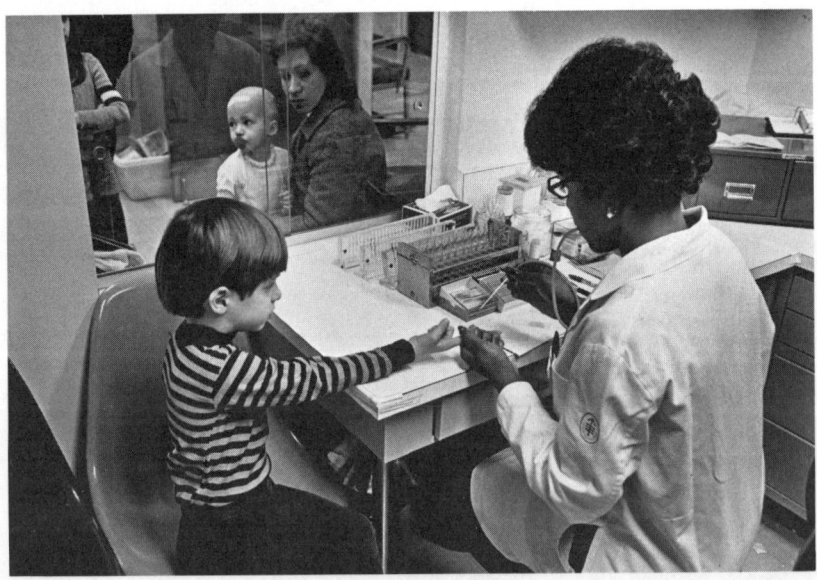

A young patient at the Memorial Sloan-Kettering Cancer Center in New York City. (COURTESY OF MEMORIAL SLOAN-KETTERING CANCER CENTER, NEW YORK)

Cancer 61

CANCERS THAT RESPOND TO CHEMOTHERAPY—AFTER SURGERY AND/OR RADIATION (WHERE SUITABLE) HAVE BEEN APPLIED

Type of Cancer	Useful Drugs	Results
Prolonged Survival or Cure		
Gestational trophoblastic tumors	Methotrexate, Dactinomycin, Vinblastine	70% cured
Burkitt's tumor	Cyclophosphamide (many others)	50% cured
Testicular tumors	Dactinornycin,* Methotrexate,* Chlorambucil*	30–40% respond, 2–3% cured
Wilms' tumor	Dactinomycin with surgery and radiotherapy	30–40% cured
Neuroblastoma	Cyclophosphamide with surgery and/or radiotherapy	5% cured
Acute lymphoblastic leukemia	Daunorubicin,* Prednisone,* Vincristine,* 6-Mercaptopurine,* Methotrexate,* BCNU*	90% remission; 70% survive beyond 5 years
Hodgkin's disease Stage IIIb & IV	HN2,* Vincristine,* Prednisone,* Procarbazine,* Bleomycin	70% respond, 40% survive beyond 5 years
Palliation and Prolongation of Life		
Prostate carcinoma	Estrogens, castration	70% respond with some prolongation of life
Breast carcinoma	Androgens, estrogens, alkylating agent,* 5-Fluorouracil,* Vincristine,* Prednisone,* Methotrexate*	20–40% respond with probable prolongation of life

Type of Cancer	Useful Drugs	Results
Chronic lymphocytic leukemia	Prednisone, alkylating agents	50% respond with probable prolongation of life
Lymphosarcoma	Prednisone, alkylating agents	50% respond with probable prolongation of life
Acute myeloblastic leukemia	Arabinosylcytosine and Thioguanine	65% remission with prolongation of life
Palliation with Uncertain Prolongation of Life		
Chronic granulocytic leukemia	Alkylating agents, 6-Mercaptopurine	90% respond with good control during most of course
Multiple myeloma	Alkylating agents	35% respond objectively; 50% have subjective relief of symptoms
Ovary	Alkylating agents	30–40% respond
Endometrium	Progestins	25% respond, chiefly pulmonary metastases
Uncertain Palliation		
Lung	Alkylating agents	30–40% respond briefly
Head and neck	Alkylating agents, methotrexate	20–30% respond briefly
Large bowel	5-Fluorouracil	10–20% respond
Stomach	5-Fluorouracil	10% respond
Pancreas	5-Fluorouracil	<10% respond
Liver	5-Fluorouracil	<10% respond
Cervix	Alkylating agents	<10% respond
Melanoma	Alkylating agents, VLB†	<5% respond
Adrenal cortex	o,p'DDD	Relief of Cushingoid syndrome
Soft tissue and osteogenic sarcoma	Adriamycin, methotrexate	20% respond
Local Chemotherapy		
Technique		
Intracavitary injection for recurrent effusion	Alkylating agents, Fluorouracil, Quinacrine	50% of effusions controlled

Type of Cancer	Useful Drugs	Results
Intrathecal injection for meningeal leukemia	Methotrexate, Arabinosylcytosine	80% improved 2 months
Extracorporeal perfusion for cancer of extremities	Alkylating agents	Irregular and uncertain
Continuous infusion for cancer of head and neck, liver and pelvis	Methotrexate-Leucovorin, Fluorouracil	Irregular and uncertain

SOURCE: *Ca—A Cancer Journal for Clinicians,* published by the American Cancer Society (July–August, 1974).
*May be used in combination.
†Vinblastine.

2. In many other cases, chemotherapy, while not yet curative in advanced metastatic disease, has delayed the progression of the disease and therefore prolonged survival.

This is true in breast cancer and cancer of the prostate, with the use of estrogen preparations in cancer of the prostate and the use of combinations of drugs and steroids in breast cancer, depending on the type of tumor and the age of the patient.

3. *Local chemotherapy was recently introduced for the treatment of precancerous keratoses and superficial skin cancers.* This form of therapy has been *proven successful in thousands of patients.* It is particularly valuable for the management of multiple extensive epitheliomas covering large portions of the body surface, which could not be adequately treated by other methods. Local chemotherapy is now being widely used as the *first practical chemical treatment for the most common neoplasms in man.*[13]

A cream containing an anticancer drug (such as 5-FU) is applied to the area containing the lesions. The tumors undergo selective inflammatory reactions which result in their disappearance without serious side effects on the normal skin or other tissues. The selective effect on tumors permits healing with minimal and usually no scar formations.[13]

Lesions that are too small to be otherwise diagnosed react and undergo resolution. Early lesions are therefore cured before they become more serious clinical problems. Thus the subsequent incidence of tumors is reduced. *Local chemotherapy therefore permits prevention, diagnosis, and cure of precancerous and malignant tumors.*[13]

The results indicate that chemical agents can be selective for the destruction of malignant cells without causing serious effects on normal cells.[13]

4. *For the first time immunological methods have been used successfully for the treatment of precancerous and malignant tumors* by inducing delayed hypersensitivity reactions in neoplasms of the skin.[13]

Prevention, early diagnosis of clinically not diagnosed lesions, and cures lasting for more than five years have been accomplished by immunotherapy in more than 50 patients with extensive premalignant keratoses, superficial basal cell carcinomas, and squamous carcinomas in situ.[13]

The immune response is induced by chemical agents which produce an allergy (delayed hypersensitivity) in the skin. This results in tumor destruction without adverse effect on the normal tissues. Immunotherapy has been shown to be associated with specific cell-mediated immunity predominantly due to hypersensitivity. The hypersensitivity reaction can be transferred from sensitized to nonsensitized patients by white blood cells.[13]

The selective curative effect of immunotherapy indicates that the body immune defense mechanisms can be induced to reject cancer without adverse effects.[13]

5. Chemotherapy (intensive treatment with drugs, often in combination) of acute leukemia, Burkitt's tumor and Hodgkin's disease is producing a *much higher percentage of long-term remissions* and probable cures than conventional therapy with single agents or low-dose combination therapy.[12]

Drugs developed in recent years which have proved useful and life-saving include vincristine, methotrexate, daunomycin, cytoxan, mercaptopurine, adriamycin and cytosine arabinoside.[12]

The *median survival time* for children with acute leukemia

has increased from just *under four months prior to 1947 to approximately three years*. Many patients have survived more than 5 years from the diagnosis of their disease—*some show no evidence of disease eight to 20 years after the first diagnosis.*[12]

XII. What Are the Leads in the Field of Cancer Research?

Today cancer is being attacked by research from within nearly every branch of science. The cancer studies are diverse; many are complex. The following highlights will indicate their scope, and some of the practical achievements:

1. Virus research

Virus studies continue to dominate the field of research on cancer causation.

There are a large number of cancers in animals known to be caused by viruses, and the evidence that they cause human cancer becomes stronger.

Evidence implicating viruses in human leukemia continues to mount. This area of research is being intensively studied with the eventual goal of the development of a preventive vaccine not only for leukemia but for other types of cancer as well.

2. Immunology

The study of the human body's resistance to disease offers cancer scientists some of the most promising leads to possible cancer control. Evidence is being accumulated on the existence of a natural resistance to cancer by healthy persons.

The role of the thymus gland in stimulating this immune mechanism is a factor under study.

3. Chemotherapy of cancer

The search for drugs that can halt or slow down tumor growth is a major undertaking of cancer research. Several thousand compounds are tested annually for anticancer activity. A group of these drugs has cured cancers in animals. About 44 drugs are now in use in treating human cancers.[4]

Ranking of Current Treatments for 16 Solid Tumors

Tumor	Cell kill potential of Chemotherapy	Cure potential of initial Surgery or radiotherapy	Tumor incidence
1. Breast	*Very High* 1. ≅60% response rate with drug combinations. 2. Good durations of remission. 3. Significant incidence of complete response. 4. Many active drugs.	*Excellent* 1. Almost all patients get curative intent treatment (i.e., primary tumor is removed). 2. Criteria exist for separating good and poor risk for cure.	Most common killer in women.
2. Ovary	*High* 1. Single agents can give 50% response rates. 2. Several agents active. 3. Combinations poorly tested.	*Generally Poor* 1. Overall 5-year survival is 20%-25%. 2. 36%-50% of women inoperable when first diagnosed.	High incidence and attacks relatively young women.
3. Lung	1. Small cell—*excellent* 2. Adenocarcinoma and large cell—*Fair to Poor* 3. Epidermoid—*Poor* 4. While response rates are reasonably high, impact on survival is minimal with possible exception of small cell.	*Poor* 1. Only 25% operable for cure with 5-year survivor rate of 25% in this group. 2. Overall 5-year survival dismal.	The single and most important cancer killer in the United States.
4. Colon	*Poor* 1. Several "active" agents but none exceed 20% response rate. 2. No successful combinations to date.	*Good* 1. ≅75% of patients amenable to curative resection. 2. Cure rate ≅50% in those undergoing curative resection.	Second leading cancer killer in both sexes. Highest incidence tumor in both sexes.

Tumor	Cell kill potential of Chemotherapy	Cure potential of initial Surgery or radiotherapy	Tumor incidence
5. Stomach	*Poor to Fair* 1. Several active drugs but none highly active. 2. Some slight successes with combinations (e.g., BCNU + 5-FU).	*Fair to Poor* 1. 25% of patients resectable for cure. 2. 25% of resected patients live 5 years. 3. Overall 5-year survival 12%.	Although incidence dropping, still No. 6 among cancer killers in United States. 21,000 new yearly cases estimated with 15,000 deaths.
6. Uterine-cervix	*Fair to Good* 1. Several active agents, but many unevaluated. 2. No combination data.	*Good* Cure rate dependent on stage: IA- 100% Both IB- 90% surgery IC- 70% and II- 50% x-ray III- 30% curative. IV- 5% 60% overall 5-year survival.	57,000 new cases yearly with 9,000 deaths.
7. Pancreas	*Poor* Two or three minimally active drugs with little impact on survival.	*Dismal* Overall only 7-10% amenable to curative resection with high surgical mortality rate and minimal survival of 5%-10%.	No. 4 in cancer killers with incidence rising dramatically
8. Head and Neck	*Good* 1. Several active agents—50% response rate for optimally used methotrexate. 2. Most drugs not studied. 3. Almost no combination data.	*Good* Both surgery and radiotherapy curative. 50% overall 5-year survival rate.	31,000 new cases yearly with ≅10,000 deaths.
9. Prostate	*Unknown*	*Generally Good* 1. Dependent on stage. 2. 51% overall 5-year survival rate.	High—45,000 new cases yearly with 18,000 deaths.

Tumor	Cell kill potential of Chemotherapy	Cure potential of initial Surgery or radiotherapy	Tumor incidence
10. Testicular	*Excellent* Curative potential against metastatic disease. Highly active combinations.	*Good* Both surgery and x-ray cure.	Rare overall, but most common tumor in young men age 28-32.
11. Sarcoma	*Fair to Good* Some degree of activity for the few drugs tested. Combinations give 40%-50% response rates.	*Variable* Depending on the many histologic types.	Generally rare.
12. Brain	*Poor* 1. One active class of drugs with minimal impact on survival. 2. Most drugs not studied. 3. No combination data.	Depends on histological type. In Grade III or IV glioma, no curative potential with surgery or x-ray alone. Overall survival at 5 years for *all types* = 28%	8,000 estimated yearly deaths from all types. Attacks the young.
13. Melanoma	*Fair to Poor* 1. Only a few active drugs with none greater than 20% response rate. 2. No successful combinations to date.	*Good* 61% overall 5-year survival rate.	52,000 estimated yearly deaths.
14. Bladder	*Almost Unknown* 1. Some activity for adriamycin and 5-FU, which are the only drugs with any kind of adequate data. 2. No combination data.	*Fair to Good* 56% overall 5-year survival.	24,000 new cases. 7,000 deaths.
15. Kidney	*None* Most drugs not tested.	*Fair* 36% overall 5-year survival	Estimated 9,000 deaths/year.
16. Esophagus	*None*	*Dismal*	Relatively uncommon.

SOURCE: National Cancer Institute, Bethesda, Md.

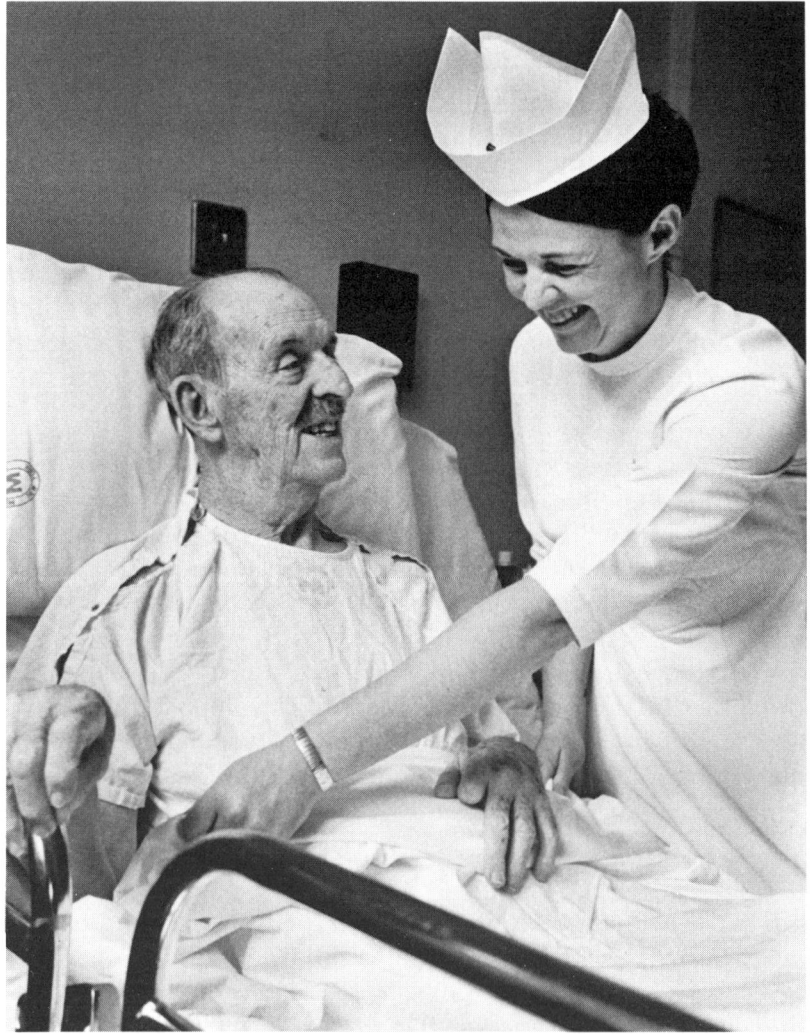

(COURTESY OF MEMORIAL SLOAN-KETTERING CANCER CENTER, NEW YORK)

4. Supportive therapy

This is designed to make cancer patients more comfortable and to control complications of the disease. Recent research has developed ways of *preventing hemorrhage* and infection in leukemia patients by transfusion of platelets.

Another potential adjunct to treatment being evaluated is the isolation of patients in a relatively germ-free environment during drug therapy.

5. Radiation treatment

This is being improved by the development of new instruments and more precise methods of irradiation to reduce undesirable side effects and deliver the radiation dose directly to the cancer-affected area. Conventional X-ray and supervoltage equipment is used. In addition to naturally radioactive radium, artificially produced isotopes such as I^{131} and P^{32} are available and have proved useful in treating some forms of cancer. Radiation is also being used in combination with other treatment. For example, in some cases of cancer, radiation before or after surgery appears to be of benefit to the patient.

6. Cancer surgery

Surgery is increasingly effective as a result of careful maintenance of the chemical balance of the patient's body, new techniques for replacing lost blood and for overcoming shock, new operating room equipment for monitoring patient responses, and a renewed emphasis on sterile operating room procedures.

New surgical techniques of perfusing anticancer drugs can sometimes be helpful in some forms of cancer. Advances have been made in reconstructive surgery, particularly following operations for cancer of the head and neck.

XIII. What Is Environmental Cancer Research?

It is the effort to identify factors in the world around us that increase the risk of developing malignant disease.

Several environmental carcinogens are known: (1) *excessive sunlight* causes skin cancer; (2) *certain industrial dyes and coal tar derivatives* used in the manufacture of rubber products cause bladder cancer in exposed workers; (3) *heavy doses of X rays and other forms of ionizing radiation* cause leukemia, bone tumors, and other types of cancer.

XIV. Do Cigarettes Help to Cause Lung Cancer? Yes!

Recently cigarette smoking (and atmospheric pollution) have been recognized as contributing factors in the development of lung cancer.

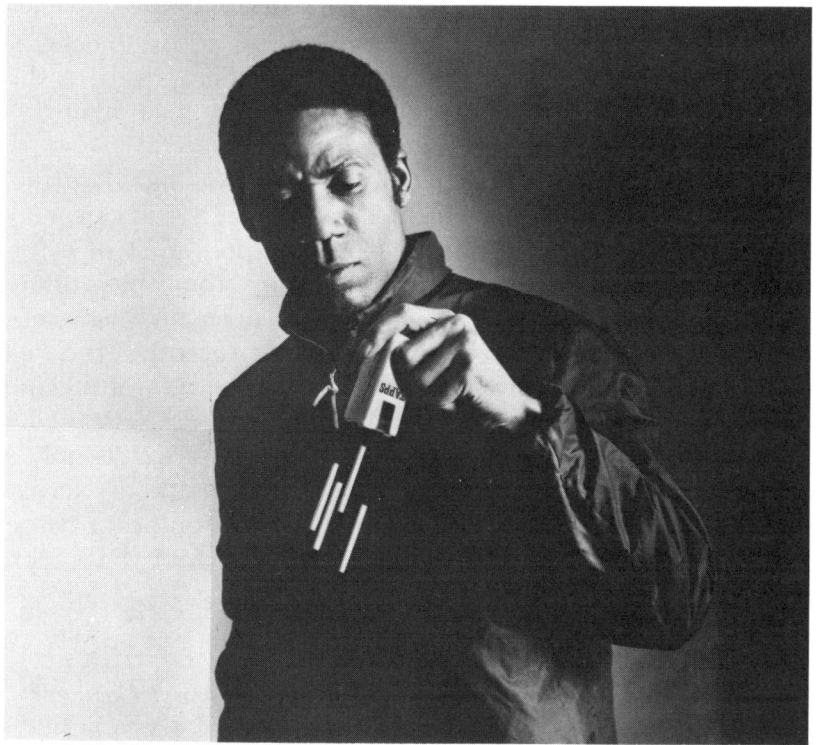

Don't let your dreams go up in smoke! (COURTESY OF AMERICAN CANCER SOCIETY, INC., NEW YORK)

(Lung cancer, the *chief cause of cancer death in men,* killed in 1975 approximately 63,500 men and 17,600 women, a total of 81,100.[2])

(In 1973, almost 20 times as many people died from lung cancer alone as from all forms of tuberculosis.[1])

The public is being warned of the health risks associated with the use of cigarettes, and many urban areas are taking steps to rid themselves of seriously polluted air.

XV. What Are Other Areas of Research?

Research on cancer diagnosis is one of the major approaches to solving the cancer problem. Because early diagnosis is almost always essential if cancer is to be effectively treated, methods are sought to detect the disease at the earliest possible moment, even before overt symptoms appear.

Improvements in techniques during the past decade have made it possible to study, with high precision, the biochemistry of the human body, and such studies may lead to the recognition of subtle changes that foreshadow malignant disease or signal its microscopic presence.

Many scientists are engaged in research on blood, urine, and other body fluids in which a cancer diagnostic clue may lie. Others are investigating the possible application of cytology to the detection of cancer of the lung, stomach, prostate gland, and other sites into which the body normally sheds cells that can be removed and examined. This procedure, the *Pap smear*, has proved highly successful in the detection of uterine cancer among large groups of women.

Mammography for the detection of breast cancer is only a few years old and now an even more precise method—xerography—has been developed, through which significant tissue changes can be detected even before a tumor has been formed.[3]

XVI. What Are the Needs in the Fight Against Cancer?

1. Large additional funds are needed by the National Cancer Institute, the American Cancer Society, and other agencies working in this area to exploit leads in research in viruses, immunology, and chemotherapy so that cancer can be eliminated.

An effort to make the conquest of cancer a national goal with funds similar to the National Aeronautics and Space Administration is necessary if the conquest of cancer is to come in the next decade.

2. *More funds are needed for the construction of cancer research center facilities.*

3. *New treatments and cures* must be found to aid the over one million people now *under treatment* for cancer, the estimated *53 million now alive* who will *have* cancer and the *35 million of these who will die* from cancer unless these new treatments, cures, or preventive measures are found and successfully put into use.

Notes

1. National Center for Health Statistics, Department of Health, Education, and Welfare, Washington, D.C.
2. 1973 and 1975 Cancer Facts and Figures. Published by American Cancer Society, New York.
3. 1972 and 1973 Annual Reports, American Cancer Society, New York.
4. Information obtained from the National Cancer Institute, Bethesda, Maryland, 1973.
5. Barbara S. Cooper, Office of Research & Statistics, Social Security Administration, Department of Health, Education, and Welfare, in personal communication January 26, 1975.
6. *Ca—A Cancer Journal for Clinicians.* Published by the American Cancer Society, New York. July/August 1973.
7. 1975 Fact Book. Published by the National Cancer Institute, National Institutes of Health, Bethesda, Maryland.
8. 1972 Annual Report, Administrator of Veterans Affairs. Roughly, 54,000 patients were discharged from VA hospitals during fiscal 1972 with a principal diagnosis of malignant neoplasms. The average length of stay of all discharged patients in the VA hospital system in fiscal 1972 was 50.4 days. The per diem cost in the medical bed sections of VA inpatient facilities in fiscal 1972 totaled $58. Thus, assuming that the 54,000 patients were hospitalized on the average 50.4 days, at a per diem cost of $58, their over-all cost of care was $158 million.
9. Department of Veterans Benefits, Veterans Administration, Washington, D.C., personal communication, March 1, 1973, from Edward R. Silberman, Director, Management & Budget Service.
10. 1973 Marketing Guide, published by Drug Topics, Medical Economics Co., Oradell, New Jersey.
11. American Cancer Society, New York, Frank Kramer, September 24, 1952.
12. James F. Holland, M.D., Roswell Park Memorial Institute, Buffalo, New York. Personal communication August 30, 1974.
13. Edmund Klein, M.D., Chief Department of Dermatology, Roswell Park Memorial Institute, Buffalo, New York.

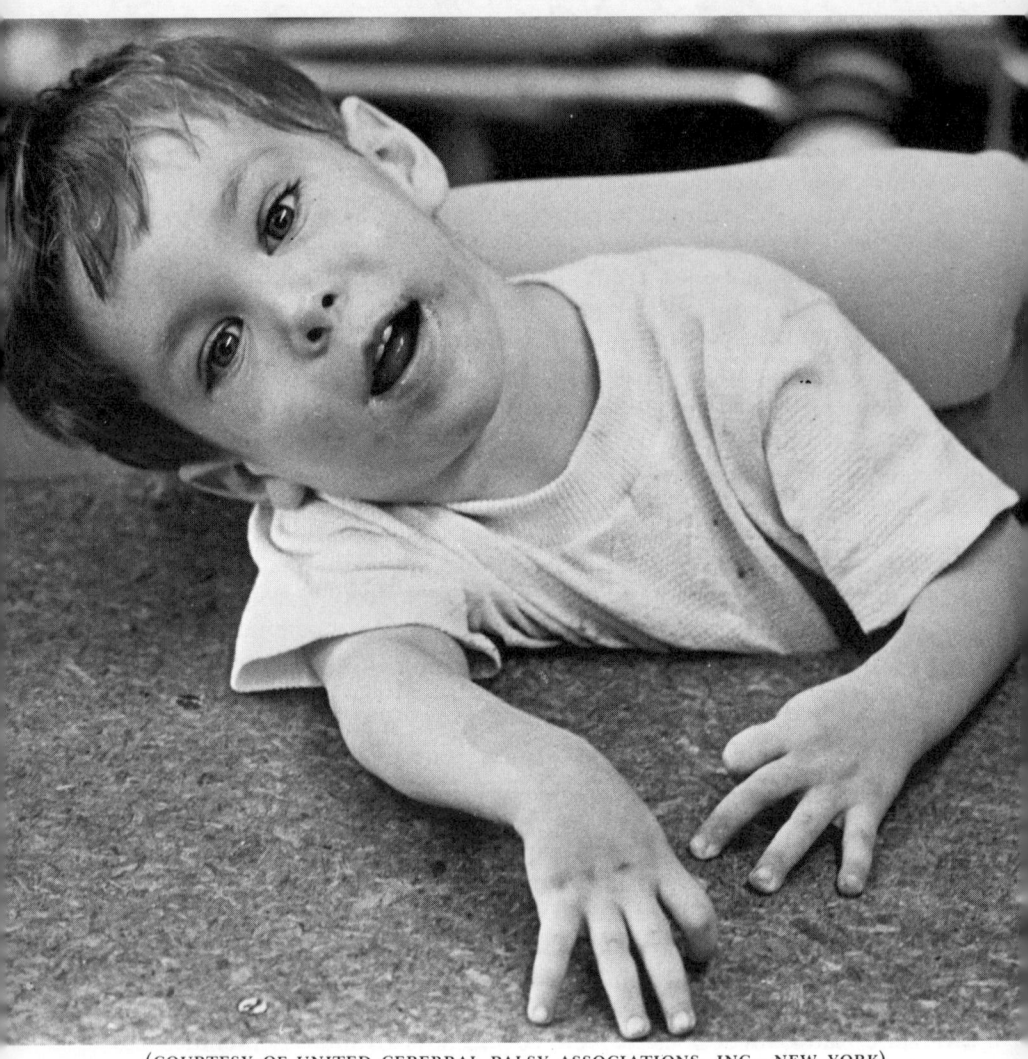
(COURTESY OF UNITED CEREBRAL PALSY ASSOCIATIONS, INC., NEW YORK)

What Are the Facts About Cerebral Palsy?

I. What Is Cerebral Palsy?

1. Cerebral palsy is the general term applied to a *group of disabling symptoms resulting from damage to the developing brain that may occur before, during, or after birth and that results in loss or impairment of control over voluntary muscles.*[1]

2. Anyone may be affected by the condition, regardless of race, economic standing, or environment, since anything that can damage brain tissue can cause cerebral palsy.[1]

3. Cerebral palsy is neither progressive nor fatal. For the most part it is not inherited.[1]

II. How Many People Are Victims of Cerebral Palsy?

An estimated 750,000 persons have cerebral palsy. *About 15,000 babies are born with cerebral palsy annually* or 1 newborn in every 200 live births.[1]

III. What Are the Characteristics of Cerebral Palsy? [1]

1. Motor involvement

The characteristic of cerebral palsy is the presence of motor involvement. These motor involvements include awkward or involuntary movements, poor balance, irregular gait, poorly articulated speech, tightness of muscles—all of which are caused by the brain's inappropriate regulation of movements.[1]

2. Associated handicaps in cerebral palsy

Although cerebral palsy denotes a person with a motor handicap, its relationship to the brain almost inevitably results in other types of handicaps as well.[1]

a. *Mental retardation:* from 50-75 percent of children and adults with cerebral palsy are retarded intellectually to some degree, mostly with mild to moderate subnormalities.

b. *Convulsions:* these may initially occur at any age.

c. *Speech problems:* especially poor articulation (a result of faulty coordination of the speech musculature) affects 70 percent or more persons with cerebral palsy.

d. *Visual disorders:* these include an eye turning in or out (strabismus) or visual impairment affecting 35 percent of those with cerebral palsy.

e. *Hearing impairments:* reported in 20 percent of persons with cerebral palsy when the disorder is due to jaundice following birth.

f. *Learning disabilities:* conceptual and perceptual problems and language disorders may occur in children with generally average or above average intelligence.

g. *Behavior disorders:* brain damage may result in less-than-normal adaptability to stress and anxiety; however, a major effect is poor parent-child relationships.

h. *Dental abnormalities:* insufficient buildup of tooth enamel during prenatal development makes the person with cerebral palsy especially susceptible to dental caries and "irregular" positioning of teeth.

i. *Contractures:* joints such as the ankle, elbow, or wrist become fixed in an abnormal or deformed position because of the excessive and unnatural pull of muscles around that joint.

IV. What Are the Major Types of Cerebral Palsy?

1. There are *six major types* of cerebral palsy, as follows:[1]

a. *Spastic:* muscle spasms are the most frequently occurring motor symptom of cerebral palsy.[1]

b. *Athetoid:* marked by constantly recurring, slow, involuntary writhing movements of the arms and legs.[1]

c. *Ataxic:* walking like a drunken person.[1]
d. *Tremor:* similar to the fine tremulousness seen in adults who have Parkinsonism.[1]
e. *Rigidity:* muscles contract slowly and stiffly, leading to clumsiness.[1]
f. *Mixed:* two or more of the above.[1]

2. The motor difficulty may involve all four extremities or it may be limited to just one; or an arm or leg on one side of the body may be disabled (the most common type).[1]

In some persons with cerebral palsy, the symptoms are so slight that except for some clumsiness they may be unnoticed. Others may be extensively handicapped, in a wheelchair, and require assistance with the most basic activities of daily living, such as feeding and toileting.[1]

V. What Are the Main Causes of Cerebral Palsy?

1. *Prematurity.*[1]
2. *Anoxia* (difficulty of the newborn in breathing).[1]
3. *Complications* of labor or delivery.[1]
4. *Jaundice* (a yellowing of the skin) of the newborn due to Rh or other blood type incompatibilities, infection, or prematurity.[1]
5. *Infections* of the brain, such as meningitis or encephalitis. Occasionally an inflammation of the brain may occur after routine cases of measles or German measles and other virus disease.[1]
6. *Poisonings,* such as lead.[1]
7. *Accidents* resulting in head trauma.[1]
8. Low birth weight independent of the duration of pregnancy.[2]

In over one-third of affected individuals, the cause at present is unknown.[1]

VI. What Are the Treatment Goals in Cerebral Palsy?

The general treatment goal for the individual with cerebral palsy is to help him function as well as he can within the limits of his basic handicap. While it may be impossible to alter the extent of his motor coordination, it is possible to train him to get the "most out of what he has." At present, therapists are using *certain treatment regimes geared specifically to improving the lack of coordination.* There is insufficient evidence to know whether the improvement frequently seen is solely the result of treatment or simply the result of growth and maturation.[1]

Drug therapy (including the tranquilizing drugs, L-DOPA, Dantrolene) is also being used to control some of the symptoms of cerebral palsy.[1]

Another major treatment objective is the *prevention of the secondary handicaps* listed above. If this is impossible, then the aim is to reduce the harmful effects these conditions cause.[1]

VII. What Are the Nonmedical Aspects of Cerebral Palsy?

1. Changing needs of cerebral palsy victims over the years

Since cerebral palsy affects the adjustment of child and family in so many ways, treatment cannot be geared solely to the child's physical needs. A *comprehensive approach to treatment includes the afflicted child as well as his family* and the treatment regime may change to meet their changing needs.[1]

As he grows older, the child with the multiple handicaps of cerebral palsy needs, in addition to medical and related therapies, *special education, vocational counseling and guidance, psychiatric and/or psychological counseling, recreational, and social programs.*[1]

Adults with cerebral palsy need facilities in which they can live independently, barrier-free transportation, work opportunities, education, legal and financial counseling, recreational and social programs—in short, what other adults need but which are usually denied to the handicapped.[1]

2. Economic problems

Providing *long-term* treatment, and particularly *residential care* when the child is severely disabled, often results in *financial sacrifices* that place a very heavy burden upon the entire family. Few families have the resources to meet these costs, making it necessary to utilize both public and private resources.[1]

Adults with cerebral palsy who *can be vocationally rehabilitated and become sufficiently independent to hold competitive jobs* often cannot find employment. They may be able only to work in noncompetitive situations such as sheltered workshops.[4]

Many, because of the severity of their handicaps, *will require partial or total lifetime care.*[1]

3. Parental problems

The *parents* of the handicapped child also *require counseling and assistance* to help them adjust to their child's condition. A local affiliate of United Cerebral Palsy Associations can help the family understand and deal with the problems of raising and maintaining a handicapped son or daughter. The affiliate can also assist parents in locating whatever additional community resources may be required. UCP affiliates often assume lifetime partnerships with the individual with cerebral palsy and his family and, in turn, families become involved in many aspects of the local agency's program.[1]

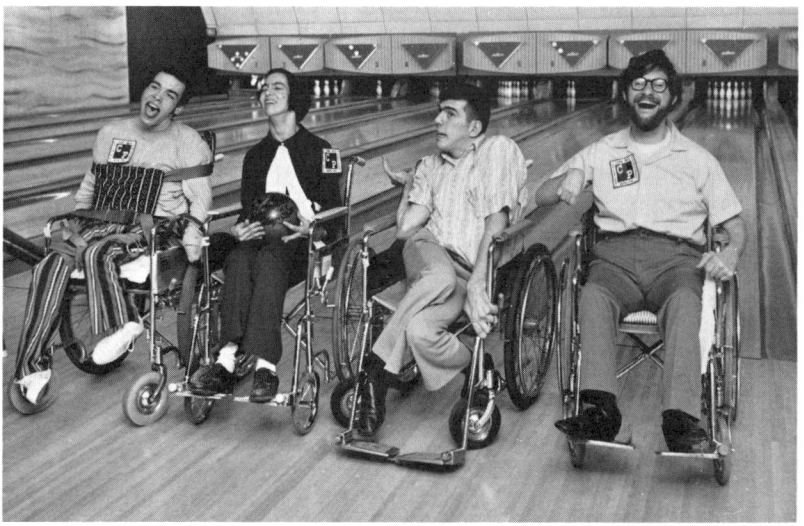

United Cerebral Palsy bowling team from Columbus, Missouri, enjoys a victory.
(COURTESY OF UNITED CEREBRAL PALSY ASSOCIATIONS, INC., NEW YORK)

VIII. What's Being Done to Help the Victims of Cerebral Palsy?

Since damage to brain tissue cannot presently be repaired, there is no cure for cerebral palsy as such. However, with early and appropriate treatment and training, individuals with the mental and physical disabilities of cerebral palsy often can and do improve. The following spectrum of services may be required.[1]

1. Medical

Specialized diagnosis, testing, and evaluation; nursing care; physical, occupational, speech, and hearing therapies; surgery; psychiatric, psychological counseling, and guidance; special dental treatment; braces, glasses, hearing aids, and other supportive and adaptive equipment; drugs.

2. Educational

Infant programs stressing the stimulation of growth and development along as normal lives as possible for babies identified early in life as having brain damage or neurological impairments.

Prenursery and nursery groups; preschool and school readiness programs; developmental and day-care programs; special education classes.

3. Vocational

Prevocational testing and evaluation; vocational guidance and counseling; job training and placement; sheltered workshops; social and personal adjustment training.

4. Social and recreational services

Camps (day and residential); group activities such as adapted sports; hobby and creative activities; family recreation activities.

5. Supportive family services

Training parents to work with their handicapped children; parent counseling and guidance; information about and referral to other social agencies (homemaker, medical and nursing, and so forth).

Cerebral Palsy 81

In recent years, a rapid expansion of diagnostic, treatment and training facilities and services for children and adults with cerebral palsy has taken place. These include diagnostic clinics, rehabilitation therapy centers, developmental nurseries, preschool and special education and training programs, sheltered workshops, home service programs. In addition, early identification of babies suspected of having brain damage or neurological impairment is being emphasized so that effective care and treatment may be started promptly.

IX. What Additional Facilities and Services Do Individuals with Cerebral Palsy and Their Families Require?[1]

Although progress has been made in helping many individuals with cerebral palsy, there remains a *great need for special facilities, services, and programs* for those persons who are so physically and mentally disabled they require lifelong care.

These include such supportive services as:[1]

1. Information, referral, and follow-along services (assuring continuity of services to meet changing needs).

2. Special living arrangements for handicapped individuals adapted to their social, physical, and intellectual capacities.

3. Protective services to assist those with multiple handicaps to obtain community services to which they are entitled and which also protect their civil and human rights. (These should include a public guardianship program, especially important as parents grow older and die.)

4. Programs that provide creative and social experiences for cerebral palsied teen-agers and adults without vocational potential.

X. What Agencies Are Working in the Field of Cerebral Palsy?

1. Federal agencies[1]

The National Institute of Neurological and Communicative Disorders and Stroke, National Institutes of Health, Bethesda, Maryland; *The National Institute of Child Health and Development,* National Institutes of Health, Bethesda, Maryland; *Bureau of Education for the Handicapped,* Office of Education, Department of Health, Education, and Welfare; *Maternal and Child Health Services,* Health Services and Mental Health Administration, Department of Health, Education, and Welfare; *Division of Developmental Disabilities Administration,* Social and Rehabilitation Service Administration, Department of Health, Education, and Welfare; *Veterans Administration.*

2. National Voluntary Health Organizations

United Cerebral Palsy Associations, Inc., and its state and local affiliates; the *National Easter Seal Society for Crippled Children and Adults,* Inc., and affiliated Easter Seal societies in every state and Puerto Rico; National Association for Retarded Children and the state and local units: Association for Aid to Crippled Children.[1]

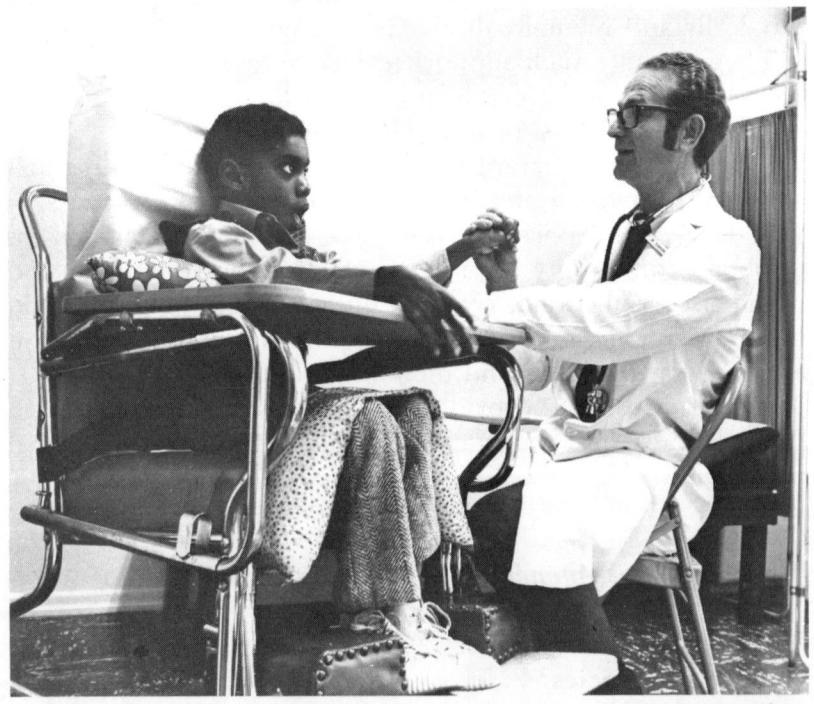

(COURTESY OF UNITED CEREBRAL PALSY ASSOCIATIONS, INC., NEW YORK)

3. Some state and local tax-supported services

State departments of health and welfare; state departments of education; state hospital schools; state vocational rehabilitation services; state services for crippled children; state departments of mental hygiene and mental retardation; developmental disabilities councils; public school programs for exceptional children.[1]

4. Professional organizations

The American Academy for Cerebral Palsy; the American Academy of Neurology; American Neurological Association; the American Academy of Pediatrics; The International Cerebral Palsy Society, and so forth.[3]

5. Civic, service, and fraternal groups

The groups that support direct service and research activities, as well as programs for recruitment and training of professional workers.[3]

XI. How Much Is Being Spent for Services for Victims of Cerebral Palsy and for Professional and Public Education?

1. In 1974, fund-raising campaigns conducted by United Cerebral Palsy affiliates across the country raised a total of $19,653,147.[1] Allocations by the National Association of the UCP Associations for the year ended September 30, 1974, were as follows:

Research, professional health education, and training	$ 896,496
Community services	1,290,297
Public health education and information	455,240
Total program services	$2,642,033

2. Other public and private agencies contribute indirectly to cerebral palsy-related work by providing facilities and services that are not used exclusively for that purpose. Funds from

public or private sources to aid crippled children, the mentally retarded, underprivileged families, veterans, and so forth, may be used for cerebral palsy management, but because they are not so labeled, it is impossible to compute how much indirect financing is being done in the field of cerebral palsy nationally.[1]

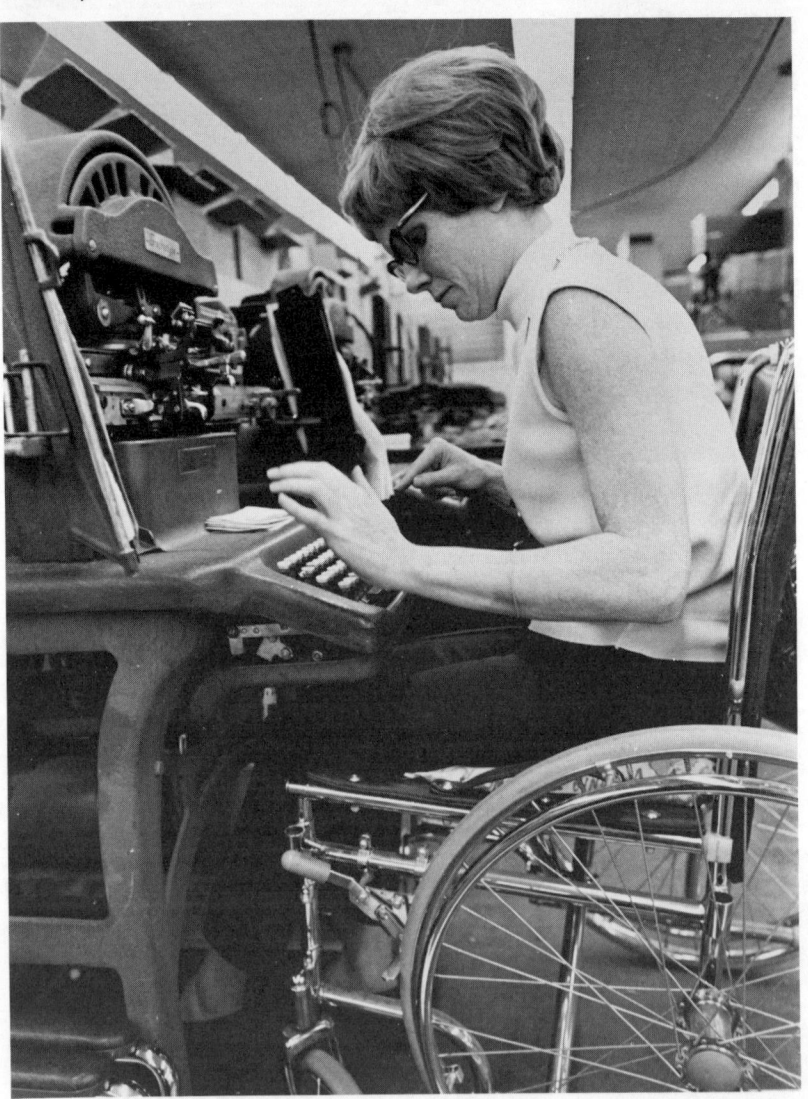

(COURTESY OF UNITED CEREBRAL PALSY ASSOCIATIONS, INC., NEW YORK)

a. For the fiscal year ending August 31, 1972, the National Easter Seal Society for Crippled Children and Adults (including its 52 state and territorial societies) had a total income of $52.9 million.[3]

XII. How Much Money Is Available for Research in Cerebral Palsy?

About *$13 million* as follows:
1. *Voluntary agencies' funds listed total $896,496.*
   a. In 1974, appropriations and expenses for research and professional health education and training of the *United Cerebral Palsy Research and Educational Foundation totaled $896,496.*[1]
   The foundation underwrites studies in a wide-ranging research attack on cerebral palsy *concentrating its priority efforts on problems directly related to prevention.*[1]
   Foundation support stresses research related to prematurity prevention through family planning and other means, blood group incompatibilities, viral diseases affecting the nervous system, problems of labor and delivery, and resuscitation of the newborn.[1]
   b. Other national voluntary health organizations such as the *National Association for Retarded Children,* the *National Foundation* and the *National Easter Seal Society for Crippled Children and Adults* have provided funds for research in fields closely related to and affecting our knowledge of cerebral palsy.[1]
   For the fiscal year ended May 31, 1974, the *National Foundation* expended $6,193,083 in support of research programs against birth defects.[6]
   For the fiscal year ended August 31, 1972, the National Easter Seal Society for Crippled Children and Adults expended $455,294 for all medical research within its area of interest.[3]
2. *Government funds listed total $12.2 million.*[2]
   a. The National Institute of Neurological and Communicative Disorders and Stroke of the U.S. Public Health Service spent in fiscal year 1973 for research in cerebral palsy an estimated $12.2 million.

3. *In comparison* with the above $13 million spent for research in cerebral palsy, the American people spent in 1972 approximately:[5]

- $496 million for chewing gum
- $276 million for women's hair sprays
- $302 million for toilet waters and cologne

4. Public awareness of cerebral palsy as a national health problem is of such recent origin that research funds in this field still fall far short of minimum needs.

XIII. What Are Some of the Problems in Cerebral Palsy That Require Research?

1. *The target areas of cerebral palsy research* may be grouped under three basic classifications:

　a. *Primary prevention* of the main cause of cerebral palsy is *prevention of prematurity*. This can be largely eliminated by widespread efforts to promote family planning to prevent too frequent pregnancies and to prevent them in very young girls. More research is needed for easier methods of contraception.

　b. *Detection*—particularly the detection at an earlier age in order to start appropriate treatment and developmental stimulation as early as possible.

　c. *Therapy* (treatment)—*both basic and clinical research are needed* in each of these areas. The basic research attempts to understand the essential mechanism of central nervous system functions. The clinical research involves study of the problems of management of cerebral palsied patients, evaluation of various methods of treatment, and planning facilities to meet their needs.[3] [4]

2. The following is a partial list of *projects that require continuing research* in the field of cerebral palsy:[1]

　a. *Prevention*
　　i. Causes of prematurity, through better means of family planning, and through hormonal and other studies.
　　ii. Studies of incompatible blood types (for example, Rh) and treatment of hyperbilirubinemia.

Cerebral Palsy

    iii. Search for viruses that may affect the fetus and to develop appropriate vaccines (for example, the German measles virus that has already been identified).
    iv. Fetal malnutrition.
    v. Complications of pregnancy, such as toxemia and diabetes.
    vi. Complications of delivery (for example, prolonged labor).
    vii. Problems of the newborn (for example, difficulties in breathing).
    viii. Studies into the causes of accidents and poisonings.
    ix. Studies to enable doctors to recognize the presence of an abnormal fetus during the first three months of pregnancy.
b. *Diagnosis*
    i. Improved techniques for early recognition.
    ii. Investigation of brain anatomy and pathology.
    iii. Improved psychological testing methods.
    iv. Improved vocational testing methods.
c. *Treatment*
    i. Interrelationships of medical, therapeutic, and education services in the total management program for the individual with cerebral palsy.
    ii. Development of new physical and occupational therapy techniques to improve motor function.
    iii. Definitive study to evaluate effectiveness of presently used physical, occupational, and speech therapy regimes.
    iv. Biomechanic studies for development of more useful prosthetics and assistive aids.
    v. Study of psychological problems of the cerebral palsied child and his family.
    vi. Studies to evaluate the most effective programs for *long-term care.*
    vii. Studies to demonstrate improved ways to *deliver services to the handicapped child and his family,* taking into account economy and efficiency—but with

emphasis on respect for the dignity of the patient.[1]

viii. Explore the possibilities of utilizing the new knowledge and techniques developed by NASA for possible adaptation or modification to help victims of cerebral palsy.

XIV. What Are the Goals in Program Planning in the Fight Against Cerebral Palsy?

1. Personnel training

Special training of medical and allied personnel (including doctors, nurses, therapists, psychologists, educators, social workers, vocational and recreational specialists) is needed to meet the need for cerebral palsy treatment and extended services throughout the United States.

A long-range goal should be the inclusion of cerebral palsy training as part of the general curriculum at medical and professional schools, so that doctors, therapists, teachers, and so forth, may receive this as part of their basic training. Also, special postgraduate training in this field is needed.[3]

Especially important also is the training of the therapeutic personnel to work in a team or cross-disciplinary relationship so that the various needs of the person with cerebral palsy may be met.

The UCP Research and Educational Foundation has attempted to fill this gap by supporting many training programs in medical centers throughout the United States. United Cerebral Palsy has supported four clinical professorships in cerebral palsy at Columbia University, New York; University of California, Los Angeles; University of Kansas, Kansas City; and Johns Hopkins University, Baltimore.[1]

2. New services and facilities

Closer attention to the problem of cerebral palsy in many communities of the nation makes evident the need for *improved and expanded facilities for prevention, diagnosis, and treatment.* Especially needed are facilities for the intensive care of high-risk newborn babies and those for severely physically and mentally handicapped persons. In addition, various types of facilities are needed in some areas such as family planning centers, outpatient treatment centers, rehabilitation centers, clinic-schools, social and recreational programs, day-care and development centers, information, referral and follow-along services, homemakers, vacation homes, meals on wheels, vocational guidance and job-placement programs, and home services for children and adults in sparsely populated rural areas.

Special services and programs also are needed to identify high-risk mothers and infants, and to *increase public understanding and acceptance of the importance of good prenatal health and family planning*. New programs and services also must be developed for cerebral palsied teen-agers and adults without vocational potential.

Required also are some centers that can integrate diagnosis, treatment, education, psychological guidance, research, and the training of personnel in a cross-disciplinary approach. Of course, services and facilities should always be based on needs in any given community, since they vary.[1]

XV. What Research Progress Has Been Made in Cerebral Palsy?

1. A method involving *multiple exchange blood transfusions* was discovered for preventing kernicterus, a leading cause of infant death (approximately 1,000 deaths annually) and of cerebral palsy.[1]

Cerebral palsy from this cause has been *reduced from 15 percent to 1 percent*.[1]

2. The more recent introduction of *phototherapy* has further enabled successful treatment of these children in many instances without the need to resort to transfusion.[7]

3. The Rh-conflict type can be wiped out in the future through *preventive use of Rh-O Immune Globulin* within 72 hours of delivery or miscarriage of an Rh-positive baby by an Rh-negative mother.[1]

4. Some newly developed drugs have been helpful in the treatment or management of cerebral palsy patients.[7]

   a. The tranquilizing drugs have been helpful in ameliorating aberrant behavior in some cases and the amphetamines have been of special value in organic hyperactivity.

b. L-DOPA has been useful in the athetoid type of cerebral palsy.

c. Dantrolene has proven useful for the relief of spasticity in cerebral palsy.

5. Accurate monitoring of premature babies, especially as it relates to oxygen levels, blood acidity, and disturbances in blood chemistry, along with appropriate remedial therapy, has greatly reduced the unusually high incidence of cerebral palsy in premature babies.[7]

6. A chemical substance called "surfactant," which enables the newborn lungs to mature and function properly, is entirely lacking in premature babies, causing respiratory distress and consequent damage to the central nervous system if the baby survives. The administration of corticosteroids has been found to increase the amount of surfactant in the lungs in animal membranes. A simple test for surfactant at birth has been developed. If cortosteroid therapy proves effective in human membranes, this test may save many babies from brain damage or death.[1]

7. Pregnancies that occur when the mother is poorly nourished, too young, too old, or when her babies come too frequently are now known to result in babies born with brain and neurological defects. *Family planning,* through contraceptives, and good prenatal and neonatal care can reduce the incidence of cerebral palsy caused by these factors.

Notes

1. United Cerebral Palsy Associations, Inc., 66 East 34th Street, New York, N. Y. 10016.
2. From National Institute of Neurological and Communicative Disorders and Stroke, National Institutes of Health, Bethesda, Md. 20014.
3. National Easter Seal Society for Crippled Children and Adults, Inc., 2023 West Ogden Avenue, Chicago, Ill. 60612.
4. *Cerebral Palsy—Hope Through Research,* a pamphlet for the public

prepared by the National Institute of Neurological Diseases and Stroke, National Institutes of Health, Bethesda, Md. 20014. For sale by the U.S. Government Printing Office, Washington, D.C.
5. "1973 Marketing Guide"—published by Drug Topics, Medical Economics Company, Oradell, New Jersey.
6. The National Foundation/March of Dimes Annual Report, 1974.
7. William Berenberg, M.D., Professor of Pediatrics, Harvard Medical School, Boston, Mass. Personal communication dated July 26, 1974.

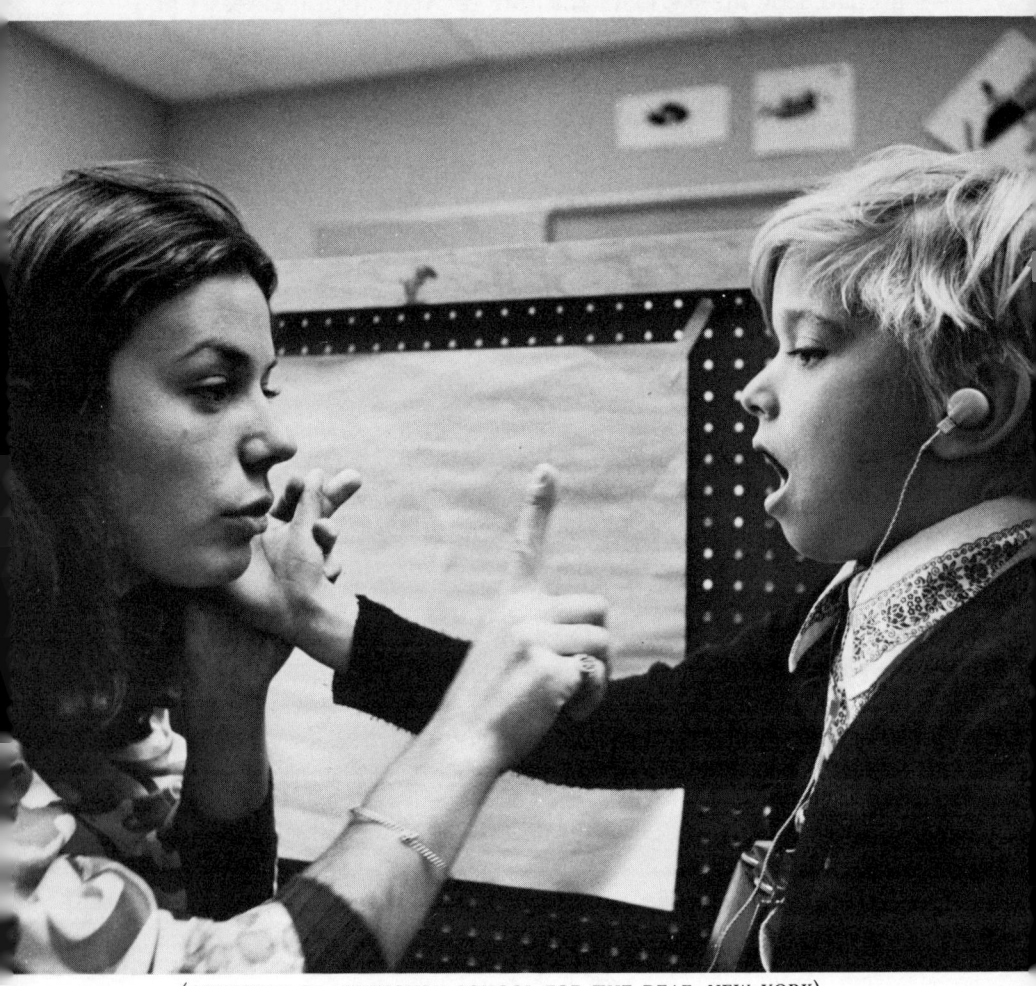
(COURTESY OF LEXINGTON SCHOOL FOR THE DEAF, NEW YORK)

What Are the Facts About Deafness?

I. How Many People Are Totally Deaf in the United States Today?

Approximately 2 million Americans lack sufficient hearing to understand speech.[1]

II. How Many People Are Partially Deaf?

1. One of every 10 people has *some degree of hearing loss,* an estimated 20,000,000 Americans.
2. The incidence of hearing loss is increasing in this country in spite of efforts to control it.[2]
3. According to the National Health Survey, there are about *11.5 million persons* in the civilian, noninstitutional population of the United States who experienced *some degree of hearing loss* which they considered serious.[3]

III. What Age Groups Have Hearing Losses?

1. More and more premature children survive a stormy early life as a result of improved pediatric practices. *The incidence of hearing problems in premature children is nearly seven times that found in normal full term deliveries.*[2]
2. The *increasing age* of our population is probably the greatest single factor for the increased incidence of hearing

93

loss. *People developing the sclerotic changes of old age have a far higher incidence* of sensorineural deafness than people in the younger groups. The degree of hearing loss seems proportional to the degree of the aging process.[2]

IV. What Is Deafness?

1. Hearing loss is generally broken down into two major categories:[4]
    a. *Middle-ear or conductive hearing loss.*
    b. *Sensorineural hearing loss,* which includes injuries to the auditory neural pathways from the end organ of the auditory nerve in the inner ear to the auditory cortex in the temporal lobe of the brain.
2. Many people suffer from combinations of middle-ear and sensorineural deafness.[4]

V. What Types of Hearing Loss Are Most Prevalent?

The most prevalent types of hearing loss according to the causes are:

1. Conductive hearing loss
    a. *Eustachian tube disfunction* often associated with adenoid disease, which results in fluid accumulation in the middle ear, and conductive hearing loss. *Allergy may cause the same type of accumulation.*[6]
    b. *Bony abnormalities*—otosclerosis (a bone proliferation that causes interference with normal movement of the innermost bone, the stapes, of the ossicular chain (the three small bones in a chain in the middle ear).[6]
    c. *Congenital deformities,* including absence or deformity of the middle ear bones and cavity.[4]

2. Sensorineural hearing loss
    a. Perinatal neural damage or developmental defects:
        i. *Erythroblastosis,* as a result of Rh or other blood incompatibility between mother and unborn in-

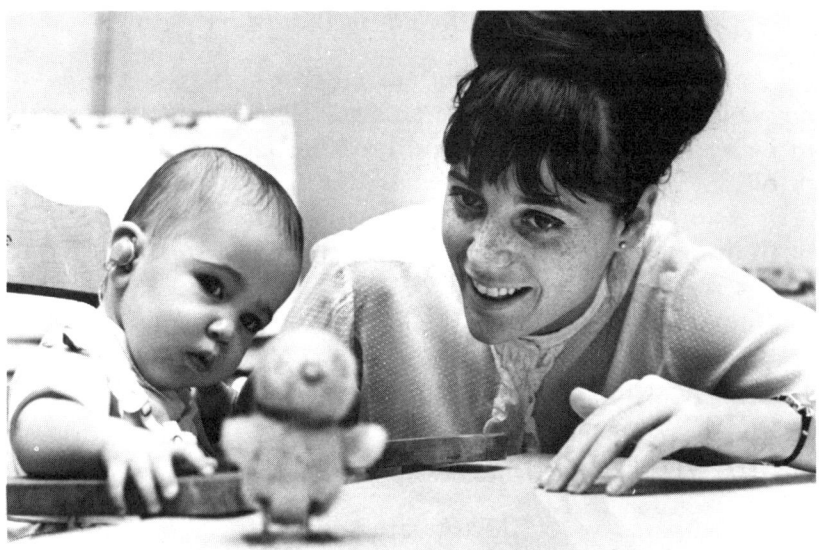

(COURTESY OF LEXINGTON SCHOOL FOR THE DEAF, NEW YORK)

fant's blood, which results in destruction of the infant's red blood cells and deposit of blood pigments in the infant tissues. *Rh sensitivity may be prevented* by giving Rh-O Immune Globulin to Rh-negative mothers after each delivery or miscarriage of an Rh-positive baby.[5]

ii. Virus infections of the mother, especially during the first trimester of pregnancy.

German measles, which has caused epidemics of babies born deaf-blind and retarded, may be prevented by vaccination. The *German measles vaccine is strongly recommended* for all boys and girls between the ages of 1 year and puberty, to reduce the possibility of exposure to German measles by pregnant women.[5]

iii. Anoxia (insufficient oxygen) at the time of delivery.[5]

iv. Brain trauma at the time of delivery.[4]

b. Aging process and vascular degenerative changes.[7]
c. The effects of some drugs.[7]
d. Prolonged exposure to excessive noise.[7]
e. Certain types of genetic disorders.[7]

VI. At What Ages Do These Disorders Occur?

1. *Sensorineural* and *central hearing loss* occurs at the *beginning and toward the end of life*. It is associated with the dangers of being brought into the world or the degenerative changes of old age.
2. The *conductive* or *middle-ear deafness* usually appears at birth or around *early school age* when children are subjected to upper respiratory infections.

Bone diseases, such as otosclerosis and osteogenesis imperfecta, begin to cause hearing loss in late puberty and may damage hearing even as late as 50 years of age.[4]

VII. How Many Doctors Specialize in Ear Diseases?

An estimated 6,000 doctors are specialists in ear, nose, and throat problems.

VIII. How Many Doctors Do We Need in the Field?

If this number could be increased to *10,000* certified specialists we would have only one otolaryngologist for every 20,000 people in this country.[4] Such a ratio would represent the minimal needs for the proper care of the population's hearing problems.[4]

Two hundred young doctors a year are being qualified in the specialty of otolaryngology. This number just about matches the number of first-year residency training positions

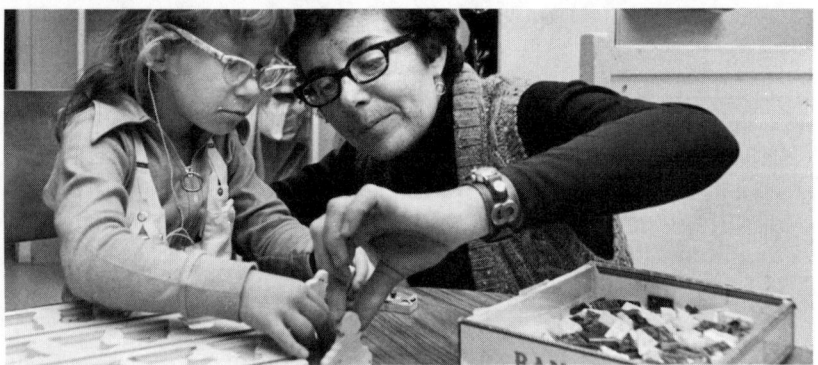

(COURTESY OF LEXINGTON SCHOOL FOR THE DEAF, NEW YORK)

open, so in order to reach the necessary goal, it is imperative that more young men be recruited into this specialty.[6]

IX. What Are the Estimated Annual Direct Costs to the Nation for the Education, Management and Compensation of People Whose Hearing Is Impaired?[8]

At least *$410,445,000*, including support of the following:

	Approximate Cost
Public residential schools for the deaf	$ 55,092,000
Private residential schools for the deaf	3,883,000
Special day programs for deaf and hard of hearing	24,190,000
Special services in regular schools	20,000,000
Preparation of special teachers	2,700,000
Captioned films for the deaf	2,800,000
Vocational rehabilitation	28,000,000
Preparation of rehabilitationists	1,200,000
Compensation for military disability	45,000,000
Audiological services for veterans	1,780,000
Community hearing and speech centers	3,600,000
Speech and hearing clinics	6,000,000
Private medical care	80,000,000
Hearing aids and their maintenance	132,000,000
Industrial claims and hearing conservation	4,200,000
Total	$410,445,000

SOURCE: *Human Communication and Its Disorders—An Overview.* A report of the National Advisory Neurological Diseases and Stroke Council of the National Institute of Neurological Diseases and Stroke, National Institutes of Health, U.S. Department of Health, Education, and Welfare, Bethesda, Md. 20014 (1969).

X. How Much Money Is Available for Research to Prevent Hearing Loss in the United States?

An estimated *$11 million*, as follows:
1. *Federal funds—$10,433,000.*[5]

The *National Institute of Neurological and Communicative Disorders and Stroke* in fiscal 1975 spent for research projects in disorders of hearing and equilibrium, and related fields of speech, learning, language, and memory, an estimated $10,433,000.

These funds were used to support 177 research grants, including five research centers and three outpatient clinics. The centers are located at the University of Chicago; Central Institute for the Deaf, St. Louis; Princeton University; the Kresge Hearing Research Institute of Ann Arbor, Michigan; and the University of Oregon, Portland. The clinics are located at the University of Pittsburgh; Northwestern University; and Stanford University, Palo Alto, California.[5]

2. About a *million dollars a year is being contributed from nongovernment sources* (private agencies, voluntary health agencies, universities) for research in hearing. This is far less than is needed.[5]

a. Of this amount, the Deafness Research Foundation made research grants and awards totaling $303,772 in 1974.[7]

XI. *Has Medical Research in Deafness Paid Off? Yes!*

1. The greatest dividend to date lies in the *microsurgery (tympanoplasty)* that has been developed to restore hearing to those individuals suffering from middle ear (conductive) deafness and mastoid infection.[6]

2. Through the years improved techniques have been developed not only for the surgical but also for medical treatment of chronically infected mastoids and middle ears. *Acute mastoid disease* has been *dramatically reduced* and almost eliminated by the use of antibiotics.[6]

3. In 1940, the fenestration operation to create a new communication into the inner ear was perfected for relief of deafness caused by otosclerosis. This operation has been almost *superseded by stapedectomy* (removal of the stapes bone which is embedded in the otosclerotic proliferation in the middle ear and the substitution of a prosthesis to serve as a stapes). This operation gives a *high return of the hearing function.*[6]

4. Recently advances have been made in the surgery for the correction of congenitally malformed external ear canals and

middle ears in order to restore hearing and to remove tumors along the auditory nerve.[6]

5. An operation, devised by Dr. William House, for the congenitally deaf, involving an electronic device, gives promise that thousands born deaf will eventually be able to hear.

6. Recent research has aided in *identifying (a) various viruses,* such as the ultraviruses, which cause infectious diseases resulting in communicative disorders, and (b) the *identification of certain drugs causing auditory damage.*[6]

7. Techniques for minimizing the effects of erythroblastosis (as a result of Rh incompatibility) have been developed.

8. Improved techniques have been developed to ensure a proper oxygen supply to the baby during and after delivery.[4]

9. New vaccines have been developed to protect pregnant mothers from some of the childhood diseases.[4] Vaccines have been developed to protect against a number of viruses (measles, German measles, Asian and Hong Kong flu).

10. New operative approaches to auditory nerve tumors have been developed.[6]

XII. What Other Advances Have Been Made Against Deafness?[7]

1. *New techniques for the examination of young children* of preschool age have been developed as well as tests *to determine the location of sensorineural damage* causing hearing impairment.

2. In industry much has been learned concerning the *control of noise hazards* causing temporary or permanent hearing impairment.

3. In the field of basic research, the *number of temporal bone banks has increased* to 41. Here collaborative studies are carried out on the lesions found in temporal bones compared with studies carried out on the same individuals during life.

Four regional temporal bone banks centers have now been consolidated into a single center—The National Temporal Bone Banks Center of the Deafness Research Foundation, located in Baltimore at the Johns Hopkins University School of Medicine.[6]

Through this consolidation, the Temporal Bone Banks Program for Ear Research now has the means to innovate new and important services. One of these is an educational program that, by offering workshops and courses on temporal bone processing, will make possible a constant upgrading of the technical skills used in this significant aspect of ear research.[6]

4. Improved techniques have been developed to study the organ of balance, resulting in improved diagnosis of a number of neurological disorders (brain tumor, Ménière's disease, skull fractures, and so forth).[4]

XIII. What Are Some Important Research Leads?

Research must be encouraged and fostered that will produce a far greater knowledge of the essential nature of deafness, particularly sensorineural deafness. In human communication all too little is known about speech or the basic lesions causing aphasia. It is fair to say that we do not yet know how we hear. Some important leads are:[4]

1. The study of the anatomy and the microanatomy of the auditory pathways.[4]
2. What happens to a sound stimulus as it travels from the inner ear up to the auditory cortex of the brain?[4]
3. The neuropathology of the central auditory pathways.[4]
4. More must be learned concerning oxygen deprivation, and specific diseases in relation to deafness.[4]
5. How effective are prostheses in severe nerve deafness?[6]
6. Evaluation of electrocochleography.[6]

XIV. What Can Be Done to Reduce the Incidence of Hearing Impairment?

1. Broad public health programs and privately supported programs of *case finding must be established to identify individuals with early hearing impairment* so that they may be benefited by

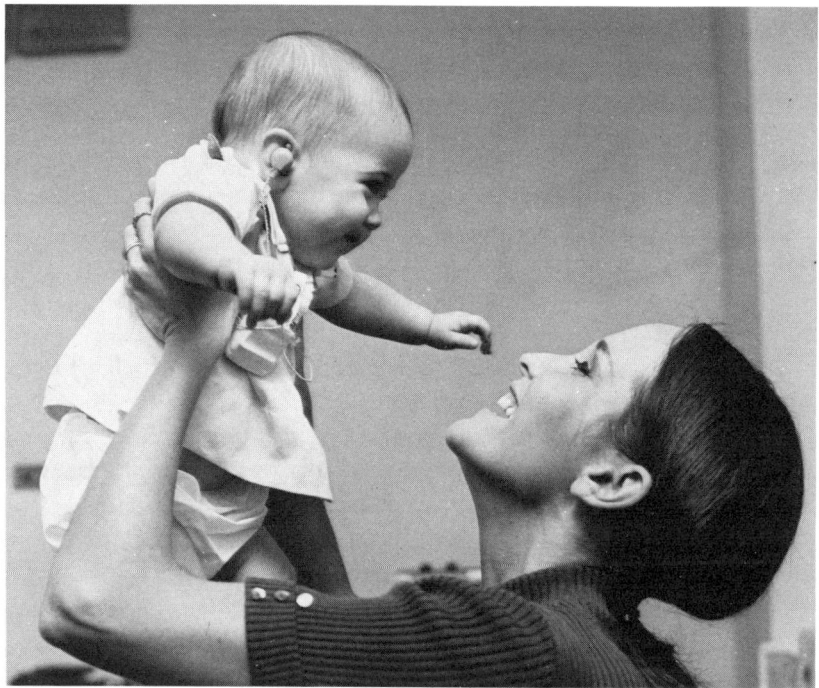

Severely hearing-impaired child at the Infant Center of the Lexington School for the Deaf in New York City. (COURTESY OF LEXINGTON SCHOOL FOR THE DEAF, NEW YORK)

early measures to control or cure the hearing loss. Such programs should extend from the maternal and child health clinics through the school systems into the industrial plants and finally into health programs for the elderly.[9]

2. Paranatal clinics should attempt to:

    a. Reduce the incidence of prenatal virus infection. The new German measles vaccine is strongly recommended for all boys and girls between the ages of 1 year and puberty to reduce the possibility of exposure to German measles by pregnant women.

    b. Establish better control of the problems of erythroblastosis and oxygen deprivation.

    c. Provide obstetrical techniques to help prevent children from receiving injuries at birth that will lead to hearing handicaps.[9]

XV. What Agencies Are Involved in Providing Service to Those with Hearing Problems?

1. The crippled children's clinics supported by the *Children's Bureau, U.S. Department of Health, Education, and Welfare*, support in many instances conservation of hearing clinics.

2. The *Division of Community Health Service of the Bureau of State Services* supports grants for community services in the communicative disorders (specifically, neurological and sensory).

3. The national voluntary agencies serving those with hearing and speech problems are:

   a. The *National Association of Hearing and Speech Agencies* which supports community care through its affiliated chapters sometimes identified as leagues for the hard of hearing.

   b. *The National Society for Crippled Children and Adults.*

   c. *United Cerebral Palsy Associations, Inc.*

   d. *The American Speech and Hearing Association* is a national organization setting and maintaining standards for professional workers in the field.

   e. The *National Association of the Deaf* is the largest of the national membership bodies serving the profoundly deaf.

   f. *The Alexander Graham Bell Association for the Deaf* serves as an international information center about deafness for professionals and parents of deaf children. Its emphasis is on the educational needs of deaf children and specifically on the teaching of speech, lipreading, and the use of residual hearing.

   g. *The Deafness Research Foundation* is the only national voluntary health agency devoted primarily to advancing ear research. In addition to its broad program of research in all forms of ear disorders, the foundation sponsors the Temporal Bone Banks Program for Ear Research in cooperation with the American Academy of Ophthalmology and Otolaryngology and the Armed Forces Institute of Pathology. There are now 41 temporal bone "banks" (ear research laboratories) throughout the country participating in the program. Because the inner-ear structures, contained in the temporal bones, cannot be examined during life, the determination of many causes of inner-ear disorder can be made only through laboratory studies of these structures after death. The foundation has conducted a public education program financed by the John A. Hartford Foundation to encourage those with all types of ear disorders to bequeath their temporal bones to advance otologic research.[7]

4. In addition to these agencies, Gallaudet College in Washington, D.C., is the nation's only college for the deaf with an enrollment of students from all over the United States and many foreign countries.[7]

5. The Research Fund of the American Otological Society makes small grants yearly to support research in the field of otology.[4]

6. The Council of Organizations Serving the Deaf is a central clearinghouse and contact point for information and combined action by national organizations serving deaf persons. The office of the Council is at 4201 Connecticut Avenue, NW, Washington, D. C. 20008.[7]

Notes

1. Preliminary estimate prepared for the government by the Deafness Research and Training Center, New York University, New York, N. Y.
2. *Hearing Loss—Hope Through Research,* publication of the National Institute of Neurological and Communicative Disorders and Stroke, Bethesda, Md. 20014.
3. *Prevalence of Selected Impairments, United States, July 1963—June 1965.* Vital and Health Statistics, Series 10, no. 48, National Center for Health Statistics, Department of Health, Education, and Welfare, November 1968. Rockville, Md.
4. John E. Bordley, M.D., Andelot Professor, Emeritus, Otolaryngology, Johns Hopkins University School of Medicine, Baltimore, Md. 21205. Personal communication.
5. National Institute of Neurological and Communicative Disorders and Stroke. Bethesda, Md. 20014, 1973.
6. Harry Rosenwasser, M.D., Director of Medical Affairs, The Deafness Research Foundation, New York, N. Y. Personal communication, August, 1973.

7. The Deafness Research Foundation, New York, N.Y.
8. *Human Communication and Its Disorders—An Overview.* A report of the National Advisory Neurological Diseases and Stroke Council of the National Institute of Neurological Diseases and Stroke, National Institutes of Health, U.S. Department of Health, Education, and Welfare, Bethesda, Md. 20014, 1969.
9. Conservation of Hearing Committee, American Academy of Ophthalmology and Otolaryngology.

What Are the Facts About Digestive Diseases?

I. How Many People Suffer with Digestive Diseases?

1. Digestive diseases include disorders of the stomach, intestines, biliary passages (gall bladder), liver, and pancreas. Their causes are various—infection, cancer, alcoholism, genetic defects, and reactions to life stress.

2. Each year, Americans spend nearly *300 million man days away from work—and 116 man days in bed*—because of acute and chronic digestive disease.[1]

3. Digestive diseases affect about *13 million* Americans.[1]

4. Digestive diseases represent the *number one cause of hospitalization* in the United States.[1]

5. Twenty-eight percent of all cancer deaths are due to cancer of the digestive organs.[2]

II. What Is the Economic Loss from Digestive Diseases?

1. The estimated economic loss to the nation is *$16 billion yearly*.[4]

2. Of all disease categories, digestive diseases rank *third* in causing economic loss, exceeded only by cardiovascular diseases and accidents.[1]

3. The economic loss to the United States due to *peptic ulcer* alone is calculated at just *$1 billion yearly*.[1]

III. How Many Doctors Specialize in Gastroenterology?

1. Of 320,903 active physicians in the United States in 1972, *only 1,839 were listed as specialists in gastroenterology*.[3]

2. In addition, 649 physicians listed their surgical specialty as colon and rectal surgery.[3]

IV. How Much Is Being Spent for Research and Training in This Area?

1. In fiscal 1975, the National Institute of Arthritis, Metabolism and Digestive Diseases spent an estimated *$24,029,000* for research in digestive diseases and nutrition.

2. Research and training funds expended by the Institute in recent years for digestive diseases alone are as follows:

                1970—$12,754,000
                1971—$13,069,000
                1972—$16,404,000
                1973—$16,165,000

Taking into consideration the economic inflation in the United States today, it can readily be seen that research funds in this area being expended by the National Institute of Arthritis, Metabolism and Digestive Diseases are decreasing.

3. Support from nongovernmental sources is meager.

    a. There is as yet no nationally organized voluntary health agency devoted to the broad problems of digestive diseases.

    b. There are no large philanthropic foundations for which digestive diseases is a major field of interest.

    c. Support from industry has been largely for applied research and development. The pharmaceutical industry estimates that $18.5 to $37 million (5 percent to 10 percent of their annual $370 million expenditure for research and development) is related to products useful in digestive diseases.

V. What Is Needed to Help Combat This Major Health Problem?

A survey of major digestive diseases reveals many urgent needs for new knowledge which can and should be met by larger-scale, better-organized research and training at the laboratory level, at the bedside, and in the community.

It is proposed that this effort be organized by the joint actions of professional societies, a national voluntary health agency, and agencies within the Federal Government made especially responsible for the problems of digestive disease.

VI. What Are Some of the Promising Research Leads in This Area?

Recent research advances include:

1. The demonstration that long-term oral administration of chenodeoxycholic acid can result in *dissolution of long-standing cholesterol gallstones.*[1]

More than 15 million people in the United States are estimated to have cholesterol gallstones, and many are surgically removed each year. An estimated 6,000 patients die each year as a result of gallbladder surgery. Chemical dissolution of gallstones may offer a desirable alternative to gallstone-related surgery and a possible means of prevention of further gallstone development in patients diagnosed as being of special risk.[1]

2. The National Institute of Arthritis, Metabolism and Digestive Diseases is currently evaluating the therapeutic and prophylactic value of current drug treatments of regional enteritis (Crohn's disease), which causes severe pain, fever, and weight loss, and frequently requires prolonged periods of hospitalization and abdominal operations involving resection or removal of portions of the intestine. The drugs being tested include *prednisone, azulfidine,* and *azathioprine.*[1]

3. The synthesis of *gastrin,* the hormone that stimulates secretion of gastric juices, has provided an important research tool for studying peptic ulcer, in which an excess of acid digestive juices is secreted.[1]

4. The administration of vitamin A may reduce or prevent development of a special type of peptic ulcer—"stress ulcer"—which develops in man as a result of severe burns or profound stress or trauma. Research results of one study suggest that

treatment with high doses of vitamin A reduces the risk of gastroduodenal ulceration in severely stressed patients.[1]

5. Biliary obstruction, whether it occurs inside or outside the liver, results in excessive accumulation of bile acids and bilirubin in the bloodstream, and is associated with persistent jaundice and, eventually, intractable pruritus (severe itching). Investigators supported by the National Institute of Arthritis, Metabolism and Digestive Diseases have shown recently that phenobarbital treatment reduces jaundice and pruritus in patients with biliary obstruction (cholestasis) in the liver.[1]

Notes

1. Information from National Institute of Arthritis, Metabolism and Digestive Diseases, National Institutes of Health, Bethesda, Md. 20014, 1973.
2. National Center for Health Statistics, U.S. Public Health Service, Department of Health, Education, and Welfare, Rockville, Md.
3. *Health Resources Statistics, Health Manpower & Health Facilities, 1974.* DHEW publication no. (HRA) 75—1509. National Center for Health Statistics, U.S. Public Health Service, Department of Health, Education, and Welfare, Washington, D.C.
4. Editorial in *Gastroenterology* 66: 152-156 (1974).

What Are the Facts About Epilepsy?

I. What Is Epilepsy?

1. Epilepsy is a disorder of the nervous system. Seizure is the chief characteristic of this disorder. Epilepsy may be defined as recurrent loss or impairment of consciousness which may or may not be accompanied by muscular movements ranging from slight twitching of the eyelids to convulsive shaking of the entire body.

Depending on the type, seizures may last from 10 to 30 seconds or from 5 to 15 minutes. The frequency of epileptic seizures can vary from one in a year or so, to several a day.

2. Epilepsy is classified from the *standpoint of origin* or from the *standpoint of kind of seizure*.
    a. *Classification by origin*
        i. *Idiopathic:* All cases in which the *origin of the seizures is unknown*, that is, there is no demonstrable structural or pathological defect of the brain and nervous system. *Seventy-five percent of cases fall into this category.* Idiopathic cases, however, are slowly becoming less in number as expanded research places more and more of them in classification ii (below)—symptomatic.
       ii. *Symptomatic:* Includes all cases in which a *definite organic cause for seizures* has been demonstrated, such as a traumatic epilepsy caused by *head injuries,* following *industrial accidents, war injuries,* or, increasingly, automobile accidents.[3]
    b. *Classification by type of seizure*[3]
       i. *Grand mal:* This attack, the most frequently

found, consists of loss of consciousness, tightening of muscles, and falling to the ground, followed by convulsive movements.

ii. *Petit mal:* This consists of a momentary blackout, during which there may be brief staring or brief rhythmic twitching of the eyelids or other facial muscles. This is most frequently seen in children.

iii. *Psychomotor:* In this form, attacks consist of clouding of consciousness with automated patterned movement often followed by brief periods of amnesia.

COMMON TYPES OF EPILEPTIC SEIZURES

	Grand Mal	*Petit Mal*	*Psychomotor*
Who	Children and Adults	Children and Adults	Children and Adults
Description	Loss of consciousness with convulsive seizure, usually falling to the ground	Brief loss of consciousness, staring, blinking, etc.	Period of amnesia often accompanied by inappropriate actions
Duration	2–5 minutes	Less than 1 minute	2–5 minutes
Frequency	One or more times daily, weekly, monthly, or annually	Many times an hour, day, week, or month	One or more times weekly, monthly, or annually

II. How Many Persons Die of or Are Affected by Epilepsy?

1. Epilepsy *per se* is rarely a cause of death, nor is it usually a significant cause of accidents. The tragedy is that epilepsy is usually a *long-term chronic disease,* with 80 percent of seizures starting in childhood or adolescence. However, epilepsy may begin even in old age.[3]

In 50 percent of the persons with epilepsy who receive modern medical treatment the disease is controllable. In another 30 percent of such cases control is partial; nevertheless, the large majority of people with epilepsy are fully employable so long as their occupations do not expose them or others to danger in case of an on-the-job seizure.[3]

2. Approximately *2 million to 4 million* persons throughout the country (1 percent to 2 percent of the population) suffer from this disorder.[2]

The Epilepsy Foundation of America estimates that 2 percent of the present population in the United States—or about 4 million persons—suffer from some convulsive disorder.³

III. What Are Some of the Causes of Epilepsy?

1. The specific cause of epilepsy is not known, although in general, it is ascribed to a disorder of brain cell function.³

2. *Injuries to the infant prior to, during, or after birth; severe head injury or brain tumor; certain common infections that can settle in the brain,* such as the organisms that cause sleeping sickness, measles, meningitis, or whooping cough—all these may result in certain forms of epilepsy.

3. For a large number of individuals with epilepsy (75 percent) there *seems to be no precipitating cause.* This is called idiopathic epilepsy (see Question I). Persons with this form may have a predisposition to seizure for reasons still undiscovered.³

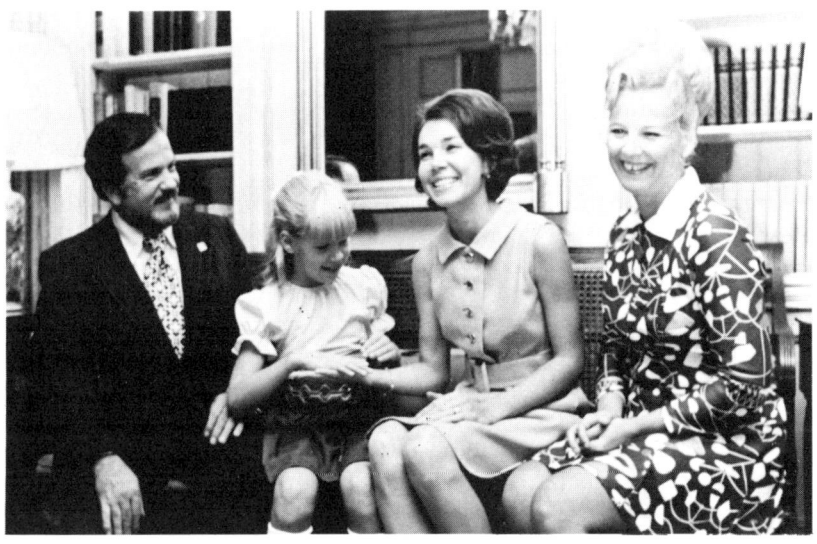

Diana Lynn Nielsen, 1972 Poster Child of the Epilepsy Foundation, visits the White House and has a chat with Julie Nixon Eisenhower, the former President's daughter. With Diana are her mother, Mrs. Lawrence Nielsen, and the Foundation's executive vice president, Paul E. Funk. (COURTESY OF EPILEPSY FOUNDATION OF AMERICA, INC., WASHINGTON, D. C.)

4. Medical opinion is divided as to the extent to which the genetic factor may cause epilepsy. Some authorities do not classify epilepsy as genetic, though there has lately been somewhat greater evidence that it may be genetic in origin.³

IV. What Is the Economic Cost of Epilepsy?

Epilepsy costs individuals, families, and the nation *over $4.25 billion annually.*⁴

Program	Annual Cost for Epilepsy
Aid to the permanently and totally disabled	$ 70,266,690.00
Aid to the blind	420,423.20
Aid to families with dependent children	53,172,876.00
Vocational rehabilitation	9,648,134.00
Social Security disability benefits	65,038,880.00
Crippled children's program	4,700,000.00
Medicaid	31,300,000.00
Medicare	125,300,000.00
Veterans Administration	89,430,210.00
Special education	85,610,270.00
Institutionalization	231,649,000.00
Unemployment wage and hour loss	1,720,224,000.00
Private medical costs	1,879,945,000.00
Research	5,895,252.00
Total	$4,372,600,735.20

V. Do We Have Any Treatment for Epilepsy?

1. Drugs have been developed that can wholly or partially control epileptic seizures in some 80 percent of selected cases; *however, great numbers of cases that could benefit by such treatment never receive it.*²

2. Over 14 anticonvulsant drugs licensed in the United States and half a dozen more experimental ones can control seizures, including: phenobarbital, diphenylhydantoin (Dilan-

tin), Tridione, Paradione, Mesantoin, Phenurone, Mysoline, Mebaral, Celontin, Milontin, Zarontin, Diamox, Diazepam, bromides, and so forth.[2]

In 1974, the Food and Drug Administration approved carbamazepine (Tegretol) as an epilepsy drug. This was the first time in 14 years that a drug for long-term treatment of epilepsy was approved.[2]

Some of these drugs in combination are more effective than when used alone. Each patient must be studied individually and given various drug trials over a period of time.

3. These anticonvulsants in most cases are *effective enough so that the person with epilepsy can assume the responsibilities* of the ordinarily healthy person (assuming the work he does would not endanger himself and others in event of seizure).

4. Gas-liquid chromatography, a rapid, accurate laboratory method, has been applied to the quantitative assay of the antiepileptic drugs. This permits clinicians to obtain knowledge of the level of the drug in the blood which is essential in the successful treatment of epilepsy patients. Gas-liquid chromatography methods permit the physician to determine the dosage levels at which an anticonvulsant drug is the most effective.[3]

5. Techniques now available for the surgical removal of the damaged area of the brain have proved useful in the control of certain seizures in a few carefully selected patients.

However, such operations are extremely few. Out of the 5 percent of today's epilepsy patients medically considered for such operations, only about 2 percent of this 5 percent are actually operated upon.

VI. Why Do Less Than 50 Percent of All Epilepsy Patients Receive Effective Treatment?

1. Both the sufferer and the public misassociate seizures with mental abnormality; and in some communities a person with epilepsy is also shunned because of the "evil" long mistakenly associated with this disorder. *The sufferer from epilepsy,* therefore, *hesitates to make his disability known* by seeking medical aid.[3]

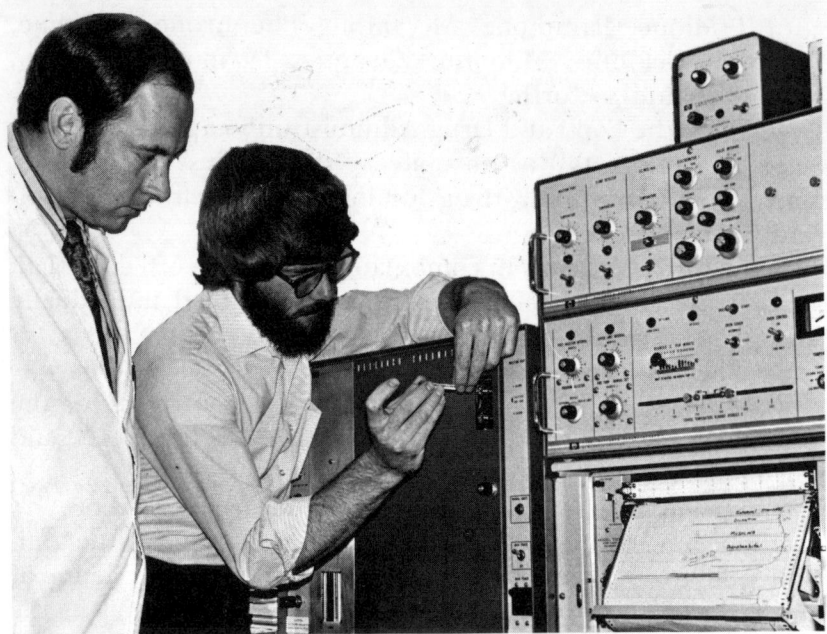

Gas-liquid chromatograph being operated by Dr. Robert K. Gerding (left) and an assistant at the Good Samaritan Hospital, Portland, Oregon. (COURTESY OF EPILEPSY FOUNDATION OF AMERICA, INC., WASHINGTON, D.C.)

2. *Public attitudes still make it difficult for the adult with epilepsy to get a job, receive an education, or have children.* The last two states with marriage prohibition laws against people with epilepsy (Virginia and West Virginia) have repealed them. However, nine states still have sterilization laws applying to persons with epilepsy, although none have been enforced for many years. Many states have inadequate Workmen's Compensation and Second-Injury Fund laws, in addition to innumerable written and unwritten administrative procedures in every state that hamper epilepsy victims.[2]

3. The 1965 U.S. Immigration Act, which became effective in December of that year, permits persons with epilepsy to enter the country on visa (including for purpose of treatment, formerly denied) or with the intention of citizenship. No longer are they classified with the insane, criminal or morally depraved.

4. Not enough specialists are capable of adequately diagnosing the disorder and treating it.

VII. How Much Is Being Spent for Research in the Causes, Treatment and Prevention of Epilepsy?

Approximately *$6 million* annually as follows:
1. The National Institute of Neurological and Communicative Disorders and Stroke, fiscal 1975 $4,317,000.[2]
2. *Epilepsy Foundation of America,* 1973   113,800.[4]
3. In addition, the *National Institute of Mental Health,* the *Rehabilitation Services Administration,* the *Veterans Administration,* the *National Science Foundation,* the *Department of Defense* also support research related to epilepsy, although the exact amounts being expended are not available.[4]

   i. In 1973, the National Institute of Mental Health spent $707,472 and the Rehabilitation Services Administration spent $101,000 for research in epilepsy.[4]

4. In contrast, it is estimated epilepsy costs more than $4 billion annually to the American economy to care for the public institutionalized patients with severe epilepsy, those thousands depending upon noninstitutional public assistance, or who are maintained by relatives in private institutions, plus the loss of productive man-hours. The majority who live outside insitutions are supported by their families.[3]

VIII. How Many Neurologists Are There in the United States?

1. According to the latest figures of the American Board of Psychiatry and Neurology, there are only 1,200 board-certified neurologists in the United States. This does not take into account neurologists who are not board-certified, or most of the nation's neurological surgeons.[3]
2. Major medical specialists treating epilepsy in the United States include:[3]

Specialty	*Number Practicing*	*Board-Certified Specialists*
Neurologists	2,969	1,200
Neurosurgeons	2,533	1,403
Pediatricians	18,251	11,998

IX. Are There Any Epilepsy Clinics in the United States?

1. *Many epilepsy centers* have been set up chiefly in large medical centers connected with universities. Excellent epilepsy treatment centers are at the Columbia-Presbyterian Hospital in New York City; Johns Hopkins in Baltimore; the University of Virginia; the University of California in Los Angeles and San Francisco; the Michigan Epilepsy Center, Detroit; the University of Wisconsin Medical School; Yale, in New Haven, Connecticut; the Consultation Clinic for Epilepsy, University of Illinois College of Medicine; the Seizure Clinic, University of Washington; and many others.[3]

X. What Must Be Done to Help the Epilepsy Patient Assume a Normal Life?

1. *Research* must be expanded both to bring about a permanent control and to improve present treatment so that the cause of seizures might be identified and preventive techniques developed.[1]

2. *Support for increased neurological training in the nation's medical schools* must be provided so that more specialists (neurologists) may be developed and more general practitioners will learn methods of handling this disorder.

3. *More clinics must be established* at key points throughout the country where practitioners can receive training for handling this problem, thus shortening the gap between modern medical discovery and patient care.

4. *Great effort must be expended at the community level to rehabilitate and employ the adult with epilepsy.* From the progressive, informed employer's viewpoint, 80 percent of all adults with epilepsy are considered "controlled," and can be counted on for reliable work performance. Nevertheless, the vast majority of employers are scarcely better informed in this regard than the general public. This is startlingly borne out by the fact that persons with epilepsy effectively rehabilitated by the U.S. Rehabilitation Services Administration make up less than 2 percent of all rehabilitants.[3]

5. *The general public must be informed about epilepsy.* Facts must replace myths, fiction. Laws must be updated and liberalized so they help integrate the epileptic into the community.

6. Paramedical groups such as nurses, psychologists, social workers, rehabilitation counselors must be educated as to modern findings and techniques in regard to epilepsy.

7. A voluntary national organization was formed in January 1968, when the Epilepsy Foundation and the Epilepsy Association of America merged to form a single, strong national voluntary agency in the epilepsy field known as the *Epilepsy Foundation of America* with offices at 1828 L Street, NW, Suite 406, Washington, D.C. 20036.[3]

The Epilepsy Foundation of America can supply the names of clinics in a particular vicinity and of especially interested doctors, as well as provide additional information about epilepsy and local epilepsy organizations.

This national association and its nationwide system of chapters are working toward a better understanding of epilepsy and in some states have successfully fought for better legislation for persons with epilepsy, but the seriousness of the present need indicates a continuing and expanded program.

8. A *professional* national association is[3] American Epilepsy Society, G.F. Ayala, M.D., Secretary, Department of Neurology, University of Minnesota School of Medicine, Box 341, Mayo-Memorial Building, Minneapolis, Minn. 55455.[3]

Notes

Grateful acknowledgment is made to the National Institute of Neurological and Communicative Disorders and Stroke, National Institutes of Health, Bethesda, Md., and to the Epilepsy Foundation of America, 1828 L Street, NW, Washington, D.C., for their helpful cooperation in reviewing and updating this chapter. Specific references are as follows:

1. *Epilepsy—Hope Through Research,* a pamphlet for the public prepared by the National Institute of Neurological Diseases and Stroke, National Institutes of Health, Bethesda, Md. 20014. Also available in Spanish.

2. National Institute of Neurological and Communicative Disorders and Stroke, National Institutes of Health, Bethesda, Md. 20014.
3. Epilepsy Foundation of America, 1828 L Street, NW, Washington, D.C. 20036.
4. *The Cost of the Epilepsies,* Epilepsy Foundation of America, Washington, D. C. 1974.

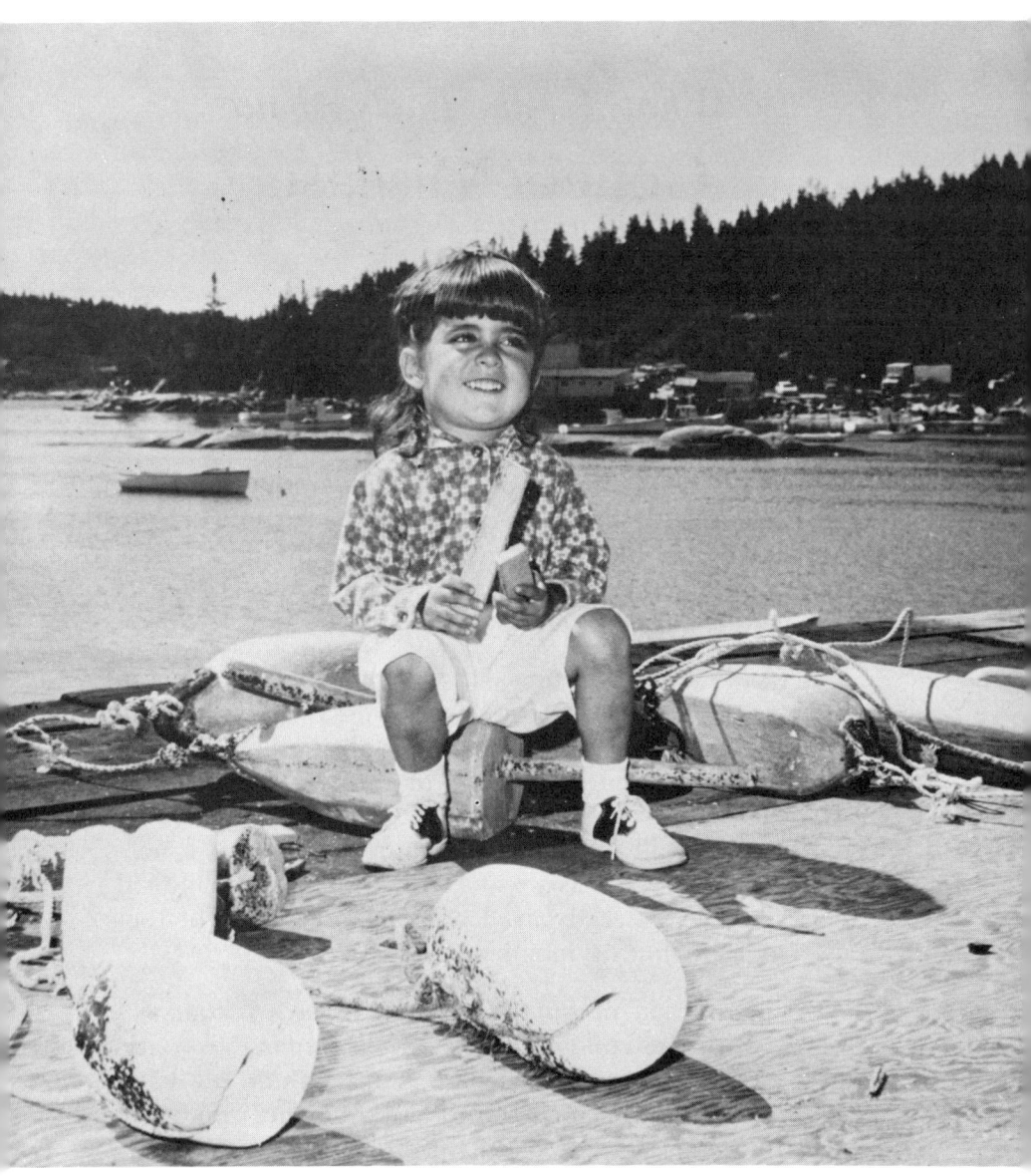

This child suffers from the inherited disorder called congenital adrenal hyperplasia. Its main symptom is premature virility in the male or masculinization in the female. These effects stem from a defect in the body's synthesis of a substance called cortisol. Other symptoms may include high blood pressure and chronic salt loss, which can be life-threatening. The condition, which is rare in the U.S., is transmitted as an autosomal recessive gene defect, meaning that both parents must contribute a gene for the disorder to occur. Favorable results often are obtained with cortisol therapy; salt therapy as necessary; and, for affected females, androgen therapy. (COURTESY OF NATIONAL INSTITUTE OF GENERAL MEDICAL SCIENCES)

What Are the Facts About Genetic Disease?

I. What Is "Genetic Disease"?

1. Diseases involving disorders of the hereditary material—the genes and chromosomes—are the oldest, most widespread, and probably the most burdensome of all human afflictions.

As one authority, Dr. J. E. Seegmiller of the University of California, San Diego, put it:

> The fact that many victims of hereditary diseases are completely unable to care for themselves and require full-time care by their relatives or become lifetime wards of the state in mental institutions or nursing homes makes the total cost to the nation far greater than that of the diseases that kill (more or less) outright, such as cancer, stroke, or heart disease, which usually affect the individuals who have already lived out major portions of their lives as contributing members of society.[1]

2. The common tie among genetic diseases is that victims are born with the conditions (or with transmissible traits for passing on the disease, which they themselves do not have, to their children) and that, if the disease does not render them sterile, they can transmit it to their offspring. Some genetic diseases are inherited in a complex manner in which several genes are involved, and some involve multiple genes plus certain environmental factors (for example, dietary ones) for the condition to express itself. These factors make the problems of assessing the burden of genetic disease in the nation today enormously difficult.

Another expert, Dr. C. J. Epstein of the University of California, San Francisco, said this:

Carried to the extreme, virtually all of human disease and deterioration can be considered as birth defects, since genetic factors are undoubtedly of importance in their origin and pathogenesis.[2]

For that reason, discussions of genetic disease are usually limited to those defects in which genetic components are well or reasonably well established; it should also be noted, however, that this list is growing constantly and is bringing more and more "nongenetic" diseases within that definition (for example, certain forms of cardiovascular problems have been found recently to result from specific genetic factors and account for approximately one-fifth of all heart attacks that occur in men under the age of 60 years).[3]

It is therefore no exaggeration to compare the genetic disease problem with the proverbial iceberg, only the tip of whose enormous mass is immediately apparent.

3. Whereas the *link of genes and chromosomes* among all genetic diseases makes a proper and accurate assessment of the problem's true magnitude extremely difficult, that link also provides medical scientists with a specific target for attacking and perhaps ultimately solving the genetic disease problem. Knowledge of the underlying mechanisms of one genetic disease can lead to the development of techniques for diagnosing, preventing, and treating it—and perhaps several other widely different but nevertheless related diseases. In fact, this principle has already been demonstrated in numerous instances, as will be shown.

II. How Serious Is the Genetic Disease Problem?

1. An estimated *15 million Americans* today suffer the consequences of birth defects of varying severity. Not all of these disorders are genetic; 20 percent are estimated not to contain a heritable component but represent the effects of agents such as infection, drugs, physical injury to the fetus, and so forth. Thus the remaining 80 percent, or 12 million Americans, carry true genetic diseases, wholly or partly due to defective genes or chromosomes.[4]

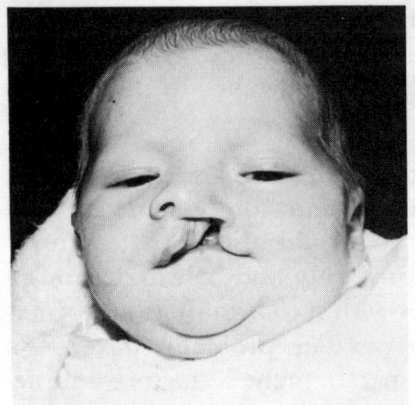 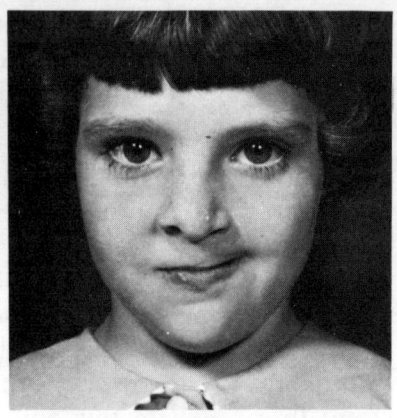

The above child, pictured at birth and at age 6, has benefited from plastic reconstructive surgery in the treatment of cleft lip/palate. Often in such cases, psychological problems in social adjustment are severe. Thought to be multifactorial (involving many genes) in nature, the syndrome appears once in each 750 births in the U.S. Thus, a total of about 6,000 affected infants are born each year. (COURTESY OF NATIONAL INSTITUTE OF GENERAL MEDICAL SCIENCES)

Other estimates of the severity of the genetic disease problem indicate that:

a. Thirty-six percent of all spontaneous abortions are caused by gross chromosomal defects (amounting to more than 100,000 per year in the United States).[5]

b. Forty percent of all infant mortality results from genetic factors.[6] [7] [8] [9]

c. Genetic defects are present in 4.8 percent to 5 percent of all live births.[5] [9] [10] [11] [12] [13]

d. Probably four-fifths of the 3 percent mentally retarded in the country are genetic.[14]

e. Thirty-three percent of all admissions to hospital pediatric wards are there for genetic reasons.[8] [15]

f. Each of us carries between 5 and 8 genes for serious (usually lethal) genetic defects, and hence stands a statistical chance of passing a serious or deadly condition on to each born child.[16]

g. Each married couple stands a 3 percent risk of bearing a genetically defective child.[17]

2. The above estimates do not take into account many of the conditions that have either been recently shown to have a genetic involvement of some sort or are strongly suspected to

have one. These include heart disease, certain forms of arthritis, diabetes, and cancer, and the most devastating and prevalent mental illnesses—schizophrenia and depressive illness.[9][13]

It can be added, too, that *10 to 12 percent* of our population is estimated to have *enzyme abnormalities* or other genetically determined deficiencies which make them hypersensitive and likely to react badly to one or another of many commonly used drugs. This hypersensitivity undoubtedly underlies a significant portion of all adverse drug reaction cases which each year account for about 5 percent of hospital admissions.[18][19][20]

3. *The costs—economic and otherwise—*of genetic disease, then, are truly enormous but also *incalculable.* How, for example, can one put a price on genetically caused spontaneous abortion? (In addition to the 36 percent caused by gross chromosomal abnormalities, there is, unquestionably, a significant but incalculable amount resulting from single lethal gene defects and from deadly mixtures of gene actions.)[5][12]

III. Why Hasn't the Genetic Disease Problem Been More Widely Recognized Than It Is Today?

1. *No comprehensive assessment* of the number, variety, and distribution of genetic and genetically involved diseases has yet been made, largely because all the data aren't available. An indication of this is that the list of recognized genetic disorders grows every year as "new" ones are discovered. This list of disorders, each of which is caused by a single defective gene (in single or double dosage), now cites nearly 2,000 and is growing at a rate of 75 to 100 yearly. The list does not include diseases caused by multiple genes or by chromosomal defects.[21]

2. Another reason for the failure of the medical profession to recognize the real magnitude of the genetic disease problem is that, until recently, genetic diseases were considered extremely rare, each one, on the average, occurring in only one in every 10,000 live births. As the figures above show, however, the aggregate of genetic diseases is extremely high—even considering just those officially recognized as such today, which would exclude such widespread conditions as

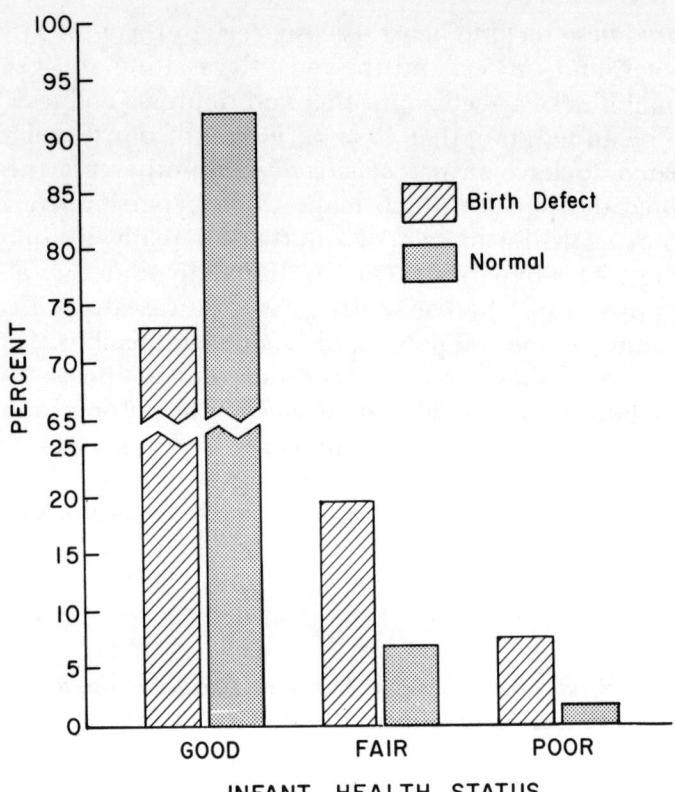

According to an infant health care study published in 1973 by the U.S. Public Health Service's National Center for Health Statistics, the prevalence of health problems in infancy was nearly five times as great among children with birth defects as among those without. In this study, birth defects (harelip, cleft palate, clubfeet, congenital heart conditions, etc.) were reported by the parents for an estimated 1.9 million children, or 8% of the U.S. noninstitutionalized children aged 6-11 years in the two-year study period 1963-65. (COURTESY OF NATIONAL INSTITUTE OF GENERAL MEDICAL SCIENCES)

heart disease, arthritis, cancer, stroke, diabetes, and mental illness. And certain genetic disorders—such as sickle-cell anemia, Tay-Sachs disease, cystic fibrosis, and thalassemia—have considerably greater impact upon particular ethnic or racial populations than the one in 10,000 for the average genetic disease. Sickle-cell disease, for example, occurs in one of 500 black children.[22][23]

3. A third and nearly as compelling reason for the general neglect of the genetic disease problem until recently is that only in the past two decades have *advances in basic science given the*

medical profession a technology for actually doing something about hereditary diseases.

It wasn't until 1956, for example, that the number of human chromosomes (46) was accurately determined. Although genetic defects are still today, strictly speaking, incurable, much can be done—and more is in the offing—toward detection, diagnosis, prevention (by genetic counseling, abortion), and treatment of these difficult medical problems.

It is now possible, for example, to diagnose some 60 serious genetic problems before birth and to identify carriers of the trait (but who do not actually have the disease) in many of these conditions. These capabilities alone give physicians and patients alternatives they never had before to make informed decisions concerning the risk of genetic disease.

In addition, a half-dozen or more techniques for treating a large number of genetic diseases have recently become available, and more are being developed every year. Nor is the prospect of true cure of a genetic disease any longer beyond realistic hope.[8 9 15 24]

IV. What Are the Effects of Genetic Disease?

1. The range of genetic diseases and their effects are all-encompassing—from rare to commonplace, from innocuous to painful, benign to deadly.
2. All ages, both sexes, and all races of man can be affected.
3. All the body's tissues and organs systems are at risk—blood, skin, bone, connective tissue, viscera, sense organs, heart and lungs, blood vessels and brain.
4. All possible forms of deleterious effects are seen in genetic disease—physical disfigurement, organ dysfunction, mental deficiency, and madness.[25]

V. How Do Genetic Diseases Produce Their Effects?

1. In the strictest sense, it is not known precisely why or how an extra number-21 chromosome produces the characteristic physical and mental effects it does in the genetic disease

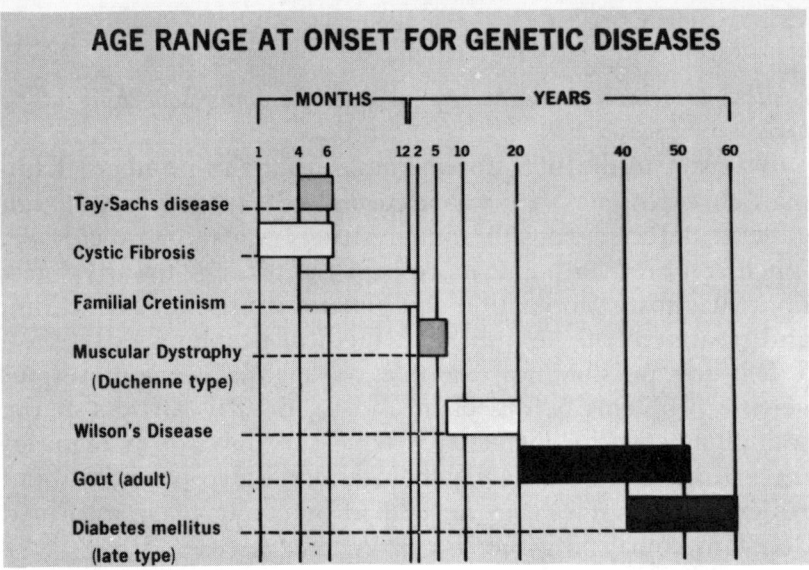

While the impact of genetic disease on the newborn is great, the clinical manifestations of hereditary defects can occur at any age from birth through maturity. (COURTESY OF NATIONAL INSTITUTE OF GENERAL MEDICAL SCIENCES)

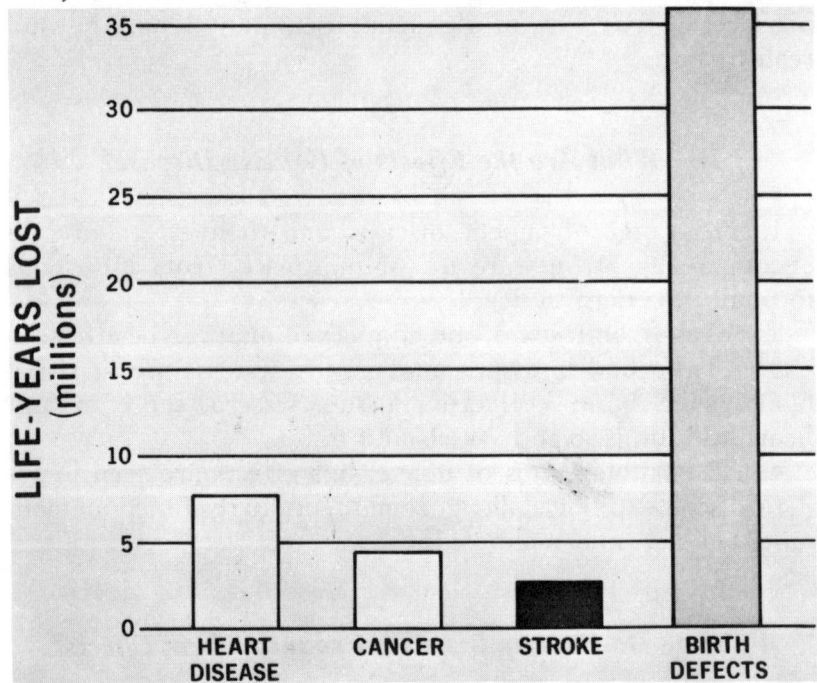

About 80% of all so-called "birth defects" are thought to be genetic in origin and constitute a leading cause of infant mortality. (COURTESY OF NATIONAL INSTITUTE OF GENERAL MEDICAL SCIENCES)

known as mongolism or Down's syndrome. Nor do we understand why an inability to metabolize galactose or milk sugar causes cataracts in infants with galactosemia, or why the buildup of amino acid phenylalanine produces gross mental retardation in children with the genetic disorder known as phenylketonuria, or PKU. We *do* know that each of these two genetic diseases results from a single defective gene, however, in contrast to an additional, entire chromosomeful of genetic material as in Down's syndrome.

2. The *recognition of specific gene defects* has given medical science the capability in a growing number of conditions:

a. To identify carriers of the trait (a one-gene dose of the disorder which does not produce the disease in the carrier but enables him to transmit it to offspring).

b. To counsel prospective trait-carrying parents on their risk of bearing a defective infant.

c. To detect a defective fetus before irreversible damage is done, and so . . .

d. To interrupt the pregnancy as some parents may desire, and thus prevent the birth of a genetically diseased individual, or, . . .

e. To treat the defective individual and so prevent expression of the disease.[8][9][15][22][24]

VI. How Are Genetic Diseases Acquired?

1. All forms of genetic disease are determined at conception and, when sterility does not result, can be passed on to subsequent generations. Whereas many genetic diseases are immediately apparent or show signs early in life, some are not expressed until later years.

2. Genetic diseases are transmitted in essentially three forms: as chromosomal abnormalities, as single-gene defects, and as complex disorders resulting from the combined action of multiple genes.

3. Significant *chromosomal abnormalities* occur in approximately one of every 250 live births, or an incidence of 0.4 percent. About three-quarters of them—or 0.29 percent of all live births—are deleterious. In addition, at least one-third of

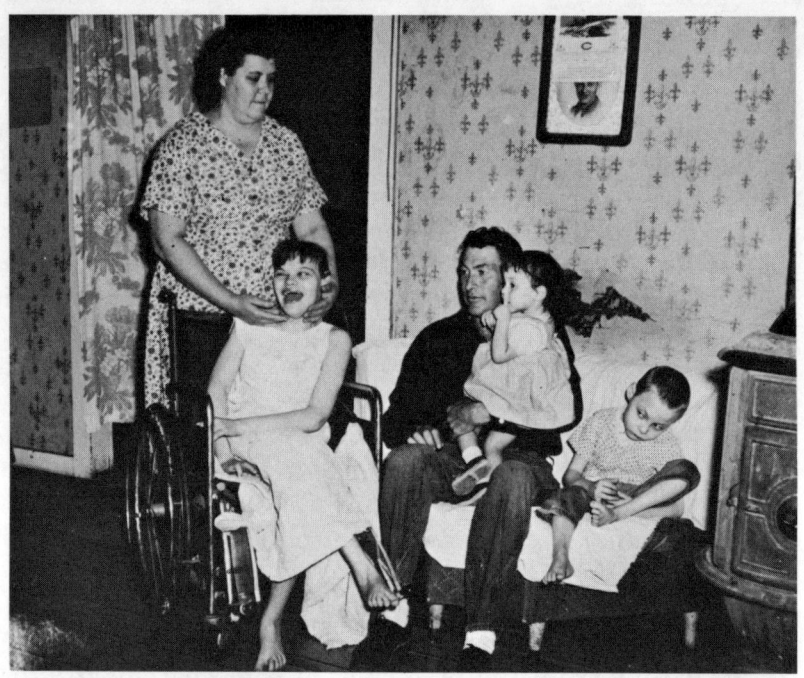

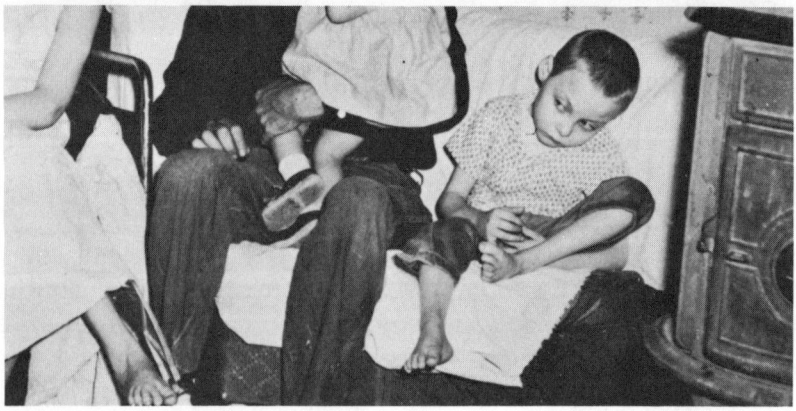

The first child born to parents (left) exhibits symptoms of central nervous system damage caused by PKU (phenylketonuria), a genetic disorder which today, in most U.S. hospitals, is routinely screened for among newborns. PKU-affected children have a defective liver enzyme and thus cannot properly metabolize the amino acid phenylalanine, a constituent of many foods. Phenylalanine accumulates in the body in a toxic form that poisons the brain cells. When PKU is diagnosed during the first few weeks of life, affected children can be maintained on a diet low in phenylalanine, which greatly minimizes brain damage. This is demonstrated in this family by their second child (closeup below), who with early diagnosis and therapy is developing normally. (COURTESY OF. NATIONAL INSTITUTE OF GENERAL MEDICAL SCIENCES)

all spontaneous abortions are probably caused by chromosomal abnormalities.[5 9 26]

Chromosomal genetic diseases include much mental retardation, multiple abnormalities such as Down's syndrome, and a variety of other extra-autosomal (nonsex chromosomal) or maldistributed sex chromosomal disorders.[5 9 26]

4. *Single-gene defects* occur in 1.8 to 2 percent of all live births. These conditions fall into three general categories: dominant, recessive, and sex-linked (or X-linked).[11 12]

a. Dominant, single-gene defects can be transmitted as disease by a single affected parent. For each of more than 940 such disorders so far discovered, there is a 50 percent risk with each pregnancy of transmitting the disease if one parent has the defective gene and a 75 percent risk if both do.

Examples include some forms of dwarfism and other physical defects and certain late-onset diseases, such as Huntington's disease, marked by progressive degeneration of the brain.[21]

b. Recessive, single-gene defects can be transmitted as disease only if both parents have either the trait or the disease. Each such condition carries a 25 percent chance of appearing in each pregnancy if both parents carry the trait.

Among the over 780 recognized recessive single-gene disorders are: sickle-cell anemia (a blood disease which mainly affects blacks), Tay-Sachs disease (a degenerative neurological disorder that leads to death in the children of its target population of largely Ashkenazic Jews), phenylketonuria, galactosemia, and cystic fibrosis (an endocrine, pancreas and respiratory illness that is the most prevalent of these disorders among whites).[21]

c. There are over *150 known sex-linked single gene disorders.* They are so named because the defect is carried on the X chromosome. The fact that women have two X chromosomes while men have but one, which is paired with another designated Y chromosome, leads to a different pattern of inheritance for those defective genes found on the X chromosome. This is based on the fact that men give their X chromosome only to their daughters, never to their sons, who always receive the father's Y chromosome. Thus, a female may have the trait for such a disorder that is recessive but not the disease because she has a normal X chromosome to balance the trait's effect. A male, however, must demonstrate the disease if he receives from his mother an X chromosome bearing the abnormal gene. The risk of affected offspring to a trait-carrying mother, then, is 50 percent with each male birth. Examples of X-linked recessive genetic disorders are hemophilia, Hunter's disease, muscular dystrophy of the Duchenne type, diabetes insipidus, the Lesch-Nyhan syndrome, and certain types of ataxia.

5. The third general category of genetic diseases (in addition to the chromosomal and single-gene defects) is the *complex or multigene disorders*. There is as yet no complete estimate of the actual number of such multifactorial diseases, although an incidence of from 1.7 to 2.6 percent of all live births has been suggested as reasonable.[10]

There is no way of determining for certain the potential risk of contracting a multifactorial disease; authorities tend to employ the "recurrence rule of thumb," which says that in a family with one affected offspring, the probability of having another is less than 5 percent. The mode of transmission is at least as complex as is the action of the genes involved in each of these multiple-gene diseases (for example, clubfoot, congenital dislocation of the hip, certain forms of diabetes). One authority, Dr. R. Wynne-Davies, has explained complex inheritance in the following way:

> In man, most traits are inherited by multiple gene systems and show continuous variation; that is, characters change imperceptibly over a wide range with no apparent discontinuity in expression—as with height and intelligence, for example.... It has become apparent that many of the common congenital malformations are also inherited in a similar manner. At first sight, this might seem improbable, in view of the all-or-none character of the disorders; an individual either has club foot or has not. There is no gradation here merging into the normal at one end of the distribution. However, it is probable that there is an underlying gradation of some factor immediately related to the deformity and all those individuals beyond a certain level (the threshold) on the normal

distribution curve will exhibit the disorder, while others will appear normal.[27]

It seems highly likely that many of the afflictions of man that appear to have a hereditary basis of some sort—conditions such as certain forms of cancer and cardiovascular disease—are transmitted in a complex way such as the above.[9,10]

6. Altogether, then, the *overall incidence of recognized genetic diseases is 4.8 to 5.0 percent of all live births.* While this seems to be a high figure for a class of diseases once thought to be extremely rare, it is important to remember that the estimate does not include such disorders that are widely thought to be at least partly genetic in origin.[5,10,11,12,13]

VII. What Is the Burden of the Genetic Disease Problem Carried by the Public and Medical Profession?

1. As previously stated, a reliable comprehensive estimate of the real cost—in tears as well as in dollars—of genetic disease is as incalculable as it is enormous. One reason for this is that the most common (innocuous, nondebilitating, and nonlethal) conditions are the least costly, and the most costly are the rarest (with some notable exceptions, such as cystic fibrosis and Down's syndrome).

2. In addition to the figures cited under Question II, reflecting the impact of genetic disease on the population (12 million Americans afflicted, and so forth), estimates have been made of the proportion of the nation's medical capability that is brought to bear on these conditions.

One figure frequently cited is that about one-quarter of all hospital beds and places in institutions for the handicapped are occupied by persons suffering from disorders that are wholly or partly genetic in nature. This may seem high, but it should include 19 percent of all such spaces occupied by schizophrenics and persons suffering mental depressive illness and the spaces occupied by approximately 80 percent of all the mentally retarded which are caused by genetic factors as well as the estimated one-third of all pediatric admissions for genetic causes.[4,6,7,8,9,14,28]

3. If the one-quarter figure still seems high, consider the recently reported finding that 20 percent of all heart attacks that occur in men before the age of 60 years are caused by one of three genes that regulate the body's fat metabolism. (Approximately another 5 percent of heart disease is attributed to polygenic causes.) The three genetic abnormalities predisposing to heart attack were estimated by their discoverers to occur in one of every 160 Americans, making them "among the most common disease-producing genes in our population."[3]

VIII. What Progress Has Been Made Against Genetic Disease by Scientific Research?

1. The very recognition of genetic disease as an important and costly public health problem was brought about by *recent advances in the basic sciences of cell biology and biochemical genetics.* As a direct—and often unexpected—consequence of these research advances, genetic medicine has begun to emerge as a new and powerful clinical discipline, equipped with a variety of means for detecting, diagnosing, preventing, and treating the hitherto enigmatic family of genetic diseases.

2. Practical capabilities of the new field of genetic medicine are constantly expanding. Currently, they include:

   a. Fetal detection of some 60 serious genetic disorders and identification of trait-carriers in more of them.[8][9][24]

   b. Capabilities for the genetic counseling of prospective parents on their risks and for intrauterine diagnosis, elective abortion, and, in some cases, treatment.[8][9][24]

   c. Screening of high-risk populations for certain genetic traits and/or diseases and of patients for possible bad drug reactions.[8][9][15][18][20][24]

   d. Development of various therapeutic techniques, such as dietary modifications (to prevent effects of PKU and galactosemia, for example), and administration of genetically deficient substances (vitamin B-12 for pernicious anemia, growth hormone for dwarfism, and so forth).[8][9][15]

   e. Removal of substances that act as toxins to the genetically afflicted (such as copper from persons suffering Wilson's disease).[8][9]

Genetic Disease

f. Immunological typing of tissues and transplantation of vital organs (for example, kidney transplants for persons with polycystic renal disease, and bone marrow for thalassemia patients and those with certain inherited immune deficiencies).[8,9,15]

g. Enhancement of enzyme actions (for example, treatment of hereditary jaundice by administration of enzyme-triggering phenobarbital).[9,29]

3. Today it is possible to treat genetic diseases of metabolism by restricting exposure of the victims to substances that they cannot metabolize, and a lesser number of others can be managed by administering the required metabolite.[8,9,15,24]

IX. If an Overall Assessment of the Economic and Social Burden of Genetic Disease Cannot Be Made as Yet, Can Any Specific Examples of Costs and Savings Possible for Individual Genetic Diseases Be Made?

1. Estimates have been made of yearly and lifetime costs of various genetic diseases, often with astonishing results.

For example, it has been estimated that the lifetime cost of maintaining a seriously genetically defective individual is $250,000 (assuming institutionalization).

Using that estimate and the fact that Down's syndrome occurs, conservatively, once in every 700 live births and that there are therefore at least 5,000 new cases every year in this country, the lifetime-committed expenditure for new cases of Down's syndrome, alone, would be about $1.25 billion yearly —a staggering sum for a single disease entity. Yet with present technology it is theoretically possible to prevent the birth of a substantial proportion, if not all mongoloid fetuses.[6,14,26]

2. Another way of calculating the toll of genetic diseases is to estimate the future life-years lost by them.

One widely cited estimate indicates that some 36 million future life-years are lost in this country by birth defects, putting the figure for recognized genetic disease (80 percent of birth defects are genetic in whole or in part) at 29 million future life-years lost, or several times as much as from heart disease, cancer, and stroke.[4]

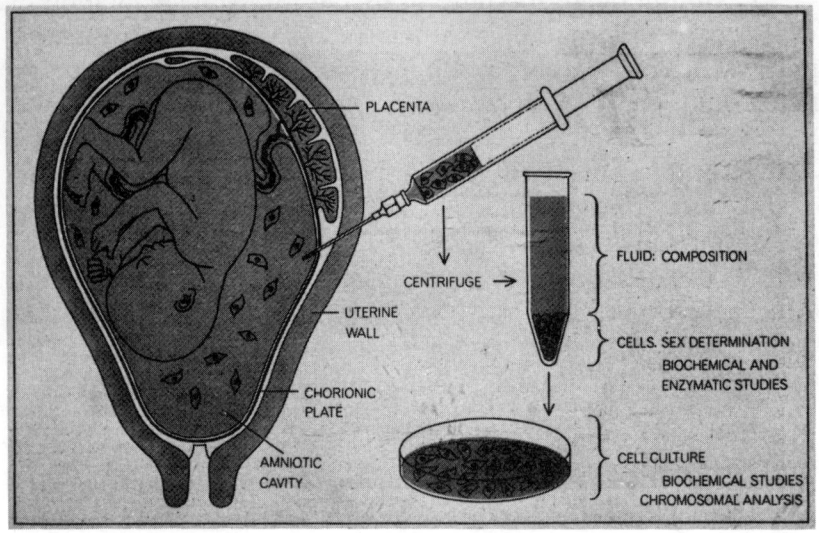

Assessment of the genetic status of a human fetus is more and more enhanced by the medical procedure called amniocentesis. It involves the withdrawal of a sample of amniotic fluid from an expectant mother's uterus by means of a hypodermic needle. The fluid contains cells shed by the growing fetus that can be cultured in the laboratory and tested for biochemical and chromosomal defects. Amniocentesis currently is applicable in some 60 serious genetic disorders. A determination usually can be reached by the 14th to 16th week of pregnancy, when therapeutic abortion is medically feasible and legally permissible in most states. (COURTESY OF NATIONAL INSTITUTE OF GENERAL MEDICAL SCIENCES)

3. Consider the costs of *Tay-Sachs disease*. Intensive care of the child over its brief life span runs about $35,000. There are about 50 cases of this disease every year in the United States. The annual cost, therefore, for this rare genetic disease amounts to $1,750,000 without detection of carriers, intrauterine diagnosis, and selective abortion of affected fetuses—all of which have now become possible through recent research advances which, themselves, did not require the expenditure of even one year's worth of Tay-Sachs disease care.[30]

4. Consider *phenylketonuria*, or PKU. This mentally retarding genetic disease occurs approximately once in every 14,000 newborn. Screening newborns for the disease costs $1.25 per test; or, approximately $17,000 is spent to detect each case. An additional $8,000 to $16,000 must then be spent for dietary treatment over a 5 to 10 year period, to prevent progres-

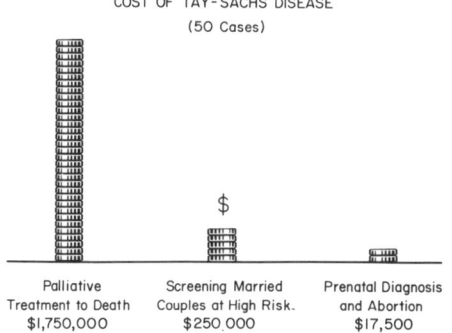

COST OF TAY-SACHS DISEASE
(50 Cases)

Palliative Treatment to Death	Screening Married Couples at High Risk.	Prenatal Diagnosis and Abortion
$1,750,000	$250,000	$17,500

(COURTESY OF NATIONAL INSTITUTE OF GENERAL MEDICAL SCIENCES)

sion of the disease's retarding effects. This brings the total cost of prevention to $33,000 per child. Untreated, severe mental retardation cared for over, say, 50 years in an institution at a cost of no more than $20 a day, would run to $365,000, or more than 10 times the cost of prevention. Add to this savings the input from the individual through earnings, taxes, and family and societal contributions.[1][31]

Such figures must be convincing, for some 48 states now require screening of newborn for PKU and certain other genetic diseases. Results? A survey of nine Western state mental hospitals revealed no cases of PKU after screening for the disease became available, but 25 cases of the disease in children too old to have benefited from the screening.[1]

Incidentally, the above-cited cost of detection and prevention of a serious genetic disease—roughly one-tenth the cost of care where detection, prevention, and care are possible—seems to hold for these conditions in general.

Screening high-risk (older) pregnant women for Down's syndrome *in utero* might prevent 1,000 cases yearly, which would otherwise cost some $300 million in lifetime care. To detect 1,000 cases, 96,000 pregnancies would have to be screened at a cost of between $15 million and $25 million, or less than a tenth of the cost of lifetime care.[32]

X. How Much Effort Is Being Put into Research on Genetic Disease?

1. The National Institutes of Health is spending approximately $100 million a year on research related to genetic dis-

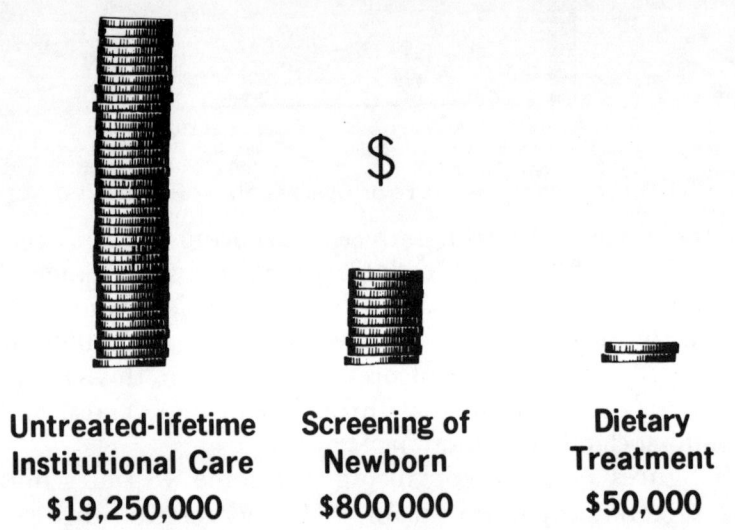

COST OF PKU (Phenylketonuria)
(50 Cases)

Untreated-lifetime Institutional Care	Screening of Newborn	Dietary Treatment
$19,250,000	$800,000	$50,000

(COURTESY OF NATIONAL INSTITUTE OF GENERAL MEDICAL SCIENCES)

ease, of which a high proportion is administered by the National Institute of General Medical Sciences. The NIGMS's initiative in genetics research and investigator training includes programs in human chromosome mapping, basic mechanisms underlying the regulation of gene action, cell biology, and other areas that are likely to give new clues to the management of genetic diseases.[33][34]

2. The NIGMS has designated 10 national centers for research in medical genetics.[34]

3. Other agencies, both public and private, are supporting genetic research; however, few of these have specified how much is being spent on genetic disease research.

In sum, however, it should be clear that expenditures for genetics research as it pertains ultimately to genetic medicine are disproportionately small compared to the savings they can produce, even in the short run, for only a small percentage of all genetic diseases. Clearly, the payoff for research dollars invested promises ultimately to be higher than that expended for practically any other line of medically oriented research, so sweeping is the horizon of genetic medicine for combating diseases.

4. Unlike other fields of medical research, the enormous payoffs already achieved and foreseen for the near future in genetic medicine come not from cures but from new techniques for diagnosis, prevention, and treatment—overall management of genetic disease.

No genetic disease has yet been cured, in the strictest sense of the word, nor is any likely to be rendered curable very soon, for this would require actual repair of the genetic defect so that it would be neither expressed as disease nor transmissible to a subsequent generation.

Even this feat, however, no longer seems beyond reach. Scientists experimenting with lower organisms have already demonstrated to some extent the feasibility of laboratory technologies for conferring healthy genes to deficient cells.

Such feats of "gene therapy" should ultimately be no less transferable to the human patient one day in the future than any of the many other basic scientific advances that have been made in the past very few years and which have now drawn world attention to man's most ubiquitous malady—genetic disease.[8 9 35]

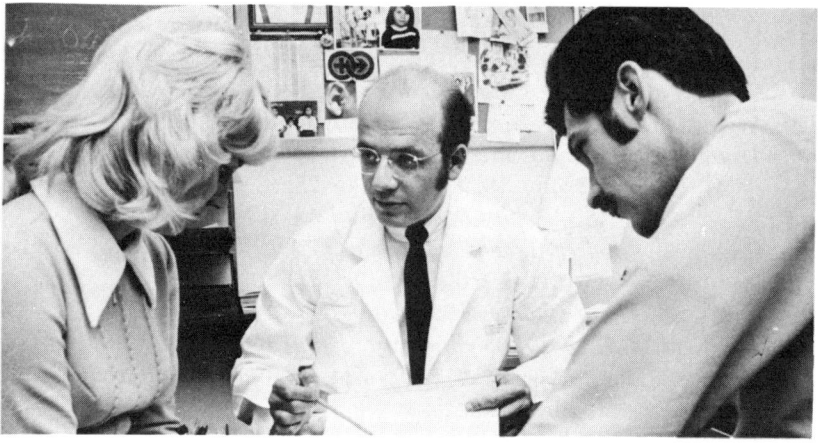

For families who risk the transmission of serious inheritable diseases—whether they are aware of it or not—genetic counseling has begun to emerge as a major gateway to the benefits of new knowledge and technologies gained through basic and clinical research. (COURTESY OF NATIONAL INSTITUTE OF GENERAL MEDICAL SCIENCES)

Notes

1. Testimony by J. E. Seegmiller, M.D., Professor, Department of Medicine, University of California, San Diego, before the Labor/HEW Subcommittee of the Committee on Appropriations, U.S. House of Representatives, June 11, 1971.
2. C. J. Epstein, "Genetic Counseling, Past, Present, Future," *Proceedings of the Wayne State Symposium on Birth Defects and Fetal Development—Endocrine and Metabolic Factors* (Springfield, Ill.: Charles C. Thomas, 1973).
3. A. G. Motulsky, et al., Report to the American Heart Association, Dallas, Tex., November 16, 1972.
4. V. Apgar and G. Stickle, *Journal of the American Medical Association* 204:79 (1968).
5. D. H. Carr, *Advances in Human Genetics* 2:201 (1971).
6. R. Y. Berini, National Genetics Foundation, testimony before the Labor/HEW Subcommittee of the Committee on Appropriations, U.S. House of Representatives, May 15, 1973.
7. Joshua Lederberg, Ph.D., Professor and Chairman, Department of Genetics, Stanford University School of Medicine, testimony before the Labor/HEW Subcommittee of the Committee on Appropriations, U.S. House of Representatives, June 10, 1970.
8. C. L. Clow, et al., "On the Application of Knowledge to the Patient with Genetic Disease," *Progress in Medical Genetics*, vol. 9 (New York and London: Grune and Stratton, 1973).
9. World Health Organization Technical Report No. 497, *Genetic Disorders: Prevention, Treatment, and Rehabilitation* (Geneva, 1972).
10. C. O. Carter, *British Medical Bulletin* 25:52 (1969).
11. A. C. Stevenson, *British Medical Bulletin*, 17:254 (1961).
12. C. Smith, *Modern Trends in Human Genetics* (New York: Appleton-Century-Crofts, 1970), p. 350.
13. N. E. Simpson, *Diabetes* 13:462 (1971).
14. Margery W. Shaw, M.D., Director, Medical Genetics Center, University of Texas Graduate School of Biomedical Sciences, Houston, personal communication.
15. C. R. Scriver, Medical Genetics Lecture, Jackson Laboratory, Bar Harbor, Maine, August 1972; *Medical Tribune* 6, no. 18 (September 18, 1972).
16. Kurt Hirschhorn, M.D., Professor and Chief, Division of Medical Genetics, Mount Sinai School of Medicine, The City University of New York, personal communication.
17. A. G. Motulsky, M.D., Professor of Medicine and Genetics, Uni-

versity of Washington School of Medicine, Seattle, personal communication.
18. D. G. Friend, *Journal of the American Pharmaceutical Association*, 4:221-225 (1964).
19. K. L. Melmon, *New England Journal of Medicine* (October 17, 1972), pp. 1361-1368.
20. B. N. La Du, et al., *Fundamentals of Drug Metabolism and Drug Disposition* (Baltimore: The Williams & Wilkins Company, 1971).
21. V. A. McKusick, *Mendelian Inheritance in Man*, 3rd ed. (Baltimore: The Johns Hopkins Press, 1971).
22. C. R. Scriver, "Screening for Inherited Traits: Perspectives," *Early Diagnosis of Human Genetic Defects*, Proceedings No. 6, ed. Harris, Maureen, Fogarty International Center, National Institutes of Health, Bethesda, Md.
23. A. G. Motulsky, "Frequency of Sickling Disorders in U.S. Blacks," *New England Journal of Medicine* 288:31 (1973).
24. A. Milusnky, et al., *New England Journal of Medicine*, December 17, 23, 31, 1970.
25. M. W. Shaw, testimony before the Labor/HEW Subcommittee of the Committee on Appropriations, U.S. House of Representatives, May 3, 1972.
26. M. Levitan and A. Montague, *Textbook of Human Genetics* (London and Toronto: Oxford University Press, 1971).
27. R. Wynne-Davies, *Modern Trends in Human Genetics* (New York: Appleton-Century-Crofts, 1970), chap. 11.
28. *Patients in State and County Mental Hospitals 1967*, Series A., no. 2, publication of the National Institute of Mental Health, Rockville, Md. 20015.
29. S. J. Jaffee, et al., *New England Journal of Medicine*, 275:1461-1466 (1966).
30. J. O'Brien, *Early Diagnosis of Human Genetic Defects*, Proceedings No. 6, 1972, ed. Maureen Harris, Fogarty International Center, National Institutes of Health, Bethesda, Md.
31. H. L. Levy, et al., "Massachusetts Metabolic Disorders Screening Program," *ibid.*
32. J. V. Neel, "Ethical Issues Resulting from Prenatal Diagnosis," *ibid.*
33. Robert S. Stone, M.D., Director, National Institutes of Health, Bethesda, Md., personal communication.
34. Ruth L. Kirschstein, M.D., Director, National Institute of General Medical Sciences, National Institutes of Health, Bethesda, Md., personal communication.
35. H. V. Aposhian, *Perspectives in Biology and Medicine* no. 14 (Autumn 1970), pp. 98-108.

What Are the Facts About High Blood Pressure?

I. Can the Treatment of High Blood Pressure Reduce the Deaths from Strokes and Heart Attacks?

Yes.

1. If all the 23 million estimated victims of high blood pressure could be screened to detect high blood pressure early, and could receive and be maintained on the drugs now available to control high blood pressure, the *overall death rate from strokes and heart attacks would decline about 20 percent.*

2. Each year, *high blood pressure is a factor in 68 percent of all first heart attacks and in 75 percent of all first strokes.*[1]

3. In a study conducted by the Veterans Administration on the effects of treatment on morbidity in high blood pressure, there were *more than twice as many deaths* related to hypertension or atherosclerosis *in the untreated group of patients* as in those patients receiving treatment for their high blood pressure.[7]

The estimated risk of developing heart failure, stroke, or other cardiovascular complication was reduced from 55 percent to 18 percent by treatment. In other words, *treatment of high blood pressure was 67 percent effective in this study in reducing the incidence* of heart failure, strokes, and other cardiovascular complications.[7] (See Chart 1.)

II. How Many People Are Victims of High Blood Pressure?

1. High blood pressure afflicts an estimated *23 million or more* American adults, or 1 out of 6 in the population.[1] (See Charts A, B, and C, pages 149-150.)

Chart 1

Treatment can ward off complications and lengthen life.
(VA Study)

Occurrence of heart failure, stroke, and kidney complications in patients with mild to moderate high blood pressure

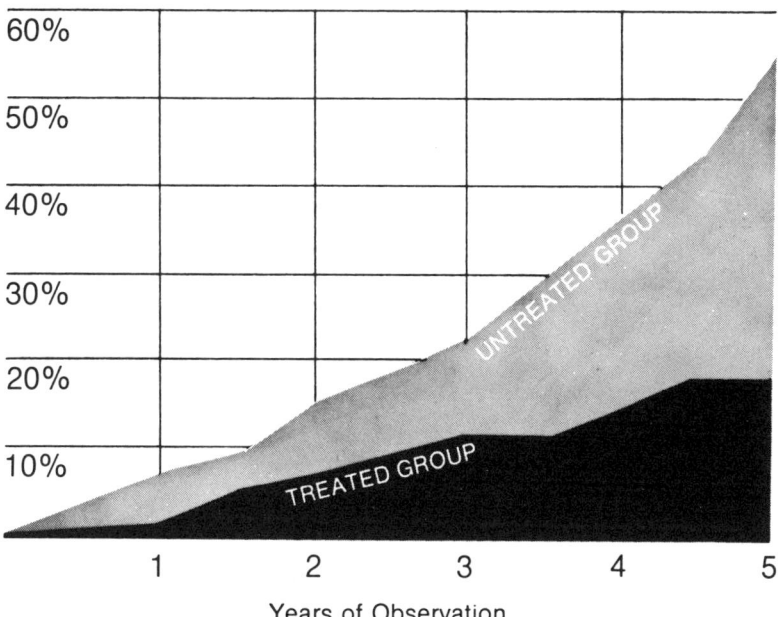

(Based on results of Veterans Administration Study cited in note 7.)

Treatment with antihypertensive drugs reduced the predicted risk of developing heart failure, or cardiovascular or cerebrovascular complications over a five-year period from 55 percent to 18 percent. Benefit of treatment showed itself early and increased steadily with time.

Chart courtesy of Health Information Services, Merck Sharp & Dohme, West Point, Pa. 19486.

2. *Only about 12½ percent* (one-eighth) of hypertensives, or 2,875,000 people, *receive adequate treatment* to control the hypertension and reduce such complications as heart failure, stroke, or kidney failure.[1] (See Chart D, page 000.)

3. *The balance of 87½ percent* of people with high blood pressure either *don't know they have it, or if they do know they have it, their treatment is inadequate or nonexistent.*[1] (See Chart D, page 150.)

> *12½%* (one-eighth) are aware of their high blood pressure, BUT are receiving *inadequate therapy.*[1]
>
> *25% (5,750,000)* know they have high blood pressure BUT are receiving *no therapy.*[1]
>
> *50% of the 23 million are unaware* they have high blood pressure.[1]

III. Do We Have Adequate Screening Programs?

1. No adequate screening programs, on a big enough scale, exist to date *to detect people with hypertension before the inevitable complications of heart disease, strokes, kidney disease, or visual problems can occur.*

IV. What Does High Blood Pressure Cost Our National Economy?

1. *Twenty-four billion dollars* was the estimated annual cost to the nation in 1967 of arteriosclerosis (heart attacks and strokes) and hypertensive disease.[2] (See Chart 2.)

2. *Since high blood pressure is a factor in such a large percentage of heart attacks and strokes, the overall estimated economic loss* represented by arteriosclerosis as well as the hypertensive diseases is probably *a more accurate measurement* of the impact of this disease on the economy than that for high blood pressure alone.

3. *Direct costs* of arteriosclerosis and high blood pressure (hospital and nursing home care, physicians' and other medical professional services, and drugs) totaled an estimated *$4.3 billion* in 1967.[2]

4. *Indirect costs due to productivity losses* because of illness and disability from arteriosclerotic and hypertensive diseases in 1967 totaled an estimated *$1.1 billion.*[2]

5. The estimated indirect economic costs to the nation measured in terms of the present value of *lifetime earnings* lost by those who died that year from arteriosclerotic and hypertensive diseases amounted to *$18.5 billion.*[2]

Chart 2

ESTIMATED ECONOMIC COSTS TO THE NATION DUE TO MORBIDITY AND MORTALITY FROM ARTERIOSCLEROTIC AND HYPERTENSIVE DISEASES, U.S., 1967[2]

Arteriosclerotic heart disease	$15,545,000,000
Stroke*	4,605,000,000
Diseases of arteries	1,082,000,000
Hypertensive diseases†	2,655,000,000
Total, arteriosclerotic and hypertensive diseases	$23,887,000,000

* Includes 20 percent not due to arteriosclerosis.
† Does not include all arteriosclerotic disease in which hypertension was involved.

V. How Is High Blood Pressure Related to Heart Attacks and Strokes?

1. In people with high blood pressure, *arteriosclerosis* of the coronary and cerebral arteries *tends to be more severe* than in normotensive persons—*leading to increased incidence of heart attacks and strokes.*[2]

2. Of the estimated 800,000 persons who have a first heart attack each year, 545,000 or *68 percent have definite or borderline high blood pressure.* (Also see Chart E, page 151.)

> 42% (335,000) have *definite* hypertension
> (95 mm HG or greater diastolic, or
> 160 mm HG or greater systolic).
>
> 26% (210,000) have *borderline* hypertension
> (below 160 systolic and 95 diastolic but
> not below 140 systolic and 90 diastolic).

68% (545,000) have definite or borderline hypertension.

32% (255,000) do *not* have hypertension (below 140 systolic and 90 diastolic).

100% (800,000)

3. Of an estimated 400,000 persons who have a first stroke each year:

54% (215,000) have *definite* hypertension
21% (85,000) have *borderline* hypertension
75% (300,000) have definite or borderline hypertension
25% (100,000) do not have hypertension

Thus, *high blood pressure is involved in 75 percent of first strokes each year.*[1]

4. Hypertension also promotes the formation of cerebral arterial aneurysms.[2]

VI. What Are the Risks of Heart Attacks?

1. The risk of coronary heart disease in men aged 30 to 59, with a diastolic blood pressure of 105 mm HG or more, is *3 times* that in men with a diastolic level of 75-84 mm HG.[2]

2. Results of the Framingham (Massachusetts) Study show that *the risk of every manifestation of coronary heart disease, including angina, coronary insufficiency, myocardial infarction, and sudden death, was distinctly and impressively related to the antecedent level of both systolic and diastolic blood pressure.*[3]

VII. What Are the Risks of Strokes?

1. In the case of *stroke, hypertensive* men of similar age and blood pressure had *nearly 10 times* the attack rate of men with *normal* levels.

As the pressure increases, the risk of stroke and heart attack also increases.[2]

High Blood Pressure

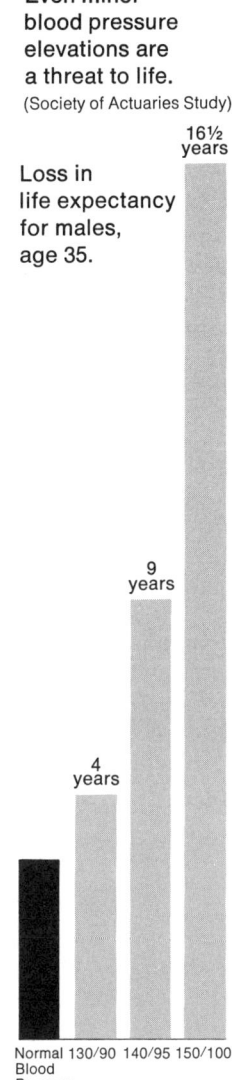

Even minor blood pressure elevations are a threat to life.
(Society of Actuaries Study)

Loss in life expectancy for males, age 35.

16½ years

9 years

4 years

Normal 130/90 140/95 150/100
Blood
Pressure

Chart courtesy of Health Information Services, Merck Sharp & Dohme, West Point, Pa.

VIII. How Many Deaths Are There from High Blood Pressure?

1. The major cardiovascular diseases caused an estimated 1,037,460 deaths in 1973.[4] High blood pressure was involved

or a contributing factor in many of these deaths, although it is impossible to estimate accurately exactly how many.

As has been stated earlier, high blood pressure is involved in 68 percent of first heart attacks and in 75 percent of first strokes, so it can be assumed that high blood pressure was a factor in over *513,000* of the 754,000 heart disease deaths in 1973, and in over *160,000* of the 214,000 stroke deaths in 1973.

IX. What Has Been the Research Progress Against High Blood Pressure?

1. As a result of the medical research breakthrough in the development of many effective antihypertension drugs, the *death rate from hypertensive disease* (as defined by the National Vital Statistics Division and not including its relationship to deaths from heart attacks and strokes) *has declined more than 65 percent* since 1950.[1]

2. While the death rate from hypertensive disease has declined, the full impact of *therapy now available* for hypertension *has not as yet sufficiently affected the death rates from other types of heart disease and strokes,* in which hypertension is involved, since many victims of high blood pressure go *undetected and untreated until the heart attack or stroke is actually experienced.*

X. How Much Is Currently Being Spent for Research in High Blood Pressure?

1. *The National Heart and Lung Institute* of the National Institutes of Health, U.S. Department of Health, Education, and Welfare, estimates expenditures for research in high blood pressure (including kidney disease) in fiscal 1974 at *$47,409,000.*[1]

Other agencies both public and private are supporting cardiovascular disease research; however, it is impossible for them to determine how much is specifically in the area of high blood pressure. (See Chart following listing estimated research expenditures in the field of cardiovascular diseases by major sources listed.)

XI. What Are the Needs in the Field of High Blood Pressure?

1. Existing medical services often fail to provide satisfactory long-term care for patients with hypertension as evidenced by the large number who either leave therapy or receive inadequate treatment. *The development and evaluation of new and more effective techniques for delivering long-term care to all hypertensive patients is urgently needed.*[6]

2. *Education of the medical profession and the public* that *even moderate hypertension should be treated* to prevent the development of heart disease (heart attacks, congestive heart failure), strokes, and kidney disease is urgently needed.

3. *More effective mass screening programs* on city, county, and national levels are urgently needed to ensure the early detection and prompt treatment of even moderate cases of hypertension. A critical need is the proper linkage of screening to long-term care.

Dr. Theodore Cooper, former Director of the National Heart and Lung Institute of the National Institutes of Health, U.S. Department of Health, Education, and Welfare, has estimated that *"a successful campaign in the public health sector for the detection and treatment of high blood pressure would result, within two to three years, in the averting of about 200,000 deaths from stroke, heart attack, kidney failure, and heart failure per year."*

4. Research to gain understanding of the disease and to develop new, improved drugs to prevent and cure high blood pressure.

Estimated Research Expenditures of Various Agencies Listed—by Type of Cardiovascular Disease

Agency	Arteriosclerosis	Hypertension	Strokes	Research in Other Cardiovascular	Total
Major Federal Funds					
National Heart and Lung Institute fiscal 1974 Obligations	$60,487,000	$47,409,000	$3,482,000	$110,462,000	$221,840,000
National Institute of Neurological Diseases and Stroke, fiscal 1975			8,578,000		8,578,000
U.S. Atomic Energy Commission, fiscal 1973				2,667,000	2,667,000
Veterans Administration, fiscal 1975			816,000	9,348,000	10,164,000
Total, Federal funds	$60,487,000	$47,409,000	$12,876,000	$122,477,000	$243,249,000
Major Private Funds					
American Heart Association and its affiliates, 1973					16,778,531
				Grand total	$260,027,531

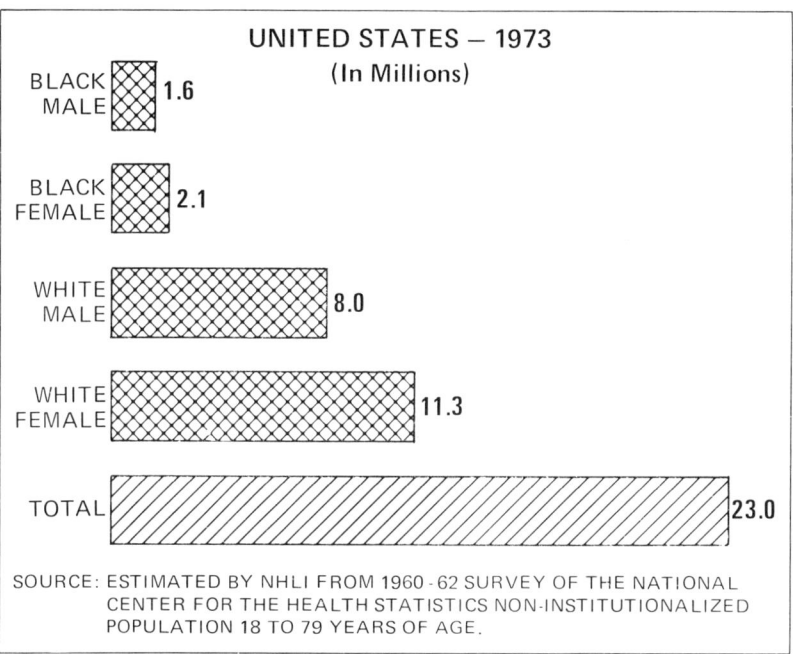

Chart A

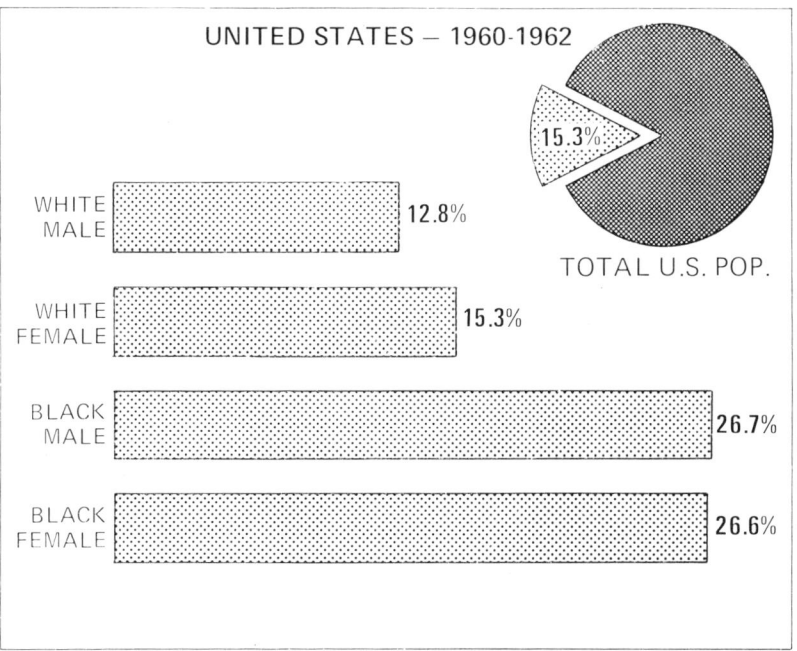

Chart B

NUMBER OF PERSONS BY AGE WITH HIGH BLOOD PRESSURE

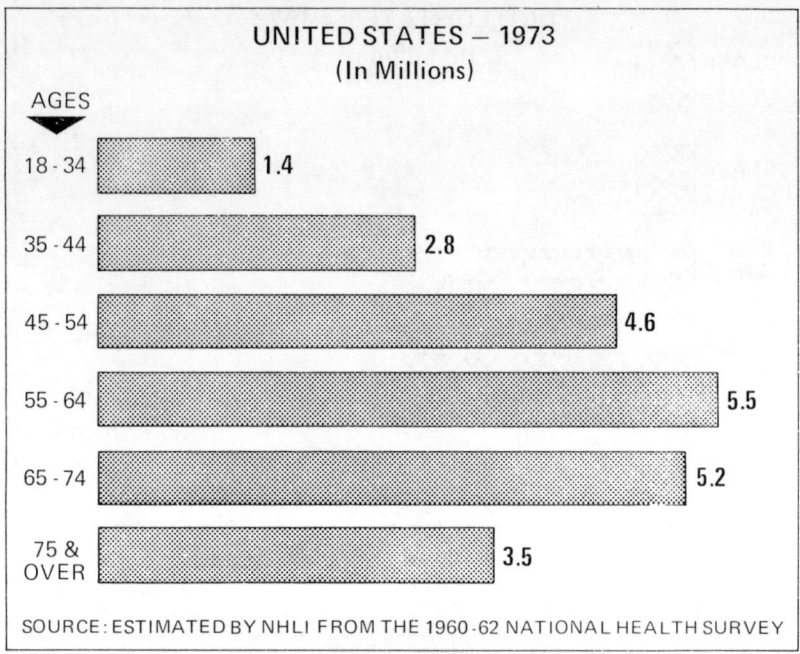

Chart C

AWARENESS AND THERAPY OF 23 MILLION PERSONS IN UNITED STATES WITH HIGH BLOOD PRESSURE

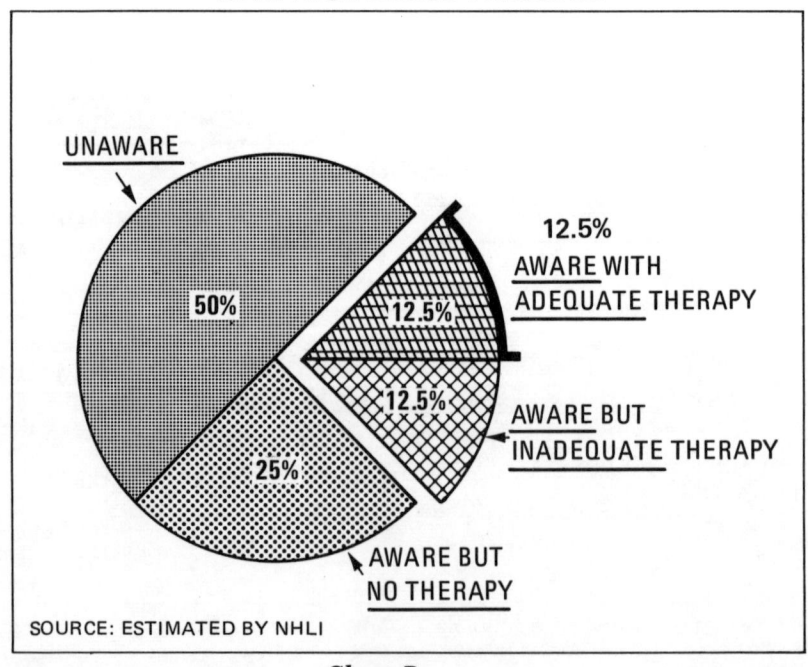

Chart D

PERCENT OF HEART ATTACKS AND STROKES WITH HIGH BLOOD PRESSURE — UNITED STATES

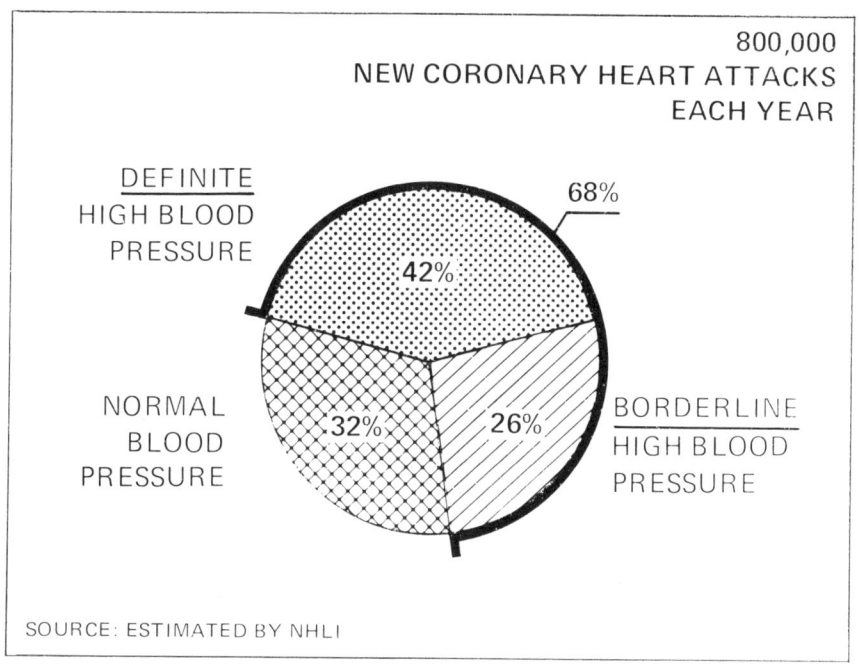

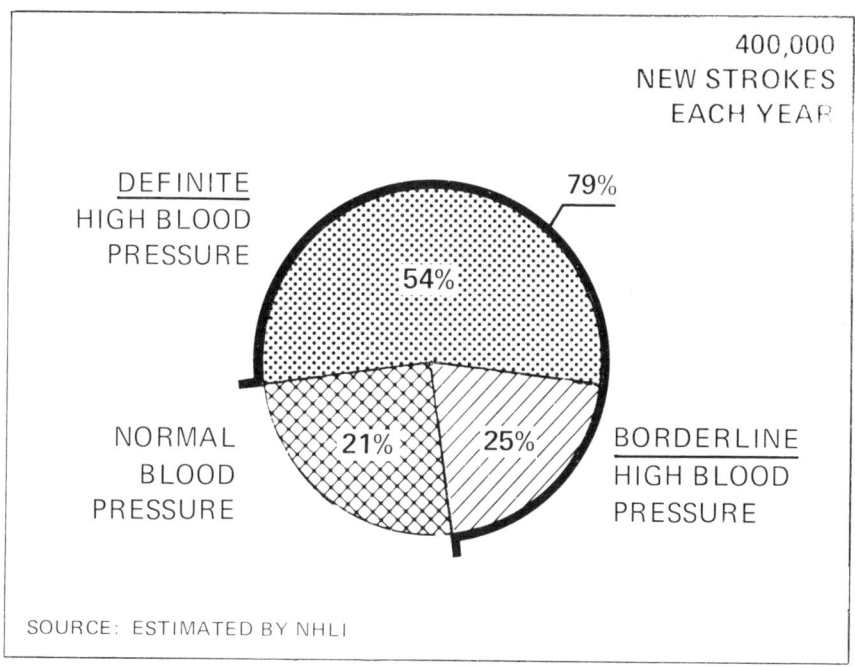

Chart E

Notes

1. Information supplied by the National Heart and Lung Institute, National Institutes of Health, Bethesda, Md.

    The estimate on the number of people with hypertension is based upon data on prevalence from the mean of three blood pressures taken in the Nat'l Health Examination Survey at one sitting, hypertension being defined as blood pressure of 160/95 mm HG or greater or evidence of hypertensive heart disease.

    Of the 23 million persons with hypertension, 4.5 million have diastolic blood pressure of 105 mm HG or greater, and 9.5 million others are at levels between 95 and 104 mm HG. The remaining 9 million have systolic blood pressure of 160 mm HG or greater but are below 95 mm HG diastolic.

2. *Arteriosclerosis*. Report by National Heart and Lung Institute Task Force on Arteriosclerosis, vol. II, June 1971, DHEW publication no. (NIH) 72-219, National Institutes of Health, Department of Health, Education, and Welfare, Washington, D.C.
3. William B. Kannel, M.D., Melvin J. Schwartz, M.D., and Patricia M. McNamara, "Blood Pressure and Risk of Coronary Heart Disease: The Framingham Study," *Diseases of the Chest* 56, no. 1 (July 1969).
4. National Center for Health Statistics, U.S. Public Health Service, Rockville, Md.
5. Lawrence B. Hobson, M.D., Deputy Assistant Chief Medical Director for Research & Development, Department of Medicine and Surgery, Veterans Administration, Washington, D.C. in personal communication, April 16, 1975.
6. "Guidelines for Detection, Diagnosis, and Management of Hypertensive Populations," report of Inter-Society Commission for Heart Disease Resources, *Circulation* 44 (November 1971).
7. "Effects of Treatment on Morbidity in Hypertension," Veterans Administration Cooperative Study Group on Antihypertensive Agents, *Journal of the American Medical Association* 213, no. 7 (August 17, 1970).

What Are the Facts About Mental Illness?

I. How Many People in the United States Are Suffering from Some Form of Mental Illness?

1. An estimated 20 million people in the United States are suffering from some form of mental or emotional illness, from mild to severe, that needs psychiatric treatment.[1]
   a. This means that about *1 in every 10 persons* is now suffering from some form of mental illness of varying degrees of severity.
2. Mental illness or other personality disturbances are usually significant *factors in criminal behavior, delinquency, suicide, alcoholism, narcotics addiction,* and, very often, in cases of divorce.
3. An estimated 1.4 million children in the United States are in need of psychiatric care.[1]

II. How Many Alcoholics Are There in the United States Today?

1. About 9 million people in the United States today are alcoholics and alcohol abusers.[2]
2. Alcohol abuse and alcoholism drain the economy of an estimated *$15 billion a year.*[2]
   a. Of this total, *$10 billion* is attributable to *lost work time* in business, industry, civilian government, and the military.
   b. *Two billion dollars* is spent for *health and welfare services* provided to alcoholic persons and their families.
   c. *Property damage, medical expenses, and other overhead costs* account for another *$3 billion or more.*[2]

153

3. Alcohol plays a major role in half the highway fatalities in the United States, and cost 28,000 lives in one recent year.

4. Public intoxication alone accounts for one-third of all arrests reported annually.[2]

III. How Many Suicides Are There Annually?

An estimated *24,440 people* committed suicide in 1973.[3]

Suicide is now the eleventh leading cause of death in the United States. Since 1962, the crude death rate from suicide has increased 15 percent.[3]

Studies supported by the National Institute of Mental Health have corroborated earlier expert opinion that the actual number of suicides is double the above figure. In addition, since it is estimated that there are 8 suicide attempts for every suicide committed, there are perhaps as many as *400,000 people who will attempt suicide this year.*[23]

IV. How Many Narcotic Addicts Are There in the United States Today?

1. There are about *68,864 known active narcotic addicts* in the United States today (as of December 31, 1970).[4]

2. In 1960, there were 32,000 arrests for violations of narcotic drug laws; in 1970, this had increased to 266,000 arrests.[4]

3. Among the leading causes of arrests in 1970, violations of narcotic drug laws ranked fourth.[5]

Leading Causes for Arrest—1970[4]

Drunkenness	1,496,400
Larceny	590,700
Disorderly conduct	572,200
Narcotic drug laws	291,600
Driving while intoxicated	281,000
Burglary	270,500
Liquor laws	218,100
Auto theft	120,100
Aggravated assault	114,200
Weapons	96,100

V. What Is the Cost of Crime and Delinquency to the Nation?

1. Antisocial conduct labeled crime and delinquency covers a wide range of behavior from truancy and petty larceny to multiple homicide and political assassination. Its monetary cost to the nation—including expenses related to law enforcement, administration of justice, and correctional efforts, as well as the cost of damage inflicted by offenders—has been estimated at more than *$20 billion a year.*
2. *Public expenditures for police, courts and corrections*—currently estimated at *more than $4 billion* annually—are borne primarily by taxpayers at the state and local level.[4] The emotional and psychological costs of crime, *which defy measurement in monetary terms,* affect in numerous ways the lives of countless innocent people.

VI. How Many People Are Being Treated for Mental Illness?

1. There were an estimated 4,190,913 patient care episodes in psychiatric facilities in the United States in 1971. These facilities included outpatient psychiatric services, mental hospitals, community mental health centers, and other psychiatric facilities.[22]

VII. What Is the Extent of Mental Illness Among Children?

1. The National Association for Mental Health estimates that *over 1.4 million children* in the United States are in need of psychiatric care.[6]
2. Of the total patient care episodes in 1971, approximately 744,000, or 18.5 percent, were accounted for by the under-18 age group.[22]
3. Of this group, 81 percent were seen on an outpatient basis and 19 percent on an inpatient basis. Of the latter, 39,000 episodes were in state and county hospitals and 46,100 in general hospitals.[5]

Distribution of Mental Health Facilities and Services by Type of Facility, United States, January 1972

Type of Facility	Number of Facilities	Number with:			Percent Distribution of:			
		Inpatient Service	Outpatient Service	Day Care Service	Facilities	Inpatient Service	Outpatient Service	Day Care Service
Total, All Facilities	3,200	1,917	2,279	989	100.0%	100.0%	100.0%	100.0%
Psychiatric hospital	482	482	338	206	15.0	25.1	14.8	20.8
State and county	324	324	238	134	10.1	16.9	10.4	13.5
Proprietary	158	158	100	72	4.9	8.2	4.4	7.3
Veterans Administration hospitals	119	110	102	49	3.7	5.7	4.5	5.0
General hospital psychiatric services	770	653	322	174	24.1	34.2	14.2	17.6
Public	158	141	86	47	4.9	7.4	3.8	4.8
Nonpublic	612	512	236	127	19.2	26.8	10.4	12.8
Residential treatment center for emotionally disturbed children	344	344	66	60	10.8	17.9	2.9	6.1
Federally funded CMHC	295	295	295	295	9.2	15.4	12.9	29.8
Day hospitals—free-standing	34	—	—	34	1.1	—	—	3.4
Outpatient clinics—free-standing	1,123	—	1,123	146	35.1	—	49.3	14.8
Public	588	—	588	79	18.4	—	25.8	8.0
Nonpublic	535	—	535	67	16.7	—	23.5	6.8
Other multiservice facilities	33	33	33	25	1.0	1.7	1.4	2.5

Source: *Utilization of Mental Health Facilities, 1971*, Analytical and Special Study Reports. series B, no. 5, National Institute of Mental Health, Chevy Chase, Md.

VIII. What Facilities Are There in the United States for the Treatment of Mental Illnesses?

1. There was a total of 3,200 mental health facilities in the United States as of January 1972 for the care and treatment of patients.[22]

IX. Which Mental Illnesses Affect the Greatest Number of People?

1. Of first admissions (no prior inpatient psychiatric care) to state and county mental hospitals in 1972.[21]

Percent	Diagnosis
26.1%	Alcohol disorders
13.9%	Schizophrenia
12.4%	Neuroses
10.5%	Personality disorders
9.9%	Brain syndromes
6.5%	Drug abuse disorders
20.7%	All other diagnoses

4. Children comprised 27 *percent of the total caseload of outpatient psychiatric services.* In contrast, 5 to 14 percent of the caseloads of inpatient facilities consisted of persons under 18 years of age.[5]

5. Of the three types of hospitals, state and county mental hospitals had the smallest proportion of children.[5]

X. What Are the Principal Diagnoses Among Resident Patients in State and County Mental Hospitals?

Of the *resident patient* population in state and county mental hospitals:

48% have a diagnosis of schizophrenia
12% have a diagnosis of organic brain syndromes associated with cerebral arteriosclerosis or senile brain disease
11% have a diagnosis of other brain syndromes
9% have a diagnosis of mental retardation

NUMBER AND PERCENT DISTRIBUTION OF ADMISSIONS WITH NO PRIOR
INPATIENT PSYCHIATRIC CARE WHO WERE ADMITTED TO STATE AND
COUNTY MENTAL HOSPITALS, BY SELECTED DIAGNOSTIC GROUPS,
UNITED STATES, 1962, 1965, 1969, AND 1972[21]

Selected Diagnostic Groups	1962	1965	1969	1972
	\multicolumn{4}{c}{Number of First Admissions}			
All Diagnoses	129,698	144,090	163,984	140,813
Alcohol disorders	19,406	24,380	42,078	36,788
Drug abuse disorders	1,652	3,549	6,343	9,093
Brain syndromes	33,978	31,345	25,548	13,910
Schizophrenia	27,266	25,374	24,540	19,607
Other psychoses	9,662	9,683	10,132	4,573
Neuroses	12,191	15,821	19,806	17,406
Personality disorders	11,850	15,295	14,620	14,784
All other diagnoses	13,693	18,643	20,917	24,652
	\multicolumn{4}{c}{Percent Distribution}			
All Disorders	100.0%	100.0%	100.0%	100.0%
Alcohol disorders	15.0	16.9	25.7	26.1
Drug abuse disorders	1.3	2.5	3.9	6.5
Brain syndromes	26.2	21.8	15.6	9.9
Schizophrenia	21.0	17.6	15.0	13.9
Other psychoses	7.0	6.7	6.2	3.2
Neuroses	9.4	11.0	12.1	12.4
Personality disorders	9.1	10.6	8.9	10.5
All other diagnoses	10.6	12.9	12.8	17.5

NOTE: Detail may not add to the total due to rounding.

These diagnostic categories account for 80 percent of the total resident population in state and county mental hospitals in 1970.[24]

XI. In What Age Groups Do Mental Disorders Take Their Greatest Toll?

1. Of total admissions to inpatient and outpatient services combined in 1971:[22]

      36% were under 24 years of age
      38% were 25 to 44 years of age

22% were 45 to 64 years old
5% were 65 or older

2. Following is a table indicating the three leading diagnoses among admissions with no prior inpatient psychiatric care who were admitted to state and county mental hospitals in 1969 and 1972 by sex and age groups.[21]

XII. What Is the Cost of Mental Illness to the United States?

1. Almost *$21 billion* was the estimated cost of mental illness to the United States in 1968 (latest available data).[17] Mental illness is one of the most costly of all diseases.
    a. About 43 percent of the cost was borne by persons other than the mentally ill and their families.[17]
The general population paid a little over $8 billion in additional taxes in order to offset the reduction in tax revenues caused by the decline of income among the mentally ill and to provide them with maintenance and treatment.[17]
    b. The costs borne by the mentally ill and their families plus their productivity losses totaled a little over $12 billion. This includes costs of care paid for by the mentally ill and their families plus productivity losses of these people.[17]

XIII. What Is the Cost of Care and Maintenance of the Mentally Ill in Public Mental Hospitals?

Estimated total maintenance expenditures of state and county mental hospitals in fiscal 1973 for inpatient services totaled $2,325,986,000.[7]

XIV. What Is the Cost of Mental Illness to the Veterans Administration?

Mental illnesses presently cost the Veterans Administration over $1.2 billion annually.

LEADING THREE DIAGNOSES AMONG ADMISSIONS WITH NO PRIOR INPATIENT PSYCHIATRIC CARE WHO WERE ADMITTED TO STATE AND COUNTY MENTAL HOSPITALS, UNITED STATES, 1969 AND 1972

Leading Three Diagnoses

Selected Age Groups	Males 1969	Males 1972	Females 1969	Females 1972

15–24	1. Schizophrenia
	2. Personality disorders
	3. Drug disorders
		1. Personality disorders
		2. Schizophrenia
		3. Drug disorders
			1. Neuroses
			2. Schizophrenia
			3.† Mental retardation
			   Personality disorders
				1. Neuroses
				2.* Schizophrenia
				   Drug disorders
				3. Mental retardation

25–34	1. Alcohol disorders 2. Schizophrenia 3. Personality disorders	1. Alcohol disorders 2. Neuroses 3. Schizophrenia	1. Neuroses 2. Schizophrenia 3.† Personality disorders Alcohol disorders	1. Schizophrenia 2. Neuroses 3. Personality disorders
35–44	1. Alcohol disorders 2. Schizophrenia 3. Personality disorders	1. Alcohol disorders 2. Schizophrenia 3. Drug disorders	1. Neuroses 2. Schizophrenia 3. Alcohol disorders	1. Neuroses 2. Alcohol disorders 3. Schizophrenia
45–54	1. Alcohol disorders 2. Schizophrenia 3. Personality disorders	1. Alcohol disorders 2. Schizophrenia 3. Personality disorders	1. Alcohol disorders 2. Schizophrenia 3. Neuroses	1. Neuroses 2. Schizophrenia 3. Alcohol disorders
All Ages	1. Alcohol disorders 2. Brain syndromes 3. Schizophrenia	1. Alcohol disorders 2.* Schizophrenia Personality disorders 3. Brain syndromes	1. Neuroses 2. Schizophrenia 3. Organic brain syndromes	1. Neuroses 2. Schizophrenia 3. Organic brain syndromes

*Tied for second place.
†Tied for third place.

1. The *estimated operating costs* in fiscal 1972 of the *VA psychiatric bed section was $429,427,000*. This does not include the costs for care of psychiatric patients in general hospitals.[8]

The average daily census of psychiatric patients in VA hospitals for fiscal 1972 was 31,422. This is 39 percent of the average daily patient load in all VA hospitals.[8]

2. In fiscal 1972, 366,186 veterans were receiving compensation and pension payments whose major disability involved a psychiatric condition. The annual value of these awards was $776,158,000.[15] The number of veterans receiving these payments has declined 41 percent since 1968.

3. At the end of fiscal year 1972, 73 mental hygiene clinics were in operation in the VA system.[8]

   a. Such clinics provided treatment to over 60,000 patients, representing over 531,000 individual interviews, and another 21,000 patients were provided fee basis mental hygiene treatment.[18]

4. Forty-day treatment centers operated by the VA provided continuing treatment to over 2,000 long-term psychiatric veterans on any given day.[8]

5. During the same fiscal year 1972, 5 new day hospital programs devoted to short-term crisis intervention treatment were started, making a total of 21 such programs now in operation. These day hospital programs provided treatment to 2,831 patients, an increase of 1,954 patients over the last fiscal year; similarly the number of patient visits climbed to over 74,000, an increase of over 29,000 since the last fiscal year.[8]

XV. *How Much Is Being Spent by Public Institutions for Care of the Mentally Retarded?*

1. The average daily resident patient population in public institutions for mentally retarded in 1970 totaled 187,897.[4] Total admissions totaled 14,985, of which 12,075 were first admissions. Net releases during the same period were 14,702.[4]

   a. During 1970, maintenance expenditures of public institutions caring for the mentally retarded totaled $871 million.[4]

XVI. How Many Psychiatric Clinics Are There in the United States?

1. As of 1972, there were *2,279 outpatient psychiatric services* in the United States.[22]
2. There were an estimated 2,316,700 patient care episodes handled by these services during 1971.[22]
3. Since 1955, the number of patients under care in clinics has increased steadily and has more than tripled since 1961 due to effectiveness of tranquilizing and antidepressant drugs.[5]
4. Of the total patient care episodes during 1971:[5]

> 632,200 (27%) were under 18 years of age
> 1,684,500 (73%) were adults

XVII. To What Extent Have Psychiatric Units in General Hospitals Been Increased?

1. Between 1964 and 1970, the number of general hospitals providing *separate inpatient psychiatric services had increased 42 percent.*[11]
There were 538 such hospitals in 1964, and 766 in 1970.[11]
2. In 1969, the average psychiatric inpatient unit had 51 beds with an average daily census of 42 patients (average occupancy rate *of 82 percent*).[11]
3. An estimated 11.8 million days of care are provided annually.[11]
4. The *average length of stay was 11 days* per discharge.[13]

XVIII. How Much Is the National Institute of Mental Health Spending in Support of State and Community Mental Health Programs?

An estimated *$468,051,000* was spent in fiscal 1975 for state and community mental health programs by the National Institute of Mental Health.[9]
Of this amount:

$199,197,000 was toward the construction and staffing of community mental health centers, public and other nonprofit, and another $26,844,000 to finance children's services

$242,010,000 was spent toward the support of community narcotic addiction and alcoholism rehabilitation programs

XIX. How Much Is Being Spent for Research on Mental Health by Major Federal Sources?

1. Approximately *$130 million* is being spent, as follows:

a. *National Institute of Mental Health,* fiscal 1975:

General mental health research	$ 82,635,000
Drug abuse research	31,558,000
Alcoholism research	9,026,000
	$123,249,000 [9]

b. The *Veterans Administration* is currently spending for psychiatric research an estimated (1975) $ 6,713,000[18]

Total Federal Funds $129,962,000

2. Although state and local governments also support research in mental health, their expenditures are not available. In 1968, state and local expenditures for mental health totaled an estimated $8.2 million.[17]

3. Estimates on other private industry and philanthropy support of mental health research are similarly not available. In 1968, they were estimated to total $12 million.[17]

4. *In contrast to the approximate total of $130 million* currently being spent *for research* against mental illness:

a. The nation spent $17 billion—OVER 130 TIMES AS MUCH—for alcoholic beverages alone in 1972,[19] about *$80 annually for each man, woman, and child. We are spending about 60* *cents annually per each man, woman, and child in the United States for research against mental illness.*

b. *Mental illness is costing the nation over $20 billion annually.* Yet our annual *research investment* to combat this toll is *less than 1 percent of this cost.* And it is only 7 *percent* of the yearly maintenance costs of our state and county mental hospitals.

XX. Has Medical Research Paid Off in the Field of Mental Illness? Yes!

Following the advent of the tranquilizing drugs in 1955, and later the antidepressants, the number of patients confined to state and county mental institutions has been reduced 61 percent—from 558,000 in 1955 to 215,573 in 1974.[7]

1. Dollar Savings[16]

Between 1945 and 1955, the overall rise in the number of patients in state mental hospitals averaged 13,000 a year.

If this average annual patient increase had continued through 1973, 234,000 more beds would have been required at a unit cost of $20,000 and an *overall cost of $4.7 billion.*

This $4.7 billion saving in bed construction costs does not include the additional reductions in patient care costs which have been realized through the reduction of hospitalized mentally ill.

Had the number of hospitalized mental patients increased during the past 19 years (1955-1974) at an average of 13,000 per year, *there would now be 805,000 patients hospitalized in state and county mental hospitals instead of the 215,573 actually there.*

These additional 544,000 patients would have cost the states in one year alone (1974) *over $5 billion.*[7]

XXI. What Is the Outlook for Patient Population Reductions by 1980?

A forecast made in 1963 to the effect that within 10 years there would be a 50 percent reduction in state mental hospital populations has now been achieved. It is now anticipated that

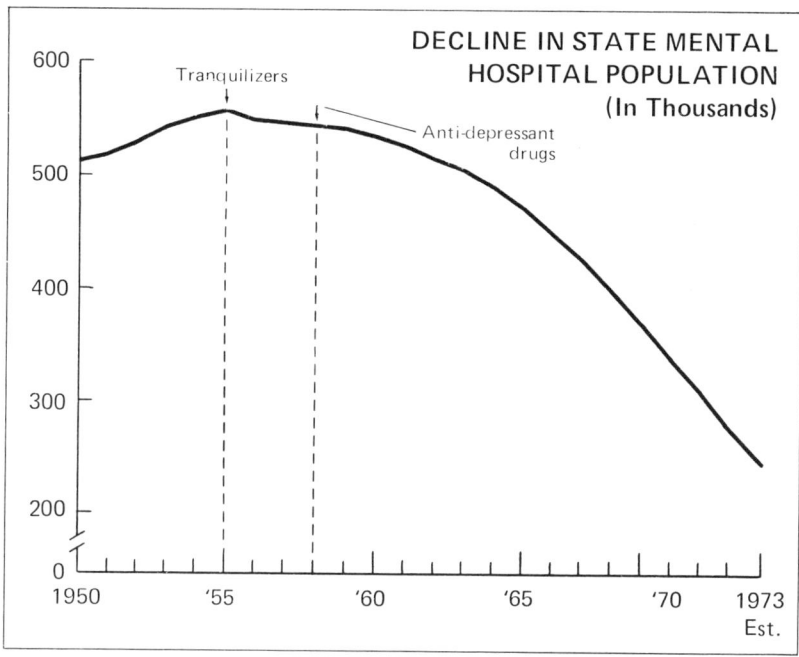

by 1980, if the present rate of decline can be maintained, there will probably be a two-thirds reduction in the hospitalized mentally ill, due to the research which resulted in new drugs. This means that the state mental hospital population will be reduced to 186,000 rather than 880,000, which would have been the projected population based on trends prior to 1955.[16]

Concomitant with the decline in state mental hospital populations is the increase in readmissions to outpatient clinics rather than to mental hospitals, so that patients remain with their families rather than going to distant mental hospitals.[16]

XXII. What Has Caused This Reduction in the Number of Resident Patients in Our State Mental Hospitals?

1. Extensive statistical documentation shows that *increased state legislative appropriations to provide intensive treatment with*

tranquilizing drugs, and antidepressant drugs, and more medical personnel to provide treatment, *have now begun to pay off* in dramatic fashion, and have finally achieved the cumulative force needed to reverse the seemingly inevitable annual rise in mental hospital populations.

a. In 1945, the average daily expenditure on each resident mental patient was $1.06; ten years later (1955) it had risen slowly to $3.06 per day. In 1965, this had *risen to $6.74.* In 1973, it increased to $25.20,[7] a 270 percent increase since 1965, *although by any hospital standard a per diem expenditure of $25.20 is grossly inadequate.*

b. In 1945, there was 1 full-time employee for every 6.8 patients in mental hospitals—an impossibly low treatment-personnel-to-patient ratio. A decade later, considerable improvement was achieved when the ratio rose to approximately 1 employee for every 4 patients (146,392 full-time employees for 558,922). By 1973, a ratio of one full-time employee for every 1.1 patients was achieved (225,227 full-time equivalent staff for 252,607 patients in the average daily census).[7]

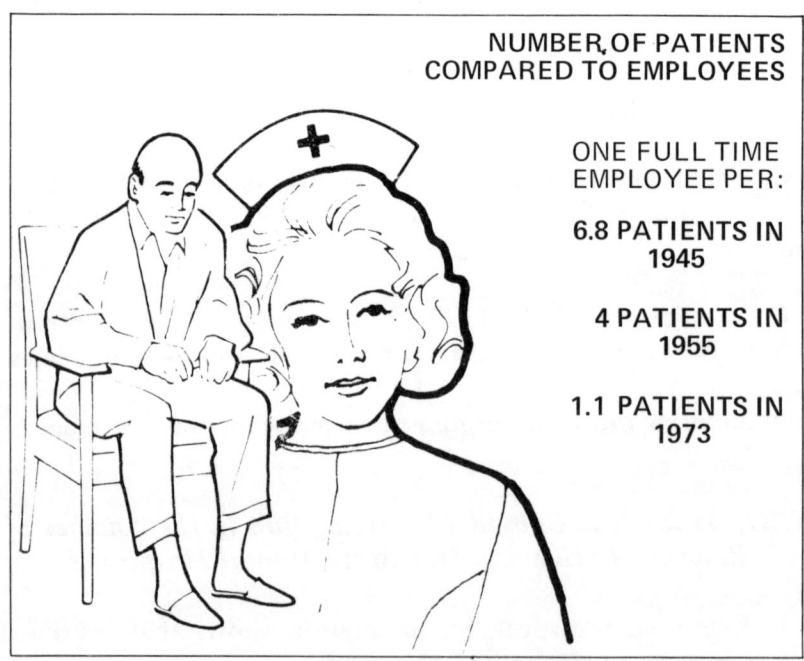

NUMBER OF PATIENTS COMPARED TO EMPLOYEES

ONE FULL TIME EMPLOYEE PER:

6.8 PATIENTS IN 1945

4 PATIENTS IN 1955

1.1 PATIENTS IN 1973

Mental Hospitals: United States 1970–1973

State	Number of Inpatients End of Year				Percent Change			
	1970	1971	1972	1973	1970–1971	1971–1972	1972–1973	1970–1973
United States, Total	337,619	308,983	274,837	248,562*	− 8.5	−11.1*	− 9.6*	−26.4*
Alabama	6,911	5,915	4,874	3,810	−14.4	−17.6	−21.8	−44.9
Alaska	184	153	110	148	−16.8	−28.1	34.5	−19.6
Arizona	864	819	579	783	− 5.2	−29.3	35.2	− 9.4
Arkansas	1,010	979	753	538	− 3.1	−23.1	−28.6	−46.7
California	12,361	10,728	8,753	9,420	−13.2	−18.4	7.6	−23.8
Colorado	1,486	1,435	1,436	1,470	− 3.4	0.1	2.4	− 1.1
Connecticut	5,346	4,712	3,803	3,635	−11.9	−19.3	− 4.4	−32.0
Delaware	1,340	1,309	1,240	1,177	− 2.3	− 5.3	− 5.1	−12.2
District of Columbia	3,804	3,405	3,000	2,921	−10.5	−11.9	− 2.6	−23.2
Florida	9,272	8,650	8,170	6,972	− 6.7	− 5.5	−14.7	−24.8
Georgia	9,996	9,472	9,954	8,604	− 5.2	5.1	−13.6	−13.9
Hawaii	527	373	260*	182*	−29.2	−30.3	−30.0*	−65.5*
Idaho	515	317	290	283	−38.4	− 8.5	− 2.4	−45.0
Illinois	17,655	15,138	12,633	10,373	−14.3	−16.5	−17.9	−41.2
Indiana	7,839	7,188	6,491	6,040	− 8.3	− 9.7	− 6.9	−22.9
Iowa	1,430	1,341	1,243	1,243	− 6.2	− 7.3	0.0	−13.1
Kansas	1,820	1,929	1,878	1,827	6.0	− 2.6	− 2.7	0.4
Kentucky	3,262	2,549	1,452	1,179	−21.9	−43.0	−18.8	−63.9
Louisiana	4,444	4,235	3,939	3,327	− 4.7	− 7.0	−15.5	−25.1
Maine	2,752	2,523	1,705	1,333	− 8.3	−32.4	−21.8	−51.6
Maryland	7,448	6,883	6,404	6,315	− 7.6	− 7.0	− 1.4	−15.2
Massachussetts	12,342	10,910	9,367	7,842	−11.6	−14.1	−16.3	−36.5
Michigan	12,966	11,469	9,392	7,563	−11.5	−18.1	−19.5	−41.7
Minnesota	3,550	3,173	2,960*	4,560	−10.6	− 6.7*	54.1	28.5
Mississippi	4,878	4,766	4,395	4,176	− 2.3	− 7.8	− 5.0	−14.4
Missouri	6,228	5,994	5,908	5,228	− 3.8	− 1.4	−11.5	−16.1

The Killers and the Cripplers

Number and Percent Change in Inpatients at the End of Year, Inpatient Services of State and County Mental Hospitals: United States 1970–1973

State	Number of Inpatients End of Year				Percent Change			
	1970	1971	1972	1973	1970–1971	1971–1972	1972–1973	1970–1973
Montana	1,199	1,167	1,104	1,066	− 2.7	− 5.4	− 3.4	−11.1
Nebraska	1,516	1,324	966	839	−12.7	−27.0	−13.1	−44.7
Nevada	263	225	224	355	−14.4	− 0.4	58.5	35.0
New Hampshire	1,983	1,873	1,659	1,446	− 5.5	−11.4	−12.8	−27.1
New Jersey	15,265	14,403	12,888	11,929	− 5.6	−10.5	− 7.4	−21.9
New Mexico	381	387	389	450	1.6	0.5	15.7	18.1
New York	65,296	58,601	50,527	44,937	−10.3	−13.8	−11.1	−31.2
North Carolina	7,352	7,055	6,531	5,805	− 4.0	− 7.4	−11.1	−21.0
North Dakota	881	701	687	632	−20.4	− 2.0	− 8.0	−28.3
Ohio	17,447	15,558	14,232	12,897	−10.8	− 8.5	− 9.4	−26.1
Oklahoma	2,939	3,088	2,843	2,691	5.1	− 7.9	− 5.3	− 8.4
Oregon	1,874	1,590	1,612	1,405	−15.2	1.4	−12.8	−25.0
Pennsylvania	25,372	22,718	20,198	19,026	−10.5	−11.1	− 5.8	−25.0
Rhode Island	1,819	1,845	1,807	1,771	1.4	− 2.1	− 2.0	− 2.6
South Carolina	5,787	5,631	5,823	5,346	− 2.7	3.4	− 8.2	− 7.6
South Dakota	1,211	1,163	1,080	942	− 4.0	− 7.1	−12.8	−22.2
Tennessee	6,346	5,888	5,417	4,918	− 7.2	− 8.0	− 9.2	−22.5
Texas	12,413	11,518	11,129	9,952	− 7.2	− 3.4	−10.6	−19.8
Utah	411	292	252	265	−29.0	−13.7	5.2	−35.5
Vermont	1,124	991	851	693	−11.8	−14.1	−18.6	−38.3
Virginia	11,171	10,575	8,578	7,877	− 5.3	−18.9	− 8.2	−29.5
Washington	2,525	2,549	2,520	1,800	1.0	− 1.1	−28.6	−28.7
West Virginia	4,252	3,950	3,844	3,475	− 7.1	− 2.7	9.6	−18.3
Wisconsin	8,113	9,123	8,334	6,792	12.4	− 8.6	−18.5	−16.3
Wyoming	449	403	353	304	−10.2	−12.4	−13.9	−32.3

Source: *Statistical Note 106*, May 1974, Survey and Reports Section, National Institute of Mental Health, Chevy Chase, Md.

Mental Illness 169

The increase in the ratio of full-time staff to resident patients has been due to the decrease in resident patients rather than any large increases in the number of staff.

c. However, the personnel shortage in state mental hospitals is still critical. In 1972, the latest year for which *detailed* information is available, there was only

> One full-time staff member for every 1.3 patients in the average daily resident patient population
> One psychiatrist for every 67 patients
> One registered nurse for every 22 patients
> One other type nurse or attendant for every 3 patients
> One social worker for every 56 patients[5]

NOTE: These ratios refer to full-time equivalent staff.

XXIII. Do the Patients in State Mental Hospitals Receive Adequate Care?

1. No. In 1973, the daily inpatient maintenance expenditure per resident patient in state and county mental hospitals in the United States was only *$25.20 per day,* or *$9,198 per year.*[7]

In the same year, Hawaii was high with $67.32 per day. Mississippi was low with only $9.99 per day.[7]

a. In contrast, the per diem costs for inpatient care in Veterans Administration psychiatric bed sections was $37.28 in 1972.[8]

b. In 1971, the expenses per patient day in non-Federal short-term general and other special hospitals in the United States, where research and surgery have brought new treatments and cure for patients, were $92.31.[10] This contrasts with $25.20, the daily inpatient maintenance expenditure per resident patient in state and county mental hospitals in 1973.[7]

> i. The average length of stay in non-federal short term general and other special hospitals in 1971 was 8.1 days.[10] By contrast the median length of stay of admissions to state psychiatric hospitals in 1971 was 41 days.[12]

COMPARISON OF LENGTH OF HOSPITAL STAYS

2,920 DAYS 8 YEARS PRIOR TO 1954 (20)

41 DAYS MEDIAN LENGTH OF STAY OF ADMISSIONS TO STATE & COUNTY MENTAL HOSPITALS 1971 (12)

8.1 DAYS AVERAGE LENGTH OF STAY IN NON-FEDERAL SHORT-TERM GENERAL AND OTHER SPECIAL HOSPITALS FOR ALL TYPES OF DISEASES 1971 (10)

STATE HOSPITALS LENGTH OF STAY IN 1954 BEFORE TRANQUILIZING AND ANTI-DEPRESSANT DRUGS vs. 1971 WHEN THESE DRUGS WERE WIDELY USED

HEALTH FACILITIES, UNITED STATES, JANUARY 1972

Discipline	All Facilities	State and County	Private Mental Hospitals	VA Psychiatric Services	General Hospitals Inpatient and Outpatient	Outpatient Psychiatric Services	CMHC	RTC*
All Staff	428,937	230,515	24,819	45,937	40,439	24,976	42,769	19,482
Total patient care staff	282,510	142,673	13,528	26,711	33,921	19,250	33,182	13,245
Professional patient care staff	131,611	41,618	7,455	14,043	22,314	17,433	20,215	8,533
Psychiatrists	21,141	5,252	1,585	1,071	6,115	3,701	2,866	551
Psychologists	14,245	2,801	402	1,173	1,775	4,589	2,943	562
Social workers	23,075	5,613	518	1,300	2,688	6,095	4,877	1,984
Registered nurses	36,511	14,114	3,217	5,144	8,422	850	4,443	321
Other professional staff	36,639	13,838	1,733	5,355	3,314	2,198	5,086	5,115
Other patient care staff	150,899	101,055	6,073	12,668	11,607	1,817	12,967	4,712
All Staff	100.0%	53.7	5.8	10.7	9.4	5.8	10.0	4.6
Total patient care staff	100.0%	50.5	4.8	9.5	12.0	6.8	11.7	4.7
Professional patient care staff	100.0%	31.6	5.7	10.7	17.0	13.2	15.3	6.5
Psychiatrists	100.0%	24.8	7.5	5.1	28.9	17.5	13.6	2.6
Psychologists	100.0%	19.7	2.8	8.2	12.5	32.2	20.7	3.9
Social workers	100.0%	24.3	2.3	5.6	11.7	26.4	21.1	8.6
Registered nurses	100.0%	38.6	8.8	14.1	23.1	2.3	12.2	0.9
Other professional staff	100.0%	37.8	4.7	14.6	9.0	6.0	13.9	14.0
Other patient care staff	100.0%	67.0	4.0	8.4	7.7	1.2	8.6	3.1
All Staff	100.0%	100.0%	100.0%	100.0%	100.0%	100.0%	100.0%	100.0%
Total patient care staff	65.9	61.9	54.5	58.1	83.9	77.1	77.6	68.0
Professional patient care staff	30.7	18.1	30.0	30.6	55.2	69.8	47.3	43.8
Psychiatrists	4.9	2.3	6.4	2.3	15.1	14.8	6.7	2.8
Psychologists	3.3	1.2	1.6	2.6	4.4	18.4	6.9	2.9
Social workers	5.4	2.4	2.1	2.8	6.6	24.4	11.4	10.2
Registered nurses	8.5	6.1	13.0	11.2	20.8	3.4	10.4	1.6
Other professional staff	8.5	6.0	7.0	11.7	8.2	8.8	11.9	26.3
Other patient care staff	35.2	43.8	24.5	27.6	28.7	7.3	30.3	24.2

SOURCE: *Staffing of Mental Health Facilities, U.S., 1972*, Analytical and Special Study Reports, Survey Reports Section, Biometry Branch, National Institute of Mental Health, Chevy Chase, Md.
*Residential treatment centers for emotionally disturbed children.

XXIV. How Many Doctors and Other Medical Personnel Are Currently Employed in Mental Health Facilities Caring for the Mentally Ill?[14]

	Total	Full-Time	Part-Time	Trainee
Psychiatrists	21,141	7,050	9,028	4,988
Psychologists	14,245	7,494	3,874	2,877
Social workers	23,075	16,303	3,824	2,948
Registered nurses	36,511	28,593	5,546	2,372
Other professional staff	36,639	26,864	7,148	2,627
Total professional patient care staff	131,611	86,309	29,490	15,812
Other patient care staff	150,899	138,098	10,164	2,637
Total patient care staff	282,510	224,407	39,654	18,449
Plus administrative and other staff (business administrators, clerical, maintenance, etc.)	146,427	133,560	12,275	592
Total all staff	428,937	357,967	51,929	19,041

Notes

1. Data from National Association for Mental Health, Arlington, Va. 22209.
2. First Special Report to the U.S. Congress on Alcohol and Health from the Secretary of Health, Education, and Welfare, December 1971.
3. National Center for Health Statistics, U.S. Public Health Service, Rockville, Md.
4. *Statistical Abstract of the U.S., 1972*, 93rd ed., U.S. Bureau of the Census, Washington, D.C.

5. Unpublished data from National Institute of Mental Health, Chevy Chase, Md.
6. 1971 Annual Report, National Association for Mental Health, Arlington, Va. 22209.
7. *Statistical Note 114,* April, 1975. Survey and Reports Section, National Institute of Mental Health, Chevy Chase, Md.
8. 1972 Annual Report—Administrator of Veterans Affairs, Washington, D.C.
9. Budget of the U.S. Government, Fiscal 1976, Appendix.
10. *Hospitals,* August 1, 1971, Guide Issue, published by the American Hospital Association, Chicago, Ill.
11. *Statistical Note 44,* March 1970, Survey and Reports Section, National Institute of Mental Health, Chevy Chase, Md.
12. *Statistical Note 74,* February 1973, Survey and Reports Section, National Institute of Mental Health, Chevy Chase, Md.
13. *Statistical Note 70,* February 1973, Survey and Reports Section, National Institute of Mental Health, Chevy Chase, Md.
14. *Staffing of Mental Health Facilities, U.S., 1972,* National Institute of Mental Health, Chevy Chase, Md.
15. Letter dated March 1, 1973, from Edward R. Silberman, Director, Management and Budget Service, Department of Veterans Benefits, Veterans Administration, Washington, D.C.
16. National Committee Against Mental Illness, Inc., Washington, D.C.
17. Ronald W. Conley, Ph.D., Margaret Conwell, Ed. M., and Shirley G. Willner, *The Cost of Mental Illness, 1968,* National Institute of Mental Health, Chevy Chase, Md.
18. Lawrence B. Hobson, M.D., Deputy Assistant Chief Medical Director for Research and Development, Department of Medicine and Surgery, Veterans Administration, Washington, D.C.
19. "1973 Marketing Guide" published by Drug Topics, Medical Economics Company, Oradell, New Jersey.
20. Testimony of Dr. Robert Felix, Director, National Institute of Mental Health, before House Subcommittee on Appropriations for Department of Health, Education, and Welfare, January 31, 1952.
21. *Statistical Note 97,* September 1973, Survey and Reports Section, National Institute of Mental Health, Chevy Chase, Md.
22. *Utilization of Mental Health Facilities, 1971,* Analytical and Special Study Reports, Series B, no. 5, National Institute of Mental Health, Chevy Chase, Md.

23. Testimony of Dr. Stanley F. Yolles, Director, National Institute of Mental Health, at hearings before U.S. Senate Appropriations Subcommittee for Department of Health, Education, and Welfare, fiscal 1970. Part 6 of the hearings, p. 899.
24. *Statistical Note 72,* December 1972, Survey and Reports Section, National Institute of Mental Health, Chevy Chase, Md.

What Are the Facts About Mental Retardation?

I. What Is Mental Retardation?

Mental retardation is a condition, often congenital, in which *normal development fails to take place as the infant grows older.* It should not be confused with mental illness, which is a breakdown of normal brain functioning, and which may occur at almost any age, in previously mentally normal people.

II. How Many People in the United States Are Mentally Retarded?

1. *An estimated 6 million Americans are mentally retarded.*[1]
   a. *The impact of mental retardation is directly felt by some 20 million family members* who share the burden and problems of care of the retarded whose inadequate intellectual development impairs their ability to learn and to adapt to the demands of society.[1] One family in 5 is affected.

2. *There are 126,000 children born every year (1 every 5 minutes) who will be diagnosed as retarded.*[1]

3. Three-fourths of the nation's mentally retarded are to be found in the isolated and impoverished urban and rural slums.[1]

4. Many mildly retarded adults manage to support themselves modestly and to stay out of trouble with the law. Although their handicaps persist, they may not be identified as mentally retarded, even if they require some assistance from welfare agencies. The more severely disabled, who cannot

175

work, are more likely to be known to state and local agencies giving aid to the disabled, yet a substantial number even in this group may be sheltered by their families and passed over in surveys.[2]

5. For these reasons, less than one-third of the estimated 6 million mentally retarded people in this country are likely to be identified as needing any form of specialized health, education, or welfare service at any one time.[2]

III. In What Age Groups Are Most Mentally Retarded to Be Found?

1. A breakdown by age of the 6 million mentally retarded is as follows:[2]

From birth to five years of age	605,000
From six to sixteen years of age	1,354,000
From 16 to 21 years of age	691,000
Total under 21 years old	2,880,000
Total over 21 years old	3,110,000
(rounded figures)	6,000,000

2. Most mental retardation originates in the prenatal period or in early childhood. However, affected preschool children are often not identified and reported. As children enter and proceed through school, their difficulty in learning becomes more apparent, with the result that the numbers reported in each grade tend to increase with age until early adolescence.[2]

Since many mentally retarded children leave school as soon as compulsory attendance laws permit them to do so, there is a corresponding decline in reported mental retardation in late adolescence. Some severely and profoundly retarded children who do not attend any schools may go unreported in those surveys which depend primarily on identification by health, education, or welfare agencies.[2]

IV. What Are the Causes of Mental Retardation?

In general *more than 100 causes are known;* others are suspected, but *many causes remain unknown.* Mental retardation results when there is [2]

1. Incomplete development or destruction of tissues of the central nervous system.
2. Lack of brain development before birth.
3. Genetic-metabolic diseases.
4. Chromosomal disorders.
5. Certain illnesses, infections, and glandular disorders during pregnancy.
6. Extraordinarily prolonged labor, pelvic pressure, hemorrhage or lack of oxygen, any of which may injure the baby's brain.
7. A child's full mental development may be arrested after birth by an accident, poisoning, glandular disturbance, chemical imbalance, or childhood disease.
8. Premature birth can lead to mental retardation and/or cerebral palsy.
9. Recent research also points to severe early emotional deprivation and other cultural and environmental factors as causes of mental retardation.

V. How Much Mental Retardation Is Due to Known Causes?

About 15 percent to 25 percent of cases have a definite known cause. They include:[2]

1. German measles, during the first trimester of pregnancy.
2. Cytogenetic disorders, such as Down's syndrome.
3. Encephalitis.
4. Gargoylism.
5. Hyperthyroidism.
6. Syphilis.
7. Jaundice due to the Rh blood factor of incompatibility, now preventable by Rh-O Immune Globulin given Rh-nega-

tive mothers after each delivery or miscarriage of an Rh-positive baby.³

8. Toxemia as a result of carbon monoxide and lead poisoning.
9. Physical trauma, including automobile accidents.
10. Prenatal injury.
11. Postnatal injury.
12. Problems in the delivery process.
13. Anoxia, which may create brain damage.
14. Metabolic disorders, such as PKU, galactosemia, and maple syrup disease, which result from improper amino acid chemistry or improper carbohydrate breakdown and absorption.

VI. How Many Public Institutions Are There for the Care of the Mentally Retarded Requiring Institutionalization?

1. In 1970 there were 190 public institutions for the care of the mentally retarded.⁴
2. *The average daily resident patient population* in these institutions in 1970 was 187,897. There was *14,985* admissions during the year, of which 12,075 were first admissions. At the end of the year, there were 186,743 resident patients on the books in these institutions. *Net releases (alive) totaled 14,702.*⁴
3. In addition, 9 percent (30,339) of the resident patients in state and county mental hospitals in 1970 had a diagnosis of mental retardation.⁷
4. In 1971, there were 2,541,552 admissions to all in- and outpatient psychiatric services in the United States.⁸

Mental retardation was the diagnosis in 59,290 (2.4 percent of these admissions).⁸

However, three-quarters of these were outpatient admissions, reflecting the fact that mental health facilities primarily play a diagnostic rather than a treatment or custodial role in the case of mental retardation.⁸

5. *First admissions* to public institutions for the mentally retarded have shown *almost a 20 percent decrease since 1965*—from 15,033 to 12,075 in 1970.⁴

6. The number of resident patients has also shown *a slight decrease since 1965*—from 187,273 to 186,743 in 1970.[4]

VII. What Is the Cost of Institutional Care?

1. Maintenance expenditures in 1970 in public institutions for the mentally retarded totaled $871 million.[4]
This is $4,635 per resident patient per year or $13 per day.
2. Only 4 percent of the mentally retarded are confined to institutions.
3. Because of the extensive services which the community must bring to bear on the other 96 percent, it is impossible to estimate the total financial burden these mentally retarded impose upon their families and communities, but it is estimated in the billions.

VIII. What Is the Federal Government Spending Overall for Services for the Mentally Retarded?

An estimated *$1.3 billion* was obligated by the Department of Health, Education, and Welfare in fiscal 1973 *for all mental retardation programs* supported.[5]

IX. How Many Diagnostic Clinics Are There in the United States for the Mentally Retarded?

1. The total number of mental retardation clinics in the United States is now 235 (1969).[10]
One hundred and fifty of these clinics (supporting some 43,000 children) are supported by the Children's Bureau of the Social Rehabilitation Service of the Department of Health, Education, and Welfare.[10]
2. There are more than 300 sheltered workshops offering training and employment for more than 12,000 retarded, youth and adults, in the United States today.[2]

X. How Many Mentally Retarded Could Be Rehabilitated if There Were Adequate Facilities?

Of the *6 million children and adults* afflicted with mental retardation:

1. *Seventy-five to 85 percent are capable of becoming self-supporting, independent* citizens both economically and socially if they receive adequate services such as special education and rehabilitation.
2. About *10 percent are capable of becoming partially* self-supporting if they receive adequate services such as:
    a. Training in self-care
    b. Medical diagnosis and treatment
    c. Day-care centers
    d. Sheltered workshops
    e. Counseling services
    f. Programs for recreation.
3. *Only a small proportion of all cases remain completely dependent.* This group of severely impaired persons requires close supervision, medical observation, and adequate personal care 24 hours a day in residential or specialized day-care facilities.[2]

XI. How Much Is Being Spent for Research in Mental Retardation by the National Institutes of Health?

1. *Over $24 million* was spent for research in mental retardation by the National Institutes of Health in fiscal 1973. The National Institute of Child Health and Human Development spent $18 million of these funds.[5]
2. Other agencies within the Department of Health, Education and Welfare, such as the Office of Education, are also supporting research in their respective areas.
3. Nongovernmental agencies such as the National Foundation, the National Association for Retarded Children, the Kennedy Foundation, and the Association for the Aid of Crippled Children also support research related to mental retardation, but the exact amounts are not known.
4. The National Institute of Child Health and Human De-

velopment provides support to 12 Mental Retardation Research Centers throughout the United States. These centers provide a multidisciplinary approach to clinical research in the complex problems of mental retardation, and the knowledge gained makes possible immediate contributions to the communities in which the centers are located.

1. University of Chicago
2. Children's Hospital, Cincinnati
3. George Peabody College of Teachers, Nashville, Tennessee
4. University of Colorado Medical Center, Denver
5. University of Washington, Seattle
6. UCLA, Los Angeles
7. Albert Einstein College of Medicine, New York
8. University of Kansas, Lawrence
9. Walter E. Fernald State School, Waltham, Massachusetts
10. Children's Hospital Medical Center, Boston
11. University of North Carolina, Chapel Hill
12. University of Wisconsin, Madison

XII. What Are Some of the Promising Leads in Research in This Area?

1. Chromosomal studies that shed light on the causes of Down's syndrome (mongolism), which affects one out of every 600 children born.
2. The great many projects in the field of genetics that promise to throw light on the transmission of hereditary defects as well as the findings related to RNA and DNA which suggest how genetic anomalies occur.
3. Biochemical studies on inborn errors of metabolism which include methods of detection and preventive treatment.
4. Researchers of the National Institute of Neurological and Communicative Disorders and Stroke have identified the weakened or missing enzyme in three inborn errors of metabolism. Two cause mental retardation—Gaucher's disease and

Niemann-Pick disease; one causes a fatal kidney ailment and neurological and ophthalmological effects—Fabry's disease. Improved tests to diagnose these disorders, or in some cases to identify carriers, have been developed.[3]

5. A simple, rapid blood test for diagnosing German measles (rubella) developed by the National Institute of Neurological Diseases and Stroke (NINDS) should help prevent retardation from that cause. The German measles vaccine is strongly recommended for all boys and girls between the ages of 1 year and puberty, to reduce the possibility of exposure to German measles by pregnant women.[3]

6. Discovery by NINDS that toxoplasmosis and salivary gland infections may outrank German measles as a hazard to the unborn children of pregnant women.[6]

7. A single injection of serum, Rh-O Immune Globulin, within 72 hours after each delivery or miscarriage of an Rh-positive baby will prevent an Rh-negative mother from developing sensitization that can cause severe mental retardation in subsequent babies. Research continues to seek help for the estimated 30,000 Rh-negative mothers already sensitized to Rh-positive babies.[6]

8. A new program by the United Cerebral Palsy Association to investigate the relationship between premature birth, mental retardation, and cerebral palsy.

9. A thorough study of the legal and ethical problems relating to the mentally retarded at several universities.[9]

XIII. What Medical and Ancillary Personnel Are Needed to Work with the Retarded and Prevent Retardation?

1. *General practitioners*—to give contraceptive information to women for proper spacing of children, for health of the mother and child.

2. *Pediatricians*—need for increasing interest of greater numbers through medical education.

3. *Neurologists.*

4. *Psychiatrists.*

5. *Surgeons*—if medicine in general gives greater recogni-

tion to the care and needs of the mentally retarded, more corrective and plastic surgery will be performed. A great deal can also be done in more acute surgical treatment—for instance, hydrocephalus, craniostenosis.

6. *Orthopedists.*
7. *Psychologists.*
8. *Speech therapists*—interest in the retarded is growing in this discipline partly as a result of speech research projects. The need for an increase of practitioners and willingness to serve the retarded is great.
9. *Nurses*—interest is increasing. The national shortage of nurses is seriously reflected in the limited number of nurses available for the retarded.
10. *Social workers*—the retarded and their families suffer particularly from a shortage of personnel.
11. *Physical therapists*—this discipline is only beginning to be used and is greatly needed particularly in a preventive role for the severely multiple handicapped retarded.
12. *Occupational therapists* can be used much more widely and effectively for educational and training as well as functional correction.
13. *Special educators for the blind* who can adapt their skills to the training of the severely handicapped blind retardate.
14. *Teachers* specially trained in teaching the mentally retarded.

Notes

1. Testimony of Dr. Gerald D. LaVeck, Director, National Institute of Child Health and Human Development, National Institutes of Health, Bethesda, Md., before Senate Subcommittee on Appropriations for Department of Health, Education, and Welfare, June 21, 1973.
2. National Association for Retarded Children, Arlington, Tex.
3. Information obtained from the National Institute of Neurological and Communicative Disorders and Stroke, National Institutes of Health, Bethesda, Md. 20014.

4. *Statistical Abstract of the U.S. 1973,* 93rd ed., U.S. Bureau of the Census, Washington, D.C.
5. Information from National Institute of Child Health and Human Development, National Institutes of Health, Bethesda, Md. 1973.
6. *Mental Retardation, Hope Through Research,* and *Mongolism (Down's Syndrome), Hope Through Research* (also available in Spanish), National Institute of Neurological and Communicative Disorders and Stroke, National Institutes of Health, Bethesda, Md. 20014.
7. *Statistical Note 72,* December 1972, Survey and Reports Section, Biometry Branch, National Institute of Mental Health, Chevy Chase, Md.
8. *Utilization of Mental Health Facilities,* 1971. Analytical and Special Study Reports, Series B, no. 5, National Institute of Mental Health, Chevy Chase, Md.
9. Robert E. Cooke, M.D., Chairman of Scientific Advisory Board, Joseph P. Kennedy, Jr., Foundation, Washington, D.C. Personal communication May 6, 1974.
10. Hearings before the Subcommittee on Health of the U.S. Senate Committee on Labor and Public Welfare on "Mental Retardation and Other Developmental Disabilities, 1969," November 10 and 11, 1969.

What Are the Facts About Multiple Sclerosis?

I. What Is Multiple Sclerosis?

1. Multiple sclerosis is most often a *chronic, progressive, and crippling neurological disease* making its initial appearance in persons *between 20 and 40 years of age.* The disease is characterized by relatively brief periods (usually four to six weeks) of increasing disability, followed by much longer periods (months to years) of stability or improvement. Its cause remains obscure.

It is typically *slow and insidious in onset, frequently difficult of diagnosis* until symptoms have progressed to the point of disability. There is *no specific diagnostic test* for multiple sclerosis.[1]

2. In multiple sclerosis there are scattered indiscriminately in the brain and spinal cord discrete areas in which *myelin* (a fatty insulating sheath normally present around most nerve fibers) *has been dissolved or destroyed.* This destructive process is called *demyelination.*[2]

3. The process through which this dissolution or destruction takes place is not known. Its result, however, is believed to be interruption or short-circuiting of the nerve impulses passing through the affected parts, thus producing paralysis, loss of sensation, or other functional alterations in those parts of the body governed by the affected nerve fibers.[3]

4. The *common symptoms* of multiple sclerosis include: *double vision, staggering and inability to keep one's balance, numbness or paralysis of parts of the body, tremor, nystagmus* (involuntary movements of the eyeball), *extreme weakness, speech difficulties, and bladder and bowel difficulties.*

II. How Many People Are Suffering from Multiple Sclerosis and Related Demyelinating Diseases in the United States Today?

1. With the present status of medical knowledge it is impossible to state a confirmed figure on the number of persons now suffering from MS and related demyelinating diseases in the United States. A reasonable estimate would be *well over 500,000, of which at least half, or about 250,000, are believed to be suffering from multiple sclerosis.*[1]

One source of difficulty in obtaining a more definite figure is that MS is extremely difficult to diagnose in its early stages, so that a survey will tend to omit many thousands of new cases. Also, many physicians are reluctant to tell minimally or partially handicapped patients that they have MS, especially if they are entering upon a period of stability or improvement.[3]

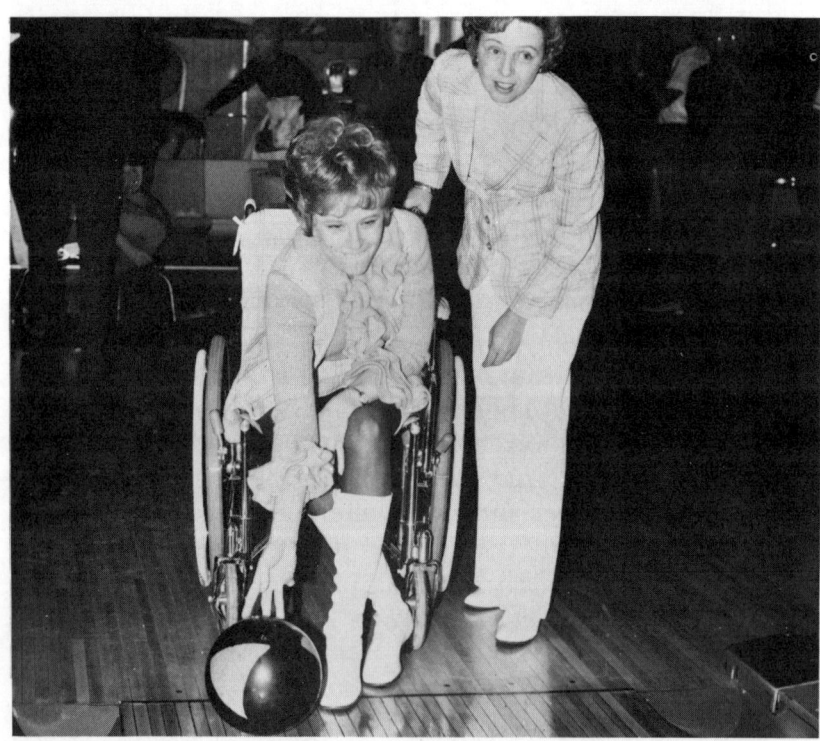

Linda Light, 1972 Poster Girl of the National Multiple Sclerosis Society.
(COURTESY OF NATIONAL MULTIPLE SCLEROSIS SOCIETY, NEW YORK)

Furthermore, typical MS pathology has been found at autopsy in persons with little or no record of neurological disease, indicating that the full spectrum of effects resulting from the MS disease process may be far wider than generally believed.[7]

The other demyelinating diseases included in this overall estimate are diffuse sclerosis, acute disseminating encephalomyelitis, Balo's disease, neuromyelitis optica, the metachromatic encephalopathies, post-infectious encephalomyelitis, acute allergic encephalomyelitis, and amyotrophic lateral sclerosis.[3]

III. What Is Being Done to Help Multiple Sclerosis Sufferers?

Multiple sclerosis was largely a neglected area until the advent of the National Multiple Sclerosis Society.

1. With the recognition that *no specific treatment is available* for multiple sclerosis, *stress has been and is being put on research to develop information on the cause and development of multiple sclerosis* so that a rational approach can be made to therapy.[3]

2. Although the medical profession is not yet able to treat multiple sclerosis directly, *the patient can and should receive careful, sympathetic, intelligent medical management* directed toward protection from intercurrent infections, maintenance of highest possible degree of general health, and amelioration of symptoms, including rehabilitative measures suited to the patient's level of disability.[3]

3. *Over 61 chapters of the National Multiple Sclerosis Society* are now *sponsoring special clinics or clinical programs* for outpatient care of multiple sclerosis patients. Many other clinics providing such care as part of their regular services have been established within the outpatient neurological services of medical schools and teaching hospitals.

All these are, however, *pitifully inadequate for the real need*. If the National Multiple Sclerosis Society or any other agency were to attempt an adequate patient care program for all the multiple sclerosis patients in this country support at the level of perhaps $200 million a year would be required.[3]

IV. How Much Money Is Being Spent for Research to Find the Cause, More Effective Treatments, and a Preventive for Multiple Sclerosis?

Approximately *$8.3 million was spent in 1974 for research* in these areas, with the funds coming almost entirely from two main sources.

1. Government funds

The *National Multiple Sclerosis Society* granted over $26 million from its inception in 1946 through 1974 for research *million* in fiscal 1975 for research dealing specifically with multiple sclerosis and related demyelinating diseases.[8]

2. Nongovernment Funds

The *National Multiple Sclerosis Society* granted over $26 million from its inception in 1946 through 1974 for research and advanced training related to multiple sclerosis. Of this total more than *$2.8 million* was actually spent in 1974.[3]

In addition, much smaller amounts are spent on MS research from time to time by other institutions and foundations.

V. How Does This Compare with Other Expenditures of the American People?

1. In contrast with the total of about *$8.3 million* being spent during 1974 for research in the field of multiple sclerosis:

    a. Estimated fiscal 1973 appropriations to the *Bureau of Sport Fisheries and Wildlife* (U.S. Department of the Interior) totalled *$75,563,000*. The mission of the Bureau is to assure maximum opportunity for the American people to benefit from fish and wildlife resources as part of their natural environment.[5]

    b. In 1972, the American public spent:

- $276,260,000 for women's hair sprays [6]
- $ 91,160,000 for nail polish and enamel [6]
- $ 81,180,000 for hand lotions and creams [6]

c. The estimated cost of patient care alone in the United States of victims of MS is more than $250 million each year.[8]

VI. How Much Is the United States Government Spending for the Establishment of MS Clinics and Services?

1. The *Federal Government is doing nothing* about establishment of MS clinics and services at this time.[4] However, the Veterans Administration does admit patients suffering from multiple sclerosis to its facilities and maintains clinics for multiple sclerosis patients. The National Multiple Sclerosis Society maintains a close and effective liaison with these VA facilities.[3]

2. The U.S. Rehabilitation Services Administration is showing increasing concern for the rehabilitative care of MS patients, and has completed a formal agreement with the National Multiple Sclerosis Society to cooperate with the society's 195 chapters, branches, and units at all levels to increase and accelerate the movement of these patients into the rehabilitation process.

In 1972, over 1,500 MS patients were admitted to local state vocational rehabilitation programs. Of these 498 were prepared for entrance into part- or full-time employment. Though obviously this is only a small proportion of those who could benefit from such services, this number still represents an increase over what was accomplished in 1970 and 1971.[3]

3. State and city health departments are not currently active in providing care and services to MS patients.

VII. How Many Doctors Specialize in Multiple Sclerosis?

1. There is *no separate specialty in multiple sclerosis* recognized by the certifying American boards. As a disease of the brain

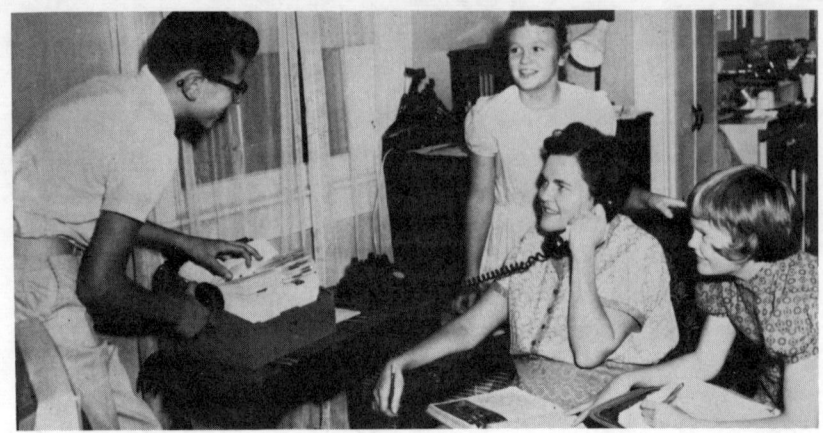

A multiple sclerosis patient, assisted by her family, developed a telephone answering service in her home. (COURTESY OF NATIONAL MULTIPLE SCLEROSIS SOCIETY, NEW YORK)

and spinal cord it is of primary concern to neurologists, and *many prominent neurologists have developed a keen interest in MS and allied neurological problems.*

a. There are at present about 2,969 neurologists practicing in the United States. According to the latest figures of the American Board of Psychiatry and Neurology, about 1,200 of these are board-certified neurologists.

2. In an effort to meet the urgent need for well-trained scientists wishing to conduct research in the several fields bearing on the multiple sclerosis problem, the *National Multiple Sclerosis Society sponsors a program of postdoctoral fellowships* for promising biomedical scientists desiring advanced training in these fields. In 1973, there were 20 postdoctoral research fellowships in force, totaling $432,837.[9] The society also sponsors a *program of summer fellowships for medical students* intended to lead them toward careers in research related to multiple sclerosis.

VIII. How Are the Known Cases of Multiple Sclerosis Apportioned Among Different Age Groups?

As some leading neurologists have stated, *MS is one of the leading cripplers of young adults* in the United States today.

It is estimated that *70 percent of all patients with multiple sclerosis are first diagnosed between the ages of 20 and 40.*

Some 15 percent are diagnosed between *the ages of 15 and 20,* and *another 15 percent between the ages of 40 and 50.*

Although seen in children as young as 4 years, onset before age 15 or after age 50 is unusual. Since, as already noted, the initial diagnosis of MS is often made years after initial symptoms, the concentration of MS onset in the young adult population is probably even greater than these figures indicate.

While the onset of MS is concentrated among young adults, the chronic and often progressive nature of this crippling condition makes it a significant problem in older age groups as well. A sixty-year appraisal of multiple sclerosis in a Minnesota community, made by scientists at the Mayo Clinic, shows that *while median age at first diagnosis is 28.3, the highest prevalence rates are for ages 50 to 69.*[3]

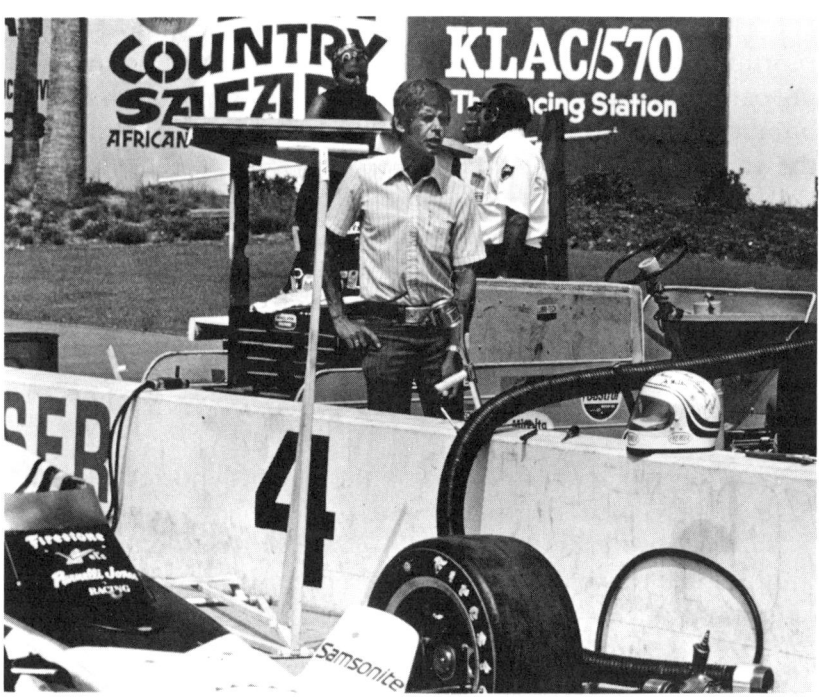

Louis Unser, former racing car driver, now has multiple sclerosis. (COURTESY OF NATIONAL MULTIPLE SCLEROSIS SOCIETY, NEW YORK)

IX. What Are the Most Vital Needs in the Fight Against Multiple Sclerosis?

1. The basic needs in the fight against MS are the discovery of the cause of the disease and the development of more effective methods of treatment and a preventive.

2. To meet these needs, and overcome the disease in the shortest possible time, *more funds are needed to support research and training programs of the National Institute of Neurological and Communicative Disorders and Stroke, and of the National Multiple Sclerosis Society.*

X. Where Can Doctors and Laymen Get Information Regarding the Treatment and Rehabilitation of Multiple Sclerosis Victims?

1. The National Multiple Sclerosis Society has published or reprinted and has available for distribution to physicians and properly qualified paramedical personnel, without charge, a number of comprehensive manuals and reprints dealing with the various aspects of the disease.

In addition, there are home care manuals available to patients with different degrees of disability. The society will supply these free of charge (when they are available) on the prescription of the attending physician.

XI. Current Directions in Multiple Sclerosis Research

1. Although multiple sclerosis was fully identified as a disease of the central nervous system *over 100 years ago,* its cause is still unknown, there is no really effective treatment, no cure, and no preventive. The increasingly intensive research on MS, sponsored in the most part by the National Multiple Sclerosis Society and the National Institute of Neurological and Communicative Disorders and Stroke, is expected to be given great impetus by the recent establishment of a National Advisory Commission on Multiple Sclerosis. The commission is ex-

pected to elicit from the scientific community a list of priorities for purposeful research on MS and make specific recommendations regarding the utilization of the nation's resources to eradicate the disease. The basic goals:[3]

    a. To have an accurate laboratory test for MS that would distinguish it from other neurological diseases.

    b. When an effective treatment for MS is finally developed, prompt diagnosis based on such a test might permit early treatment before the disease has had a chance to inflict permanent damage to the brain or spinal cord.

2. Is multiple sclerosis a *progressive disease almost always ending in complete disability?*

We know now that this is not entirely true. It would seem from postmortem studies that some persons develop lesions characteristic of MS without ever showing clinical signs of the disease. There are also patients who have relatively few attacks and, except for these brief periods, live an essentially normal life. Even in those patients who become progressively more disabled with the passing of time, the exacerbations, or periods of worsening, seldom last longer than a month or six weeks, while the remissions, or periods of improvement or stability, may last for months or even years.[3]

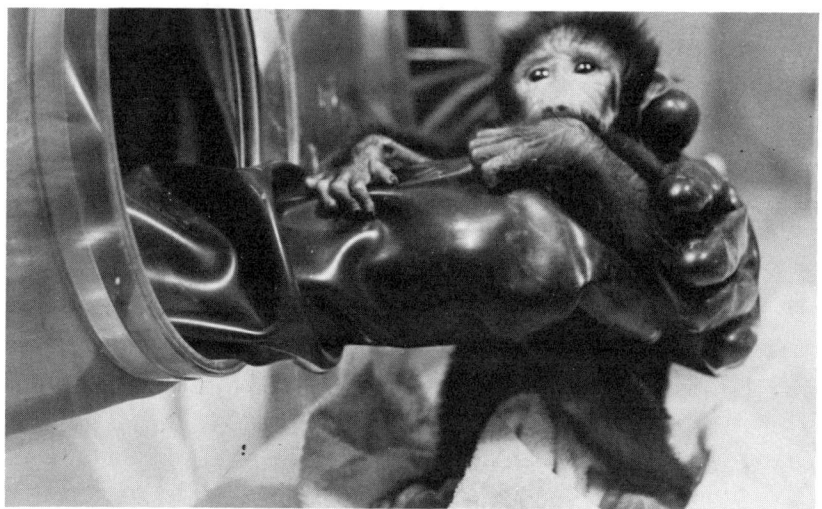

Germfree monkey being used for multiple sclerosis research. (COURTESY OF NATIONAL MULTIPLE SCLEROSIS SOCIETY, NEW YORK)

These facts suggest that the body may be almost able to control, with its own defenses, further progression of the MS disease process. This in turn suggests that only a relatively slight amount of additional help may be required to stop progression of the disease. Should this be so, the demands on research would be far less awesome than once believed.[3]

3. The rapidly growing body of knowledge about *immunological responses* in multiple sclerosis is an important source of new leads. Since the early 1960s, scientists have known that there is a factor present in the blood of MS patients that can destroy the myelin insulation around nerve fibers when nerve cells are grown in the test tube. It has been shown also that other factors in MS patients can block the transmission of impulses in nerve fibers growing in the test tube, even before there is any detectable loss of myelin. Most important is the finding that in cultures washed out and refed, the damaged myelin sheath regrows.[3]

Current immunological research on multiple sclerosis includes work on the following problems:[3]

a. If MS involves an autoimmune reaction against nerve tissue, what is the antigen that provokes this reaction? In experimental allergic encephalomyelitis (EAE), a disease that resembles MS in some respects, the antigen that induces an autoimmune attack on the experimental animal's central nervous system (CNS) is itself a very small protein found in the myelin.

Several scientists are now conducting intensive investigations into the nature and behavior of this substance, called encephalitogenic basic protein, in both animals and man. One goal of this research is the determination of the possibility that MS patients might be desensitized to the MS antigen much as the allergic patient may be desensitized to different allergens.

b. It is possible that some change in the immunologic system may precede a bout of the disease. If this is found, it may be possible to arrest further progression of the multiple sclerosis process through neutralizing the immunologic change before further damage ensues.

4. Since MS is marked by loss of myelin, and by its replacement by scar tissue, some scientists are trying to clarify the biochemical and biophysical steps involved in the deposition,

maintenance, and destruction of myelin. Although this and the even more basic research now being conducted will probably not of itself produce a solution to the MS problem, it may provide the underlying knowledge upon which such a solution could be based.

5. Is there a multiple sclerosis virus? Another important area of investigation related to multiple sclerosis is the search for an MS virus. Several investigators believe that MS may be caused by an unusual kind of virus, called a "slow virus." Unlike the better-known viruses, which produce obvious illness soon after they enter the human body, slow viruses produce observable disease only years after the infection has occurred. Two diseases of the human central nervous system, kuru and Jakob-Kreutzfeldt disease, are known to be caused by such viruses.[3]

There is also the possibility that MS is produced by an unusual manifestation of a common virus. It has been shown, for example, that in a few people measles virus can linger for years after the patient's apparent recovery, to erupt finally in a fatal disease called subacute sclerosing panencephalitis (SSPE).[3] A higher than usual level of measles antibodies in MS makes this virus suspect in this disease. In 1972, three independently working research groups using special culture methods found an influenza-like virus in the brains of MS patients. Further investigative work is in progress to determine if it is in fact related in any way to the cause of MS.[3]

Notes

1. Douglas McAlpine, Charles E. Lumsden, and E. D. Acheson, *Multiple Sclerosis—A Reappraisal,* 2nd ed. (Edinburgh and London: Churchill Livingstone, 1972).
2. George A. Schumacher, *Multiple Sclerosis,* reprinted from *Conn's Current Therapy,* 1970 ed. (Philadelphia: W. B. Saunders Co., 1970).
3. Personal communications, Director of Medical Programs, National Multiple Sclerosis Society, 257 Park Avenue South, New York, N. Y. 10010.

4. *Multiple Sclerosis Research,* Current State, Future Hopes, A Progress Report, National Multiple Sclerosis Society.
5. Budget of the U.S. Government, fiscal year 1974.
6. *1973 Marketing Guide,* published by *Drug Topics,* Medical Economics Company, Oradell, N.J.
7. Roland P. Mackay and Asao Hirano, "Forms of Benign Multiple Sclerosis," *Archives of Neurology* 17:588-600 (December 1967).
8. Information from National Institute of Neurological and Communicative Disorders and Stroke, National Institutes of Health, Bethesda, Md. 20014.
9. 1973 Annual Report, National Multiple Sclerosis Society, New York, N. Y.

What Are the Facts About Muscular Dystrophy?

I. What Is Muscular Dystrophy?

1. Muscular dystrophy is the name given to a group of chronic, noncontagious progressive diseases that are characterized by wasting and consequent weakness of the voluntary muscles. Though the rate of progression varies in the various types, most of the voluntary musculature finally becomes involved. As weakness increases, patients are confined to wheelchairs and, eventually, to bed.[1] [2]

II. What Is the Cause of Muscular Dystrophy?

1. Although the precise cause of muscular dystrophy has not yet been determined, some investigators believe that it is due to *an inborn error of metabolism,* the lack of some specific enzyme or enzyme system essential for the conversion of foods into tissues and energy.[3]

2. *A high percentage of patients come from families with a history of muscular dystrophy.* The hereditary defect may be transmitted by either parent; in the most common (Duchenne) type of dystrophy, however, it is carried as a recessive trait by clinically unaffected females and transmitted almost exclusively to their male progeny.[2]

3. Muscular dystrophy may appear without previous family history, as the result of a change, called a "mutation," in the

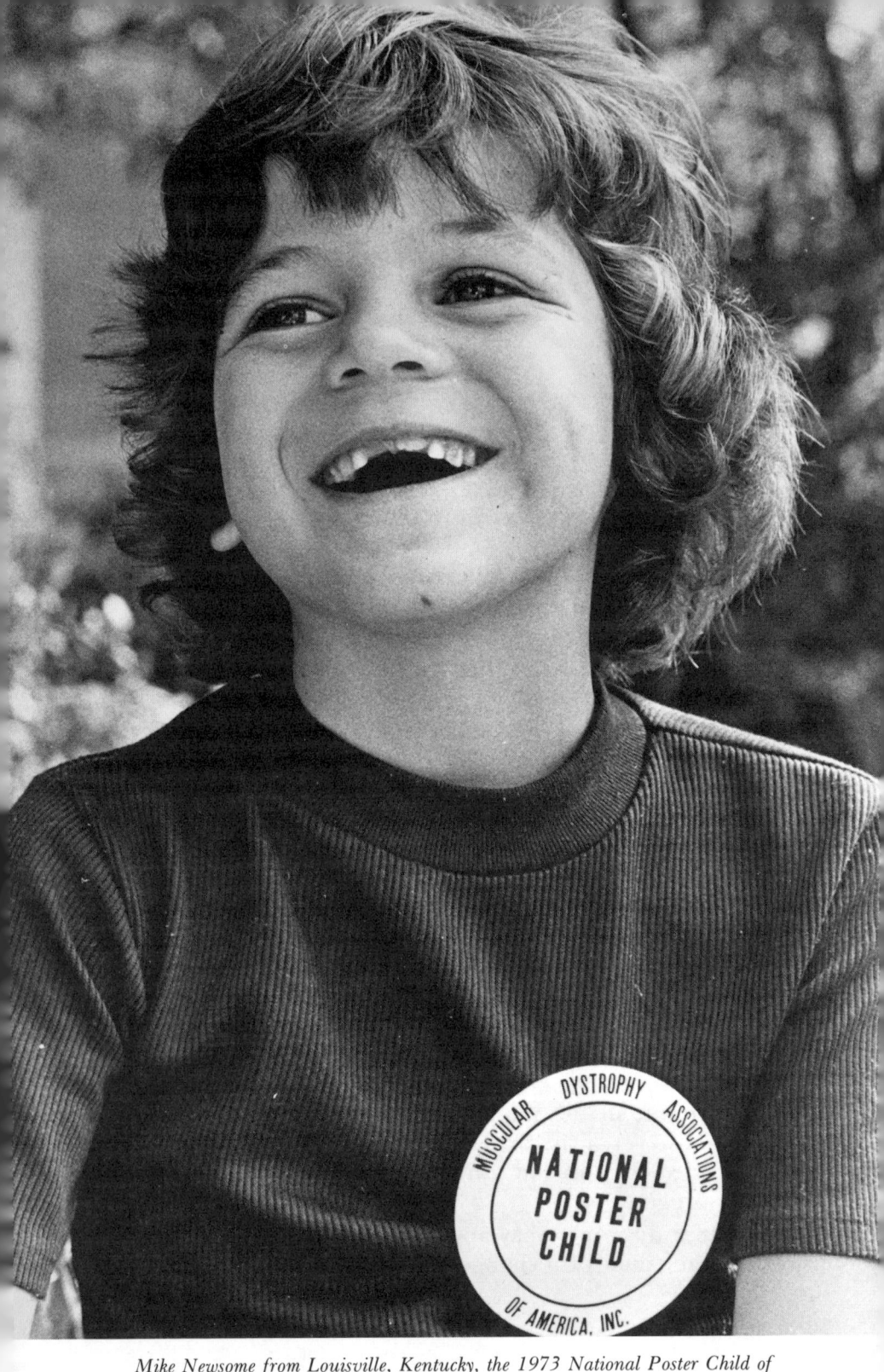

Mike Newsome from Louisville, Kentucky, the 1973 National Poster Child of the Muscular Dystrophy Associations of America, Inc. (PHOTO BY M. LEON LOPEZ, CHICAGO DAILY NEWS. COURTESY OF MUSCULAR DYSTROPHY ASSOCIATIONS OF AMERICA, INC., NEW YORK)

genetic material. Once such a mutation occurs, it becomes hereditary. The *mechanism of transmission,* however, varies in the different types of the disease.[3]

4. Hereditary muscle disease, closely resembling human muscular dystrophy, has appeared in a number of animal species, notably mice and chickens. Both these species are under intensive investigation, thus allowing scientists to perform controlled experiments which are impossible to carry out with human beings. Scientists have already derived a great deal of valuable information from animal models.[2]

5. Muscular lesions, similar to those found in muscular dystrophy, can also be induced in animals by maintaining them on a diet deficient in vitamin E.

Such lesions are reversible if sufficient quantities of the vitamin are restored to the diet, especially in combination with minute quantities of the trace element, selenium.[3] Vitamin E has not proved effective in the treatment of patients nor in animals suffering from *hereditary* muscle disease, indicating that the genetic defect prevents the body from metabolizing the vitamin efficiently.[3]

6. A recently announced development—whose potential significance for human victims remains to be assessed—was the report that *the morbid process in genetically dystrophic chickens has been reversed for the first time by the administration to them of a vegetable oil.*[4] The treatment is currently being tested on genetically dystrophic mice and the results, though not as definitive, are promising.[4]

While the oil seems to have no direct effect on the disease itself, it stimulates the regenerative capacity possessed by skeletal muscle tissue to the point that the destruction of existing cells is almost balanced by the creation of new ones, thus restoring to treated animals their functional ability.[4]

7. One promising animal model for Duchenne MD that may give clues to the cause of the disorder indicates that muscle damage may be produced by abnormalities of the small blood vessels within the muscles. If the hypothesis is confirmed, therapy might well be directed toward an entirely new goal—improvement of the microcirculation in muscle.[11]

III. How Many People Are Suffering from Muscular Dystrophy in the United States?

1. *At a conservative estimate, more than 200,000 men, women, and children* in the United States are suffering from muscular dystrophy.[5] The disease is not at present reportable and a nationwide census has never been attempted. In the State of Utah the prevalence has been estimated at 1 to 500.[5]

2. *Nearly two-thirds of the known muscular dystrophy victims* in the United States are *children between the ages of 3 and 13.* Of these, almost all will die before adulthood.[5]

IV. Does It Kill Its Victims?

1. Muscular dystrophy in itself is usually not fatal, although there are instances in which the involvement of the heart muscle precipitates death. As a rule, however, death is the result of intercurrent maladies, generally of a respiratory nature. The weakness and wasting of the chest muscles gradually lessen respiratory power; the most common cause of death is a direct interference with lung action.

2. To a muscular dystrophy patient a trifling cold may be a grave disease, as his wasted muscles make him unable to raise mucus, and there is a danger of suffocation.[1]

V. What Are the Symptoms of Muscular Dystrophy?

1. Symptoms in children are *frequent falling, difficulty ascending stairs, a peculiar side-to-side waddling gait, great difficulty in rising from a lying or sitting to a standing position, apparent increase in the size of the affected muscles,* particularly in the calf, and contractures (leading to distortions) of the affected muscles. While the contractures may cause suffering, pain is not a feature of the disease itself.[1]

2. In adult patients, *the earliest muscles affected are those of the*

shoulders, upper arms, thighs, and back, and, in certain forms of the disease, the face. In the case of the latter, the patient has a "transverse" smile and cannot whistle or drink through a straw. *There is no pain.*[1]

3. The facial symptoms may be noted in early childhood. Weakness in the shoulder girdle and upper arms is often noted during adolescence. The lower limbs are also ultimately affected.

VI. What Is the Present Status of Therapy?

1. The substance mentioned on page 199—which successfully reversed the morbid process in genetically dystrophic chickens and mice—has not yet been tested on human beings. Such clinical experiments must await further understanding of its metabolic action and possible side effects. For the present, therefore, it must be said that there is still *no effective treatment* for muscular dystrophy. To date, none of the wide variety of diets and drugs administered to patients has shown any significant lasting effect on the course of the disease.[3]

2. New substances and devices are reported at frequent intervals, but to date all have followed a similar pattern—*they consist of uncontrolled studies,* using subjective criteria on a handful of patients. Commonly these reports are publicized in the popular press with only slight and insubstantial data offered in support of the claim.[3]

Whenever suggestive favorable evidence is available in support of any substance or procedure, clinics in various parts of the country cooperating with Muscular Dystrophy Associations of America, Inc., join in testing the therapeutic efficacy.[3]

3. *Physical therapy* has proved of *limited value* in delaying contractures but does not otherwise affect the course of the dystrophic process.[6]

4. *Antibiotics* prolong the lives of many children who would otherwise succumb to respiratory infections, but have no curative effect on muscular dystrophy.[7]

VII. What Are the Main Types of Muscular Dystrophy?

1. There are four *main types* of muscular dystrophy:
    a. *Pseudohypertrophic type (Duchenne MD).* This is by far the most prevalent form. It *commences in childhood between the ages of 3 and 10,* and its course is more rapid than any of the other types. Three times as many males are affected as females. It is hereditary in the majority of cases.[5]
    b. *The juvenile form (limb-girdle)* has its onset in childhood or adolescence, its progression is slower, and patients may reach middle age. This form is hereditary, and both sexes are equally affected.[5]
    c. *The facio-scapulo-humeral form* commences in early adulthood and affects the facial muscles, shoulders, and upper arms.[5]
    d. The mixed types are a group of conditions that have their onset between the ages of 30 and 50. Not inherited, *they can strike anyone,* often causing death in from 5 to 10 years.[5]

VIII. What Progress Has Been Made in Diagnosing Patients with Muscular Dystrophy?

1. Medical understanding of muscular dystrophy has increased greatly in the past few years. It is now possible, through biochemical tests, to diagnose the disease long before the appearance of clinical symptoms.[2] Such tests, and others—notably, the analysis of biopsy samples—are also useful in identifying female carriers of the most severe type of dystrophy.[8]

IX. What Medical Facilities Are Available for the Care of Patients?

1. Because the average practitioner is not too familiar with new diagnostic techniques, the Muscular Dystrophy Associa-

tions of America, Inc., has produced a film—*Differential Diagnosis of Muscular Dystrophy and Related Conditions.* This film is specifically designed for training physicians and medical students to differentiate between dystrophy and the many disorders with which it is often confused. (The production of the film was financed by a grant from the Neurological and Sensory Disease Service, an arm of the U.S. Public Health Service.[3])

2. Muscular Dystrophy Associations of America, Inc., was also responsible for establishing a network of MD clinics in large metropolitan areas and other strategically located centers. The number of these clinics increases from year to year. In 1974, the association was supporting 136 clinics throughout the nation.[9] These clinics provide the following services:

a. Diagnostic facilities to ensure adequate differential diagnosis of patients referred to clinic.

b. Competent medical advice on special problems of the dystrophic patient.

c. Physical therapy treatments under medical supervision.

d. Medical social service assistance for personal and family problems.

e. Testing of newest drugs or therapeutic procedures on organized groups of patients under conditions of clinical control. At present, numerous research projects are in progress and as researchers continue to evolve new drugs and diagnostic techniques, these will be made available to all cooperating clinics.

f. *Cooperation with the patient's personal physician.*

3. In areas where local clinics have not been established, portions of this program are available through MDAA's affiliated chapters. The program covers not only patients suffering from all types of muscular dystrophy but also those afflicted with the following related conditions: the different forms of spinal muscular atrophy found in the infant, the juvenile and the adult; amyotrophic lateral sclerosis; peroneal muscular atrophy; benign congenital hypotonia, and the myosites.

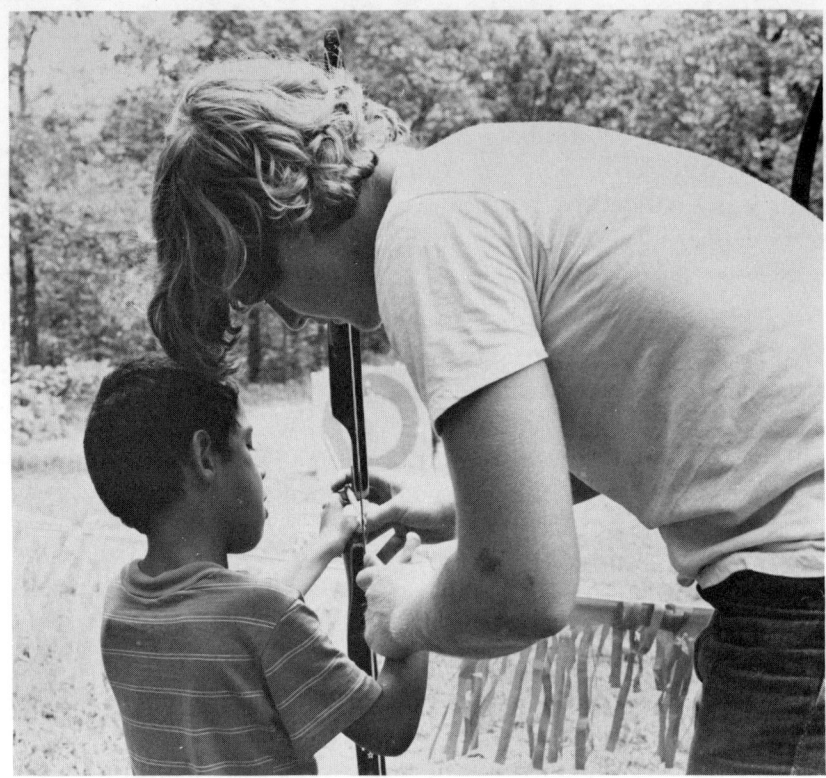

The Muscular Dystrophy Associations of America operate a number of summer and winter camps for children and adults with muscular dystrophy. (COURTESY OF MUSCULAR DYSTROPHY ASSOCIATIONS OF AMERICA, INC., NEW YORK)

X. Is Any Direct Assistance Given to Patients?

1. Muscular Dystrophy Associations of America, Inc., through local chapters, assists in the purchase and repair of *wheelchairs, hospital beds, braces, lifts and other appliances.*
2. In many areas chapters conduct education and recreation programs and provide transportation for patients.

XI. What Material Is Available for Professional and Public Education on Various Phases of Dystrophy?

1. Of primary professional interest are the *medical conferences* which are sponsored by Muscular Dystrophy Associations

of America, Inc. Frequent medical and scientific conferences are called by the association, and between these full-scale conferences, symposiums are held as convenient.[9]

2. The association has catalogued its library of information. Two bibliographies of this material are available: *Professional Publications* and *Publications of General Interest*. The association also finances the compilation of medical abstracts and distributes these on request at no charge.[9]

3. Literature of general interest is also available from local chapters.

XII. How Extensive Are the Research Programs in Muscular Dystrophy?

Approximately *$12.9 million* is being spent annually for research in muscular dystrophy, as follows:

1. For the year ended March 31, 1974, *Muscular Dystrophy Associations of America, Inc.*, expended *$6,613,934* for research into muscular dystrophy and pertinent areas of basic science through grants and awards to universities and medical centers in this country and abroad.[9]

2. *The National Institute of Neurological and Communicative Disorders and Stroke* of the U.S. Public Health Service spent an estimated *$6,314,000* on muscular and neuromuscular disorders in fiscal 1975.[11]

3. In contrast to what is currently being spent for research in muscular dystrophy, Americans spent in 1972:

- $69,480,000 for makeup bases[10]
- $64,880,000 for suntan lotions and oils[10]
- $63,050,000 for bath salts, tablets, oils[10]

XIII. What Are the Needs in the Fight Against Muscular Dystrophy?

1. Funds for research

More funds for research into the cause and treatment of muscular dystrophy, to prevent the deaths of the many children now afflicted, are needed by the National Institute of Neurological and Communicative Disorders and Stroke and Muscular Dystrophy Associations of America, Inc.

2. Education

Research leads to greater understanding of the needs of the muscular dystrophy patient, through an understanding of his psychology, his abilities, and his limitations. It is possible to enable the affected individual to play a useful part in the community. Our new understanding, obtained through scientists, *needs to become widespread among physicians, nurses, and all people* associated with muscular dystrophy cases, so that the "hopeless" prognosis *will not lead to a patient's unhappiness and despair.*[6]

3. Funds for patient care

More funds are needed to help the estimated 200,000 people in the United States afflicted with muscular dystrophy to obtain education and recreational opportunities, *orthopedic appliances, physical therapy, social services, or psychiatric assistance in adjusting to their progressive condition.*

Notes

1. A. T. Milhorat, M.D., "Progressive Muscular Dystrophy," *The Crippled Child* 29:6 (August 1951).
2. Carl M. Pearson, M.D., "Muscular Dystrophy—Review and Recent Observations," *The American Journal of Medicine* 35, no. 5, pp. 632-645.
3. Muscular Dystrophy Associations of America, Inc., 1790 Broadway, New York, N.Y.
4. Ethel Cosmos, Jane Butler, and Ade T. Milorat, M.D., "Hereditary Muscular Dystrophy in Chickens, Effect of Safflower Oil and Hexahydrocoenzyme Q4 on Structure and Enzymic Activity of Muscle." Excerpta Medica International Congress Series No. 175, *Progress in Neuro-Genetics*, vol. 1 of the Proceedings of the Second International Congress of Neuro-Genetics and Neuro-Ophthalmology, Montreal, September 1967.

5. *Muscular Dystrophy—The Facts,* publication of Muscular Dystrophy Associations of America, Inc., 1790 Broadway, New York, N.Y.
6. Arthur S. Abramson, M.D., *An Approach to the Rehabilitation of Children with Muscular Dystrophy,* published by Muscular Dystrophy Associations of America, Inc., 1790 Broadway, New York, N. Y., 1953.
7. National Institute of Neurological and Communicative Disorders and Stroke, National Institutes of Health, Bethesda, Md. 20014. A pamphlet for the public, *Muscular Dystrophy, Hope Through Research,* is available from the Institute. Also available in Spanish.
8. Ade T. Milhorat, M.D., and Loretta Goldstone, "The Carrier State in Muscular Dystrophy of the Duchenne Type—Identification by Serum Creatine Kinase Level," *Journal of the American Medical Association* 194:130-134 (October 11, 1965).
9. Annual reports, Muscular Dystrophy Associations of America, Inc., 1790 Broadway, New York, N.Y.
10. *1973 Marketing Guide,* published by *Drug Topics,* Medical Economics Company, Oradell, N.J.
11. From the National Institute of Neurological and Communicative Disorders and Stroke, Bethesda, Md.

What Are the Facts About Parkinsonism?

I. What Is Parkinsonism?

The term Parkinsonism is applied to a *group of progressive, disabling symptoms of the nervous system* which include muscular rigidity, tremors, and loss of automatic, associated movements. The typical Parkinson patient shows a stooped posture, loss of equilibrium while walking, a low-amplitude, monotonous speech, and, in rare cases, some deterioration of mental faculties.

Strictly speaking, Parkinsonism is not a disease, but rather a combination of the above symptoms which result from a variety of processes capable of producing dysfunction in the basal ganglia, as well as its connections. At postmortem examination, changes are consistently found in the substantia nigra, globus pallidus, locus caeruleus, as well as in several of the motor nerve centers in the medulla.

II. How Many People Have Parkinsonism?

The exact incidence and prevalence is unknown, but estimates indicate there are a million to a million and a half victims of this disease in the United States.

III. What Are the Chief Types of Parkinsonism?

1. *Parkinson's disease* (paralysis agitans or idiopathic Parkinsonism) is a slowly progressive disease usually beginning in the

fifties or sixties with tremor first appearing in one limb and usually spreading to other parts of the body within a few years. Loss of facial expression, a poverty and general slowness of movement gradually make their appearance and, with further progression, disturbance of gait and posture develop which may ultimately confine the patient to bed or a wheelchair existence. This type accounts for the majority of cases of Parkinsonism.

2. *Post-encephalitic Parkinsonism* typically presents some of the symptoms of Parkinson's disease plus additional symptoms, including oculogyric (causing movements of the eye) crises, weakness of the muscles controlling swallowing and various ocular palsies.

3. *Symptomatic Parkinsonism:* a host of conditions, including brain tumors, head injuries, malaria, syphilis, and certain chemicals, may, on rare occasions, so damage the basal ganglia and brain stem as to produce a Parkinson-like state. A number of rare disorders of the nervous system may present some resemblances to Parkinson's disease in addition to other symptoms.

4. *Pseudo-Parkinsonism* may be induced by many of the tranquilizing drugs employed in modern psychiatric treatment. The condition disappears when the offending drug is discontinued.

IV. What Is the Cause of Parkinsonism?

1. The causes of Parkinson's disease are still unknown. Certain forms may result from a still *undetected virus,* and a few metallic poisons have been suspected. Recent work has shown that depletion of certain *chemicals involved in nerve excitation* accompanies Parkinsonism, but how the depletion occurs is still not clearly understood. *A hereditary factor* has been suggested.

2. Post-encephalitic Parkinsonism is believed to be a sequel to a particular type of encephalitis, "encephalitis lethargica," which occurred chiefly in the 1920s. Although the cause was not found, encephalitis lethargica very probably was due to a

virus. Parkinsonism only rarely follows other types of encephalitis.

3. Arteriosclerosis may be associated with and perhaps may aggravate Parkinsonism but is not a direct cause of Parkinsonism.

V. What Is the Prevalence of Parkinsonism?

1. Epidemiological studies in New Zealand, Australia, England, Minnesota and Sweden all indicate an overall prevalence rate of about 1 case per 1,000 population; however, estimates from U.S. voluntary agencies suggest a prevalence of 1 case per 200 population. Since it is chiefly a disorder affecting older persons, the prevalence rate increases dramatically in the older age groups.

2. Males and females are approximately equally affected.

VI. What Is the Mortality of Parkinsonism?

1. In 1969, *3,208* deaths were listed as due to Parkinson's disease, but the number of persons with Parkinsonism dying each year is believed to be about 5 times greater than this figure. Strictly speaking, Parkinsonism is not in itself a direct cause of death, but it may predispose the individual to other diseases, notably pulmonary conditions, and thereby shorten life expectancy. Mean survival from onset to death is approximately 20 years.

VII. Is There Any Cure or Treatment for Parkinsonism?

1. No cure is known, but new drugs have brought great progress against the disease.

Recently, *a major advance has been made through successful trials of the amino acid, levodihydroxy-phenylalanine (L-DOPA). Reports show that up to 75 percent of the patients treated experience substantial benefits.*

Dr. George Cotzias and his associates are the first to have shown the usefulness of this drug in Parkinson's disease.

One problem with L-DOPA has been that slow administration leading to the massive doses necessary for adequate penetration of the brain was not followed, causing intolerable side effects. A way around this problem has been found. Enzyme inhibitors, which slow the breakdown of L-DOPA in the body, allow much greater penetration; a consequent reduction (up to 80 percent) in dosage, permitting faster administration with reduction or elimination of peripheral side effects.[1]

2. A variety of brain operations have been tried over the past 30 years with the aim of destroying nerve centers necessary for the maintenance of tremor and rigidity without producing paralysis or other undesirable side effects. Many different parts of the brain have been attacked, several of which yield similar results. The most favorable target to date seems to be a particular area of the thalamus. The operations performed today are relatively safe and have effectively suppressed tremor and rigidity in the majority of cases selected for surgery. Other disabling symptoms are not relieved and the course of the disease does not appear to be altered. However, L-DOPA treatment is largely replacing surgery.

VIII. What Is Being Spent for Research in Parkinsonism?

1. The *National Institute of Neurological and Communicative Disorders and Stroke* of the U.S. Public Health Service spent an estimated *$3,158,000* on Parkinson's disease research and related chronic neurological disorders of aging in fiscal 1975.

2. The Parkinson's Disease Foundation, 640 West 168th Street, New York, N. Y. 10032, is a voluntary health agency specifically interested in the disease. Since the foundation was established in 1957, it has expended over $2 million to support research in this field.

IX. What Is Needed in the Fight Against Parkinsonism?

1. *Additional research funds should be made available* to the National Institute of Neurological and Communicative Disorders

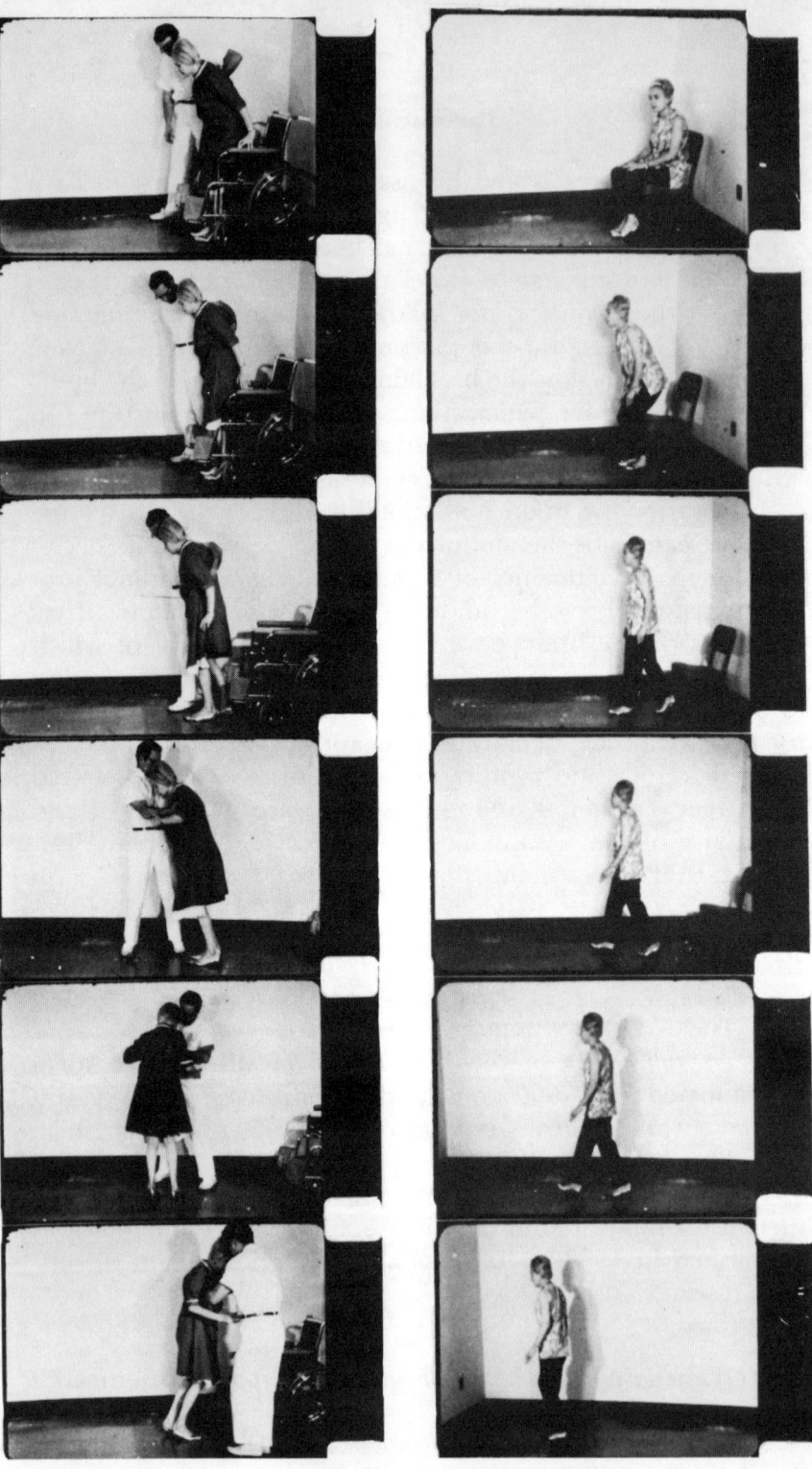

A Parkinsonian patient before and during administration of L-Dopa.

(COURTESY OF DR. GEORGE C. COTZIAS, BROOKHAVEN NATIONAL LABORATORY, NEW YORK)

and Stroke and to the voluntary agencies willing to undertake research for cures in this field.

2. *Further development of specialists* in this field is needed and further training of the general practitioner.

3. *Convalescent centers* should be developed in key cities throughout the country. These would serve not only to care for completely incapacitated Parkinson patients not helped by L-DOPA, but would also act as research-demonstration centers, where clinical testing of new agents could be done, and where proper treatment could be demonstrated to physicians, especially those from rural areas.

X. What Are the Current Research Leads?

Parkinson's disease is no longer regarded as a hopeless condition.

1. Research is currently being conducted on the potential of new chemotherapeutic agents, as well as on the control of L-DOPA's side effects.

2. The roles of viruses, arteriosclerosis, and heredity are under scrutiny.

3. Investigation into the chemistry of nerve cells holds great promise in yielding valuable information, as well as increasing knowledge of the brain's motor centers.

4. Anatomical studies with new and more sophisticated scientific instruments are also important in helping to reveal structural changes in the brains of Parkinson patients.

Notes

Grateful acknowledgment is made to the National Institute of Neurological and Communicative Disorders and Stroke, National Institutes of Health, Bethesda, Md. 20014; and the Parkinson's Disease Foundation, Columbia University College of Physicians and Surgeons, 640 West 168th Street, New York, N.Y. 10032, for their help in compiling and updating this chapter.

1. Work of Dr. George C. Cotzias, Memorial Sloan-Kettering Cancer Center, New York, N. Y.

What Are the Facts About the Population Problem?

I. What Is the Population Problem? How Many People Are Here Now?

1. The population of the world now totals an estimated 3 billion, 860 million (1973).[1]

2. It took all of history, until about 1830, for the world's population to reach 1 billion. In 1930, 100 years later, world population reached 2 billion. In 1960, only 30 years later, world population reached 3 billion.[2]

3. The current rate of population growth is 2 percent per year, or 76 million per year.

If this rate of growth continues, we will reach a world population of almost 7 billion by the turn of the century (twice the world's population today).[2] In other words, *we will double today's world population in just 35 years.*

4. *More than 80 percent of this increase* will occur *in the developing nations.*[1] The developing nations are already suffering an acute imbalance between births and deaths. Throughout much of Asia, Africa, and Latin America, successful efforts at economic development find their *gains diluted by ever-increasing numbers of people.*

   a. *Most of the additional population* will, therefore, come into the world with *limited prospects of adequate food, shelter, education and employment.*[1]

5. In 1972, approximately 125,000,000 babies were born worldwide and 49,000,000 people died, a net increase of some 76 million people in just one year.[3]

6. Modern medicine and advances in nutrition have cut the

214

death rates throughout the world, producing a fantastic population growth rate. Death rates for both children and adults have fallen sharply in recent years due in some part to successful assistance in combating such ancient killers as malaria, cholera, typhus, typhoid, and smallpox.[4]

II. What Are the Problems Associated with the World Population Explosion?

1. Inadequate food production

In the developing countries, where the population is increasing most dramatically, *food production* is rising at an average rate of *2.7 percent annually*. But the present *minimum food demand considered sufficient* to supply adequate diets *is increasing at an even faster rate—4 percent annually*.[4]

If this gap is not closed through increased food production and decreased population growth, the great majority of people will be *undernourished* and unschooled, economically unproductive and living in hovels.[4]

2. Economic hardships

    a. The rate of population growth in the world today creates a *child dependency level which the productive age groups cannot support*. Currently the percentage of dependent children (under 15 years old) in the less-developed countries runs between *40 percent and 50 percent of the population*. In the United States this figure is about 30 percent.[2]

    b. In many developing countries, industry is increasing, creating more work, but *employment cannot expand fast enough* to supply the growing number of people who need jobs.

    c. School construction, the supply of classrooms, books, and teachers cannot keep up with the flood of children who should be learning to read and write.[4]

    d. Housing, water and sewage systems, health facilities remain inadequate for the increasing numbers of people needing these services and facilities.

3. The Indian Government estimates that the 13 million people added to the Indian population each year need:[4]

> 126,500 extra schools
> 372,500 schoolteachers
> 2,500,000 houses
> 1,300,000 tons of food
> 4,000,000 jobs

The inability to meet these demands resulted in *10 million unemployed* in 1965—despite the creation of 31 million additional jobs between 1952 and 1965.

There were *63.8 million children out of school*—despite a 300 percent expansion in education facilities in that period.[4]

4. In the developed world, per capita income (gross national product for 1970 in U.S. dollars) was $3,085 as compared with $231 in the developing world.[5]

III. What Organizations Are Working in the Field of Population and Family Planning on an International Scale?

1. As of 1972, the burden of assistance has been borne by
   a. Private organizations like[6]

   International Planned Parenthood Federation
   Ford Foundation
   Rockefeller Foundation
   Population Council

   b. Bilateral programs, such as those set up by the Swedish and United States governments, Denmark, Holland, Japan, Norway, the United Kingdom.[6]

2. Commitments of the major agencies to population programs in 1972 were about *$260 million,* not including $142 million by the Department of Health, Education, and Welfare (excluding the National Institutes of Health), and $25 million by the Office of Economic Opportunity (OEO) for U.S. family planning programs.[6][8]

Population Problem

3. The United Nations' Fund for Population Activities (UNFPA) was established by the Secretary General in 1967 to support an expanded UN system program in the field of population. It is financed by voluntary contributions from over 45 countries and is administered by the administrator of the United Nations Development Program.

IV. To What Extent Is Our Population in the United States Increasing?

1. The population of the United States is now about *210 million* (including Armed Forces overseas).
2. The U.S. *growth rate is less than 1 percent annually*. At the present rate, in only 25 years, our population will increase from its present 210 million to 259 million.[11]

    a. Growth rates in the less-developed countries are significantly higher:[8]

        Latin America—2.8% per year
        Africa—2.6% per year with a high death rate
        India—2.5% per year
        Pakistan—3.3% per year

3. There were an estimated *3,141,000 live births* in the United States in 1973.[13] The birth rate has been declining:

Rate per 1,000 Population

Year	Rate
1962	22.4
1963	21.7
1964	21.0
1965	19.4
1966	18.4
1967	17.8
1968	17.5
1969	17.8
1970	18.4
1971	17.2
1972 (est.)	15.6
1973 (est.)	15.0

V. How Many Children Are Wanted?

1. Among low-income poorly educated parents surveyed in 1970, *56 percent of their children were unplanned and 31 percent were unwanted.*
2. Among the poor and poorly educated surveyed: an average of 3.0 children were wanted, yet these parents expected an average of 3.9.[8]
3. At least 15 percent of births to married couples were unwanted, according to a 1970 National Fertility Study, and an additional 24 percent were unplanned or mistimed.[7]
4. Due to the lack of distribution of reliable contraceptive information, 600,000 legal abortions were reported in 1972 and an estimated 800,000 to a million were performed in 1973.[7]
5. There have been an estimated 400,000 to 800,000 unwanted births each year during the last decade and 1 out of every 4 pregnancies was terminated by abortion.[7]

VI. What Are the Economic Aspects of Increased Population in the United States?

1. Increasingly, we may expect our increase in numbers to burden, rather than accelerate, our economy.
   a. Industrial productivity and the standard of living rather than the number of people determine purchasing power.
2. Increased expenditures—mostly public funds—needed to supply schools and colleges, health facilities, housing, water supplies, transportation, power, and so forth, for the expanding population will mean a substantially higher tax burden and bigger government.[9]
3. This year over 3 million new babies will be born in the United States and between 15 percent and 20 percent of all tax revenues will have to be spent simply to give them basic services.[9]

VII. What Is the Relationship Between Large Families and Poverty?

1. *Over one-seventh of all children* in the United States under 18 (15 percent) are being *reared in poverty.*[16]
2. Over *one-fifth of the children in families with 5 or more children* (21 percent) are being reared in poverty.[16]
3. *Among whites,* about one-ninth of all children (11 percent) and over *one-seventh of children in families with 5 or more children (15 percent) are reared in poverty.*[16]
4. Among blacks, over 40 percent of all children and *44 percent of children in families with 5 or more children are being reared in poverty.*[16]

VIII. How Many American Women Want and Need Family Planning Services?

1. About *6.2 million American women* in 1972 18 to 44 years of age (about 16 percent of all women in this age span) need family planning services, *but cannot afford them.*[17]
2. *About 2 million women* in these income groups are *currently receiving effective family planning help* from all public and private agencies combined, and another 1.2 million now are served by private physicians through government subsidies.[17] This means that only 50 percent of the target population is now being reached.
3. Thus *about 2 out of 3 of the 6.2 million women* who need family planning assistance *are still not receiving these services* from public and private agencies.[17]
4. Most of these 6.2 million women live in cities; and based on the original estimate of those needing family planning services:

    30% live in small towns in rural areas
    7.5% live on farms
    62.5% live in cities

5. Most live in or near poverty areas.[2]

IX. What Was the Estimated Cost of Providing Family Planning Services to the Estimated 6.6 Million Women Who Will Be in Need of These Services in 1975?

1. *$434,000,000* was the amount estimated to be needed to provide family planning services (at a per capita cost of $66 per woman per year) to the 6.6 million women to be reached by 1975.[18]

X. What Would the Economic Benefits Be of More Adequate Family Planning Among the Poor?

1. It has been estimated that the cost of saving a mother and society from having an unwanted child amounts to approximately *$628 per unwanted birth averted.*[19]
2. Another study has estimated that among the 9,078,000 poor and near-poor women 15 to 44 years of age in 1970 there were *318,000 unwanted births.*[20]
3. Thus, if all 318,000 unwanted births could have been averted, the cost would have been $200,000,000, but the savings and economic benefits would have been substantially greater. (Figures for savings and benefits not available.)[20]

XI. How Are Welfare Costs Affected by Our Expanding Population?

1. Ignorance about birth control has led not only to a higher rate of childbearing among the poor and uninformed than is experienced by the population generally, but contributes to the *enormous human and financial costs consequent upon the growing rate of illegitimate births.*
2. The rate of *illegitimate births has more than tripled* in the past 30 years, from 7 per 1,000 unmarried women of childbearing age to 26 per thousand in 1970.[13] The rate of illegitimacy among blacks is about 30 percent, the white rate about 5 percent.[21]
3. More than 3 times as many women in the 25-34-year age

group have illegitimate babies as compared to 30 years ago.[21]

4. Our Aid for Dependent Children (AFDC) program has almost tripled in the last decade. The program included 2.4 million children in 1960; 5.4 million children in 1969; 7 million in 1970; 7.7 million in 1971;[21] and 11.5 million in 1973.[22]

In 1955, total payments to AFDC recipients were $633 million; in 1969 this had increased to $3.6 billion; in 1971 to $6.2 billion; and in 1973 to $7.2 billion.[22]

5. Federal grants to states for child welfare services to establish, expand, and strengthen services for the protection and care of homeless, dependent, and neglected children totaled $46 million in fiscal 1973.[22]

XII. What Is Being Spent Nationwide to Provide Birth Control Services?

1. Federal appropriations for the delivery of family planning services, excluding research efforts, totaled *$163 million* in fiscal 1973, as follows:

Department of Health, Education, and Welfare Family Planning Projects	$161 million
Department of Defense	$ 2 million

Participating in the Department of Health, Education, and Welfare family planning activities are the Maternal and Child Health Service, the National Center for Family Planning Services, the National Center for Health Statistics, Indian Health Service, National Institute of Mental Health, Community Health Services, Federal Health Program Services, certain public assistance efforts under the Social and Rehabilitation Service, the Food and Drug Administration, and the Office of Education.

2. In 1971, the operating expenditures of Planned Parenthood's 190 affiliates totaled *$29.8 million,* primarily for the operation of family planning centers and similar services.

   a. Of this total, $12.4 million was received by the affiliates in the form of government grants and contracts.

XIII. What Must Be Done to Meet This Challenge?

1. Research on a far larger scale must be supported on the biological and medical aspects of human reproduction so improved methods of fertility control are developed.
2. The American people must be informed of the enormous problems inherent in unchecked population growth here as well as abroad.
3. A sense of responsibility must be developed concerning marriage and parenthood, including the responsibility of bringing into the world only those children whose parents are prepared adequately to care for and educate.
4. Existing knowledge about birth control *at low or no cost* must be made available to those who need and wish such information and guidance.

XIV. What Is Currently Being Spent for Research in This Area?

1. An estimated $72 million is currently being spent for research in this area.
2. Of this amount, about $52 million represented Federal appropriations in fiscal 1973.[10]
For fiscal 1973, $39.8 million was spent by the National Institute of Child Health and Human Development.[8]
3. The balance, about $20 million, was provided by the major private agencies which include the[6][8] Ford Foundation, Rockefeller Foundation, The Population Council, which receives support from the Ford and Rockefeller foundations, and the Planned Parenthood Federation. Research on contraception is also carried out by several pharmaceutical manufacturers.

XV. What Are Other Countries Doing About Their Population Problems?

1. By 1971, 81 percent of the people in the developing world lived in countries whose governments had a population

policy or supported family planning programs without any policy.[8][15]

   73% lived in countries that had an anti-natalist policy
   10% lived in countries that supported family planning programs without any policy

   2. Only 17 percent were in countries with neither a policy nor program support.[8][15]
   3. Of countries in the developing world,

   28 had an official policy
   26 officially supported family planning activities
   63 (balance) had little interest in or support for family planning activities[8][15]

   4. In Asia, where the largest nations, highest densities, and oldest civilizations are found, a large majority of the people live in countries whose governments are committed to a reduction in the growth rate.[15]
   5. In Africa and Latin America, on the other hand, the two continents with the highest growth rates, fewer than half the people live under governments that are committed to a reduction in the growth rate.[15]

XVI. What Are Some of the Research Leads to Help Families Have Babies by Choice and to Help Slow Down the Population Explosion?

   1. Among possible new potential methods of contraception now being researched or developed are the following:
      a. Improved pills.
      b. A type of sterilization completely harmless and reversible.
      c. Pills taken less frequently than is now necessary.
      d. Injections to be given once a month or every few months.[12]
      e. Improved IUD devices.
   2. Much of the research is in the social sciences to assess

implementation of birth control programs and to deepen our understanding of the motivations and attitudes associated with family planning.

XVII. Has Medical Research Paid Off in This Area? Yes.

1. The *world's first effective birth control pill,* perfected by Dr. Gregory Pincus of the Worcester Foundation for Experimental Biology and Dr. John Rock of Harvard, has been a *major step toward voluntary population control.*[12]
2. The intrauterine device (IUD) has been widely accepted and found to be an effective and inexpensive new method of contraception.[12]
3. Other devices have been and are being developed and improved in the effort to find new cheap and effective means of controlling fertility.

XVIII. How Many Maternal and Infant Deaths Occur in the United States Each Year?

1. In 1973 there were *470 maternal deaths* (deaths from deliveries and complications of pregnancy, childbirth, and the puerperium).[13]
2. In the same year, *55,300 infants under one year of age died.*[13] Of these, *about 73 percent failed to complete the first 28 days of life.*[13]
3. Fetal deaths in 1970 totaled 52,961 (gestation period 20 weeks or more).[13]
4. For 1972, 600,000 legal abortions were reported.[7]

XIX. Has Medical Research Paid Off in Reducing Maternal and Infant Deaths? Yes!

1. Between 1944 and 1973, the maternal mortality rate has been *reduced 93 per cent*—largely due to antibiotics. In the dec-

ade 1963-1973 alone, the maternal mortality rate dropped 58 percent.[13]

    a. The probability of dying from conditions associated with deliveries and complications of pregnancy, childbirth, and the puerperium has been reduced in 1973 to 1 maternal death for every 6,683 live births. In 1940, the risk was 1 maternal death for every 266 live births.[13]

  2. Between 1944 and 1973 *infant mortality rates* were *cut 56 percent.*[7]

    a. Mortality has declined much more rapidly among infants surviving the first 28 days of life than among infants less than 28 days old. This is due in part to the sharp reduction in mortality from influenza and pneumonia, from gastro-intestinal diseases, and from other communicable diseases—all of which affect chiefly the age group 28 days to 11 months.

XX. What Is the Role of the Planned Parenthood Federation?

  1. Planned Parenthood Federation of America, Inc., is the leading national voluntary agency working in this area. Its objective is to make effective family planning available to all, so that *each new infant can be a wanted child born by choice and not by chance to responsible parents.* In addition, the federation has made it its goal to alert the American people to the gravity of the world population crisis and to the need for expanded public and private programs to cope with it.

  2. The federation is made up of 190 local affiliates, organized in 42 states and the District of Columbia.[14]

XXI. How Much Does Planned Parenthood Raise and How Are These Funds Spent?

  1. Total revenues of Planned Parenthood and its affiliates in 1972 were $41.5 million. Of this total, $9.3 million represented patients' fees.[14]

2. Expenditures by the national office alone in 1973 were as follows: [14]

Program Services	
Service to affiliates	$1,744,769
Service to field of family planning	2,304,547
International assistance:	
International Planned Parenthood Federation	12,214
Family Planning International Assistance	2,665,467
	$6,726,997
Supporting Services	
Management and general	1,982,964
Fund raising	654,378
	$2,637,242
Payments to Affiliated Organizations	
Planned Parenthood Federation, Victor Bostrom Fund	566,788
Other	1,016,064
Other affiliates	254,695
	$1,837,547
Total expenditures	$11,201,786

XXII. Significant Legislation

1. New legislation was enacted by the President on December 24, 1970, which helped to provide urgently needed research and services in family planning.[12]

The Family Planning Services and Population Research Act of 1970 (PL 91-572) provides:

a. *Comprehensive voluntary family planning services* (consultations, examinations, means of contraception, follow-up supervision, and referral to other medical services) for all persons in the United States who want but cannot afford them.

b. *Research* to develop better methods of contraception,

further knowledge in the biomedical and behavioral sciences, improve the delivery of family planning services, and develop and disseminate data on population growth.

2. The Family Planning Services and Population Research Act of 1970, which expired on June 30, 1973, was renewed for one year. Renewal legislation contained in HR 14214, the "Health Revenue Sharing and Health Services Act of 1974," sustained a Presidential veto in December 1974 and will have to be reintroduced in the new session of Congress.

Notes

1. Population and Family Planning, report of the President's Committee on Population and Family Planning, November 1968. U.S. Department of Health, Education, and Welfare, Washington, D.C.
2. Federal Government Family Planning Programs, Domestic and International. Report and Recommendations of Republican Task Force on Earth Resources and Population, U.S. House of Representatives. Reprinted in *Congressional Record,* December 29, 1969.
3. Population Reference Bureau, 1755 Massachusetts Avenue, NW, Washington, D.C. 20036. 1973 World Population Data Sheet.
4. *The Population Challenge—U.S. Aid and Family Planning in the Less-Developed Countries.* Publication of the Office of the War on Hunger, Agency for International Development, Washington, D.C. 20523.
5. *Population Program Assistance,* December 1972. Agency for International Development, Washington, D.C.
6. *World Population, A Challenge to the U.N. and Its System of Agencies,* Report of a National Policy Panel established by the United Nations Association of the United States of America, May 1969.
7. Speech by Frederick S. Jaffe, Center for Family Planning Program Development, New York, at the Council on Foundations Annual Meeting, San Antonio, Tex., May 8, 1974.
8. Information from the National Institute of Child Health and Human Development, National Institutes of Health, Bethesda, Md., 1973.

9. *The Poverty of Abundance—American Business and the World Population Crisis,* publication of Planned Parenthood–World Population, New York, N.Y., 1965.
10. Special Analyses, Budget of the U.S. Government, fiscal year 1974.
11. Population Estimates, Series P-25, no. 496, February 1973. U.S. Bureau of the Census, Washington, D.C.
12. Information obtained from Planned Parenthood–World Population. New York, N.Y., 1974.
13. National Center for Health Statistics, U.S. Public Health Service, U.S. Department of Health, Education, and Welfare, Washington, D.C.
14. Information from Planned Parenthood–World Population, New York, 1974.
15. Reports on Population/Family Planning, No. 2, July 1970. Issued by the Population Council and the International Institute for the Study of Human Reproduction, Columbia University, New York.
16. Characteristics of the Low-Income Population, 1971. Current Population Reports, Series P-60, No. 86, December 1972. U.S. Bureau of the Census, Washington, D.C.
17. Data and Analyses for 1973 revision of the U.S. DHEW Five Year Plan for Population Research and Family Planning Services, December 1972. Center for Family Planning Programs Development.
18. *Comprehensive Report—Cost Study of a Sample of the Grantees of the National Center for Family Planning Services,* U.S. Department of Health, Education, and Welfare, 1972, Westinghouse Population Center, Columbia, Md.
19. "Center for Family Planning Program Development." Unpublished paper by Frederick S. Jaffe, January 1973.
20. *Family Planning Services in the United States.* Paper by Frederick S. Jaffe prepared for the Report of the U.S. Commission on Population Growth and the American Future, 1972.
21. U.S. Bureau of the Census, *Statistical Abstract of the United States,* 1972, 93d ed., U.S. Bureau of the Census, Washington, D.C.
22. Budget of the U.S. Government, fiscal year 1974, Appendix.

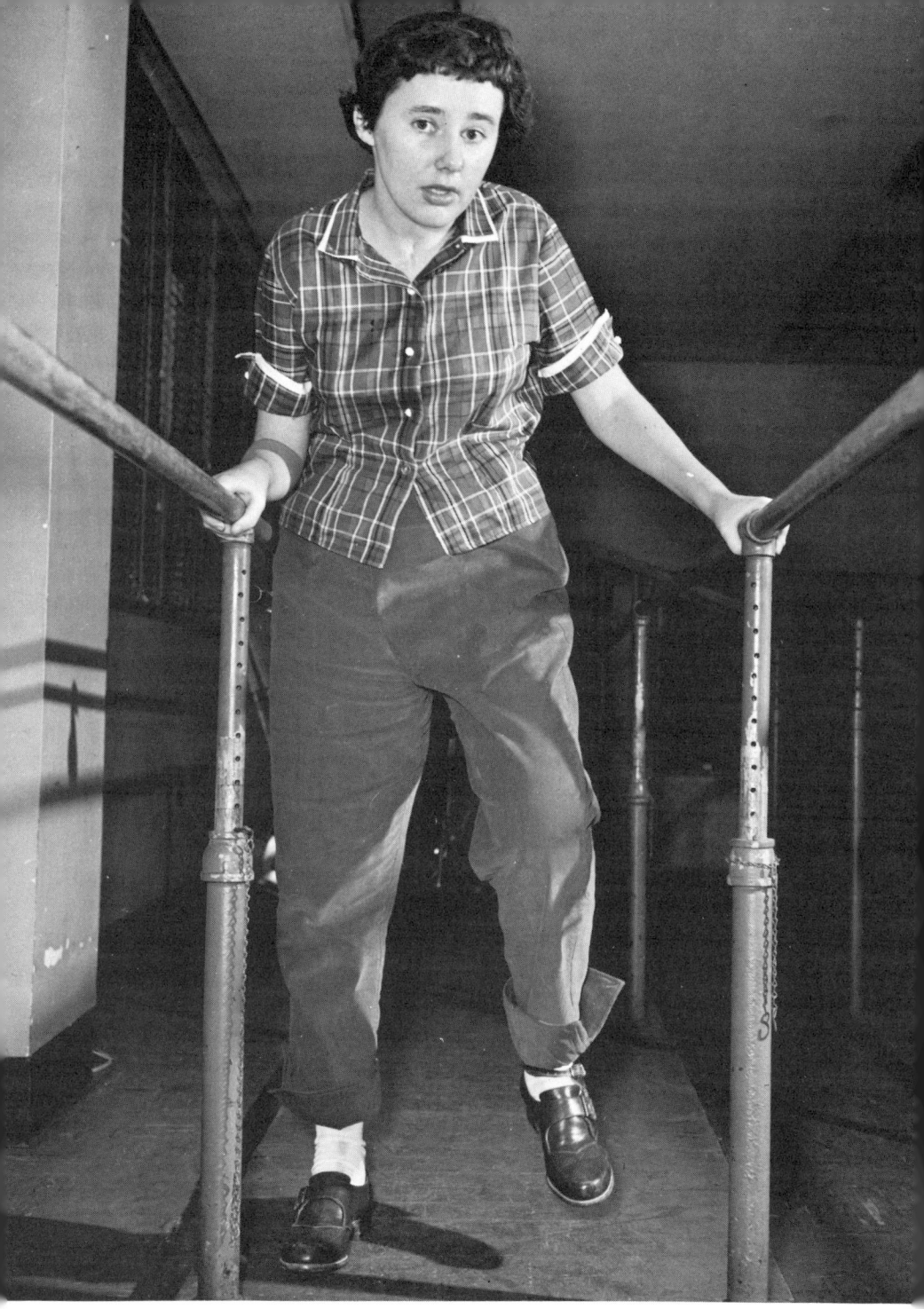

(COURTESY OF NEW YORK UNIVERSITY INSTITUTE OF REHABILITATION MEDICINE, NEW YORK)

What Are the Facts About
Disabled People in This Country?

I. What Are the Leading Disabling Conditions in the United States Today?

1. Heart and circulatory conditions, including hypertension, arthritis and rheumatism, back and spine impairments, account for over 54 percent of the activity limitation reported in a recent National Health Survey.[2]

II. Is Disability Only a Problem of Old Age?

No. Of the 23,237,000 people reporting activity limitation because of chronic conditions:[2]

    7,293,000 or 31.3% were under 45 years of age
    7,987,000 or 34.4% were 45 to 64 years of age
    7,958,000 or 34.3% were 65 years of age and over

III. What Do Illness, Injury, and Disability Cost the Nation Annually?

1. National health expenditures in 1972–73 were estimated to total *$94 billion.*[3] However, these expenditures *do not include indirect costs*—the loss of output to the economy represented by illness, disability and premature death.

2. In 1968 (latest year information available), the total economic costs of illness, disability and death were estimated at *$120 billion.*[4]

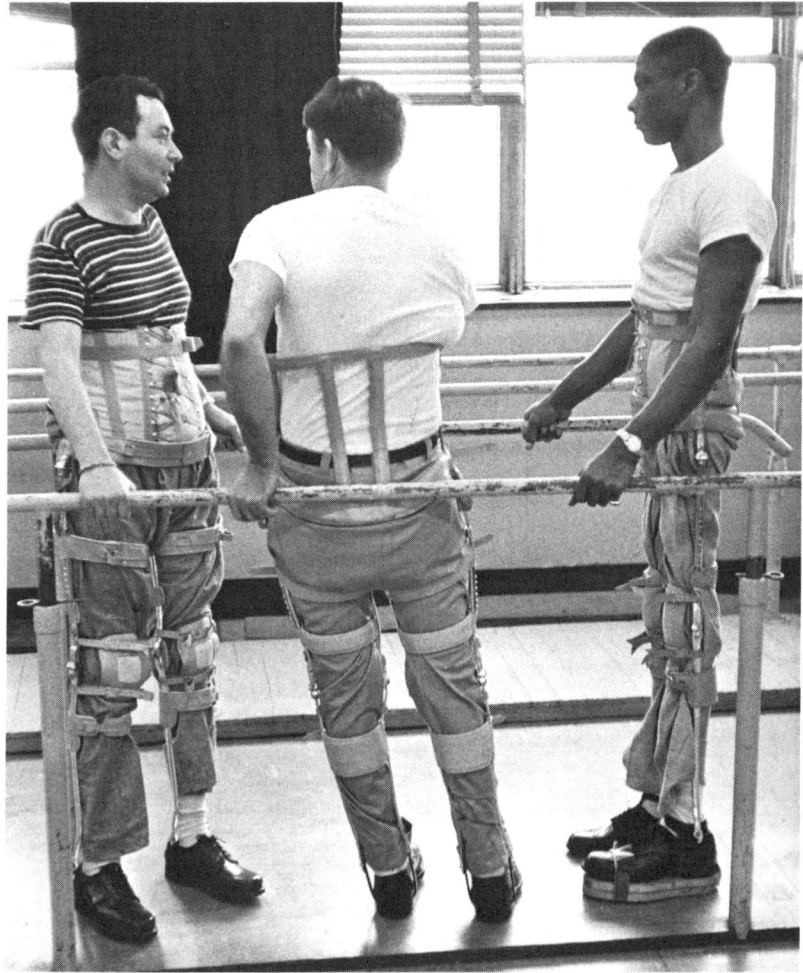

Patients at New York University Institute of Rehabilitation Medicine in New York City. (COURTESY OF NEW YORK UNIVERSITY INSTITUTE OF REHABILITATION MEDICINE, NEW YORK)

a. *Direct costs of illnesses* (expenditures for prevention, detection, treatment, rehabilitation, research, training, and capital investment in medical facilities) were estimated at *$49 billion.*

b. *Indirect costs of illness* (loss of output to the economy because of illness or disability) were estimated at *$15 billion.*

c. *Indirect costs* represented by loss of output to the economy through *premature death* were estimated at *$55.5 billion.*

The Killers and Cripplers

Average Number and Percent Distribution of Persons with Limitation of Activity by Chronic Condition 1969—1970

	All Degrees Activity Limitation	With Limitation in Amount or Kind of Major Activity	% Distribution of Activity Limitation
Heart and Circulatory			
Heart conditions	3,609,000	1,915,000	15.5
Hypertension without heart involvement	1,059,000	667,000	4.6
Cerebrovascular	604,000	166,000	2.6
Other conditions of circulatory system	907,000	435,000	3.9
Arthritis and rheumatism	3,265,000	9,934,000	14.1
Impairments of back and spine	1,613,000	990,000	6.9
Impairments of lower extremities	1,515,000	693,000	6.7
Visual impairments	1,115,000	439,000	4.8
Mental and nervous conditions	1,033,000	489,000	4.4
Asthma with or without hay fever	1,010,000	517,000	4.3
Other musculoskeletal disorders	914,000	559,000	3.9
Diabetes	865,000	442,000	3.7
Paralysis	817,000	283,000	3.5
All other conditions	4,911,000		21.1
All persons with activity limitation	23,237,000	12,302,000	100.0

IV. How Many Disabled People in the United States Are Eligible for the Federal-State Program of Vocational Rehabilitation?

The Federal-State Vocational Rehabilitation Program is a public service to prepare physically or mentally handicapped persons for employment and *place them in suitable jobs.* It is administered by especially constituted rehabilitation agencies in 54 states and territories, with financial aid and leadership from the Rehabilitation Services Administration of the Social and Rehabilitation Service in the Department of Health, Education, and Welfare.

In the United States today, there are an estimated 5 *million disabled persons* who need, want, would benefit from, and are eligible for vocational rehabilitation services under the Federal-State Vocational Rehabilitation Program to enable them to work in the competitive labor market, in sheltered employment, or in their own homes.[1]

Each year an estimated 800,000 disabled persons become

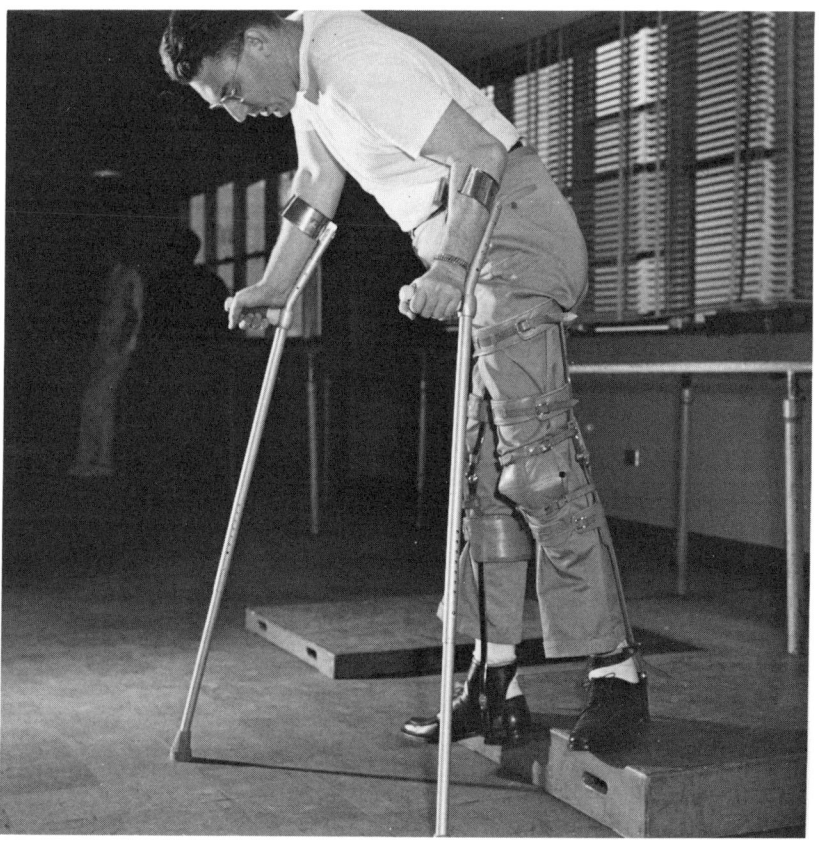

Learning to climb and descend practice curbs in the gym. The curbs are graduated in height from 2 to 4 inches. The patient is descending a 4-inch curb. The height of the average curb in New York City is 8 inches. (COURTESY OF NEW YORK UNIVERSITY INSTITUTE OF REHABILITATION MEDICINE, NEW YORK)

eligible for services under the Federal-State Vocational Rehabilitation Program.[1]

V. What Is the Federal Government Spending to Help Rehabilitate the Disabled?

1. The *rehabilitation programs* of the Social and Rehabilitation Services of the Department of Health, Education, and Welfare received estimated appropriations in fiscal 1973 of $1,029,113,000.[7]

2. These programs provide services to mentally and physically handicapped people so they may prepare for and engage in remunerative employment or employment in the home to the extent of their potential.

3. Under a formula matching basis, the states also contribute to these programs.[7]

VI. What Other Financial Help Is the Federal Government Providing to the Disabled?

1. *Public assistance programs* of the Social and Rehabilitation Services for aid to the blind and aid to the permanently and totally disabled in fiscal 1973 are as follows: [7]

Aid to the blind	$ 106,961,000
Aid to the permanently and totally disabled	1,489,096,000
Total	$1,596,057,000

2. In addition, the blind and permanently and totally disabled also receive medical assistance.[7]

VII. How Many People Were Rehabilitated in Fiscal Year 1971?

1. The 291,272 disabled persons rehabilitated to useful employment in fiscal 1971 set a new record for a single year's achievement under the Federal-State program. This was an increase of 9 percent over the 266,975 rehabilitated in fiscal

1970. This growth in the number of persons rehabilitated annually reflects intensified efforts by both Federal and state governments to meet the needs of larger numbers of disabled persons.[1]

2. In fiscal 1972, 326,138 were rehabilitated under this program.[7]

VIII. What Is the Major Long-Term Economic Benefit of Vocational Rehabilitation in Relation to Its Cost?

1. In the fiscal year ending June 30, 1971, 291,272 persons were rehabilitated under the Federal-State Vocational Rehabilitation program, and 59,336 of these were receiving some public assistance grants or were in tax-supported public institutions at the time they were accepted for services.[1]

   a. Of these 59,336 persons, *32,486 had been receiving public assistance grants* at the estimated rate of *$51 million* per year.[1]

   b. With their rehabilitation completed, the 32,486 clients will *earn an estimated $104 million in the first year after rehabilitation.*[1]

2. *What Is the Gain in Man-Hours?*

The 291,272 persons rehabilitated in fiscal year 1971 contributed an estimated *356 million man-hours of work* to our nation's production in the year after their rehabilitation. They had been contributing about *91 million man-hours of work on an annual basis at the time of acceptance for services.*[1]

3. *What Is the Improvement in Earnings?*

The *first-year earnings* of the 291,272 persons rehabilitated during fiscal year 1971 through the Federal-State Vocational Rehabilitation Program *exceeded the annual basis of their preservice earnings by an estimated $652 million.*[1]

IX. What Is the Estimated Cost of Rehabilitating All People Who Are Eligible for the Federal-State Program of Vocational Rehabilitation?

The *cost of rehabilitating the 5 million disabled persons who are eligible* for vocational rehabilitation services in the Federal-

State Program would be *about $10.8 billion,* based on fiscal 1971 basic support costs of approximately $2,200 per rehabilitated case in the vocational rehabilitation program.[1]

It should be noted, however, that this cost would not be met solely by the Federal-State Program of Vocational Rehabilitation but would be borne to some extent by other public and private sources which are already providing assistance to some of these disabled persons.[1]

X. Who Serves the Disabled?

1. *The Federal-State Program of Vocational Rehabilitation* administered by Rehabilitation Services Administration of the Social and Rehabilitation Service of the Department of Health, Education, and Welfare. Basic support grants are allocated to states according to a formula based on population and per capita income. Expenditures are at the matching rate of 80 percent for the Federal Government and 20 percent for the state.

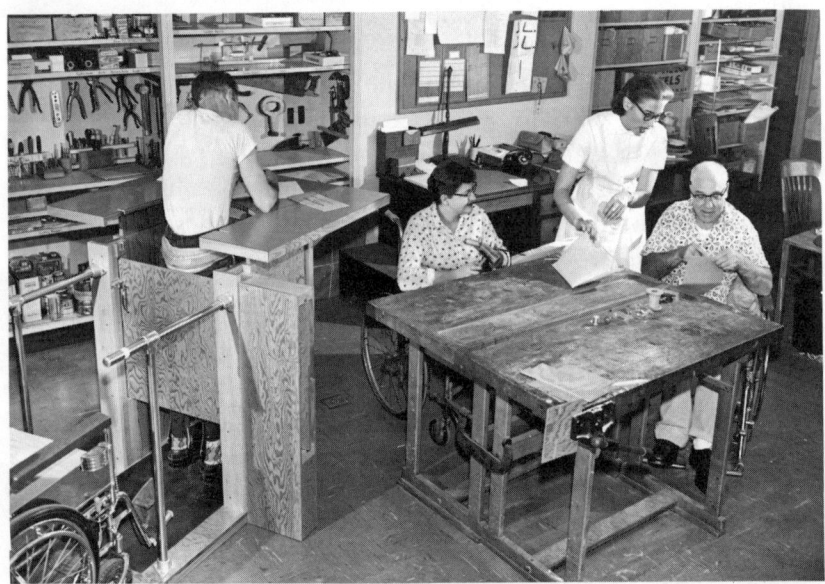

Training of the physically handicapped. (COURTESY OF NEW YORK UNIVERSITY INSTITUTE OF REHABILITATION MEDICINE, NEW YORK)

2. *Other public programs* are administered by The President's Committee on Employment for the Handicapped, the Children's Bureau of the Social and Rehabilitation Service, the Department of Labor, Veterans Administration, the Department of Defense, and state and local welfare departments and hospitals.

3. *A number of voluntary organizations* serve the handicapped directly or indirectly and in varying ways. Some render actual services or arrange for and underwrite the costs of services; others are engaged principally in support of research and public education. Well known among these groups are the National Foundation, the National Society for Crippled Children and Adults, National Tuberculosis Association, American Cancer Society, Epilepsy Foundation of America, American Diabetes Association, National Multiple Sclerosis Society, The Arthritis Foundation, American Foundation for the Blind, American Hearing Society, Goodwill Industries, National Industries for the Blind, United Cerebral Palsy, the National Rehabilitation Association, and the Muscular Dystrophy Associations of America, Inc.

XI. What Facilities Are Available for Rehabilitation?

1. *Rehabilitation centers,* which are institutional-type facilities bringing together the medical, vocational, psychological, placement, social, and other services needed to plan and carry out a program of rehabilitation. Examples of centers of the general type are the Woodrow Wilson Center at Fisherville, Virginia; the Hot Springs Rehabilitation Center in Hot Springs, Arkansas; the Georgia Rehabilitation Center at Warm Springs; the Institute for the Crippled and Disabled in New York, New York; the New York University Institute of Rehabilitation Medicine in New York City; the Kessler Institute of Rehabilitation, West Orange, New Jersey; and the Rehabilitation Institute of Chicago.

2. *Rehabilitation centers for the blind,* as for example, Industrial Home for the Blind, Brooklyn, New York; North Carolina Rehabilitation Center for the Blind, Butner, North Caro-

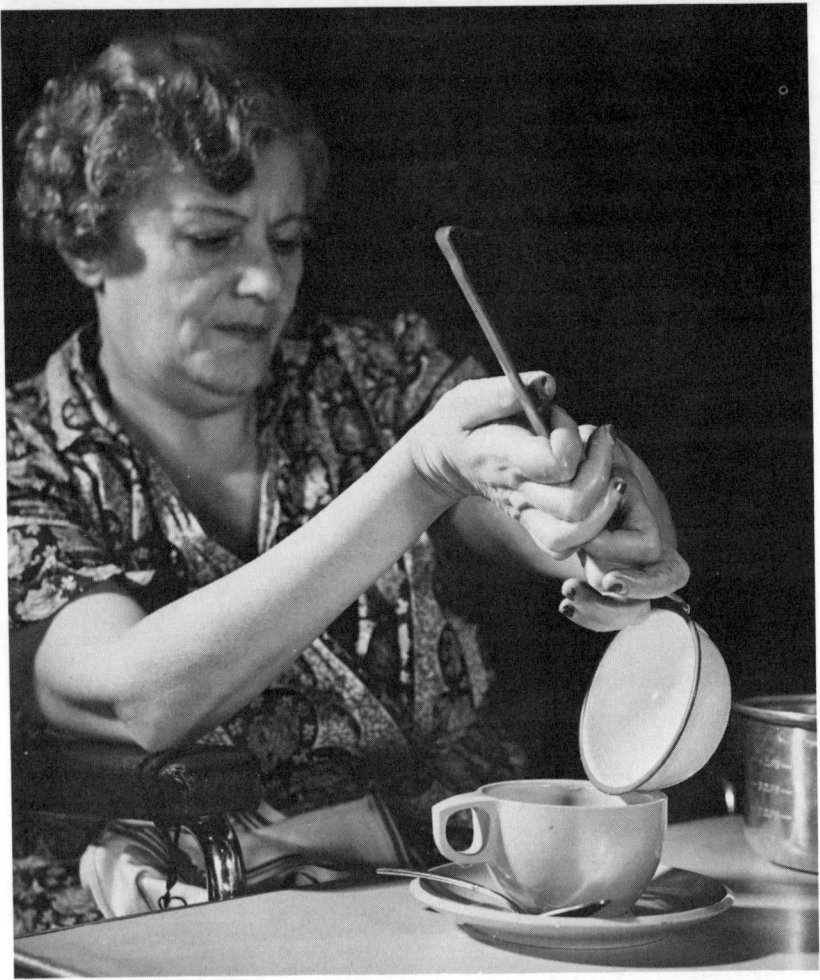

(COURTESY OF NEW YORK UNIVERSITY INSTITUTE OF REHABILITATION MEDICINE, NEW YORK)

lina; South West Rehabilitation Center, Little Rock, Arkansas; Kansas Rehabilitation Center for Adult Blind, Topeka, Kansas; St. Paul's Rehabilitation Center for the Blind, Newton, Massachusetts; Minneapolis Society for the Blind, Inc., Minneapolis, Minnesota; Adjustment Training Center, Florida Council for the Blind, Holly Hill, Daytona Beach, Florida.

3. *Sheltered workshops* were developed to meet the need for special facilities in which disabled people can be prepared for work in regular industries. For those unable to meet the de-

mands of competitive employment, the workshop may provide extended employment where the disabled may produce according to their capabilities. It is estimated there are about 1,200 sheltered workshops in the United States. Goodwill Industries of America, Inc., has local units in many communities —150 sheltered workshops and 41 affiliated branch workshops in the United States and 23 located in 9 foreign countries. National Industries for the Blind has approximately 85 affiliated workshops. Other sheltered workshops include: The Altro Workshop in New York City, facilities operated by the Volunteers of America, approximately 40 workshops for the blind unaffiliated with the NIB and workshops operated by other voluntary groups, such as the National Society for Crippled Children and Adults, the Jewish Vocational Service, and local associations for retarded children.[6]

4. *Hospitals with special services.*

5. *Speech and hearing clinics*—the April 1972 issue of *American Annals of the Deaf* lists 577 speech and hearing clinics in the United States and Canada.

Hearing societies, crippled children's programs, and other special educational services have speech and hearing clinics not included here.

6. *Model regional spinal cord injury systems,* which are research and demonstration projects providing new knowledge in rehabilitating the spinal cord injured through effective evacuation, sophisticated acute care, and high-level rehabilitation management and vocational rehabilitation. These projects are partially supported by the Social and Rehabilitation Service through the Vocational Rehabilitation Act. The seven projects are located as follows: Good Samaritan Hospital, Phoenix, Arizona; University of Washington, Seattle, Washington; University of Alabama Medical Center, Birmingham, Alabama; Northwestern University, Chicago, Illinois; New York University Medical Center, New York, New York; Woodrow Wilson Rehabilitation Center, Fisherville, Virginia; Texas Institute for Rehabilitation and Research, Houston, Texas.[1]

XII. How Many People Are Trained in Rehabilitation Methods and What Is the Need?

	Number of Professionals and Educational Training Facilities	The Needs
Physiatrists	About 800 physiatrists in the United States are diplomates of the American Board of Physical Medicine and Rehabilitation.	It has been estimated that an *additional 750 specialists could be used at once. The need will increase.*
Physical therapists	The American Physical Therapy Association has a membership of 16,500 physical therapists at present. The 71 approved schools, with certificate baccalaureate and master's degree programs, graduate approximately 2,000 persons a year.	Currently another 4,500 physical therapists are needed by hospitals alone, and there is a *total need for 13,500 additional physical therapists* for replacements or expanding programs. By 1975, about 1,300 graduates a year are expected.
Occupational therapists	There are an estimated 14,000 registered occupational therapists in the United States today. In 1972 the 39 approved schools of occupational therapy had a student enrollment of about 5,000.	By 1975, there will be need for 54,000 additional occupational therapists.
Social workers*	It is estimated that there are 170,000 social workers in practice, of whom about 57,000 are Master of Social Work graduates of schools of social work in the U.S. and Canada, and an enrollment of approximately 15,000 Master of Social Work candidates and 24,000 Bachelor of Social Work candidates.	Average annual openings over next 10 years for social workers will total about 18,000 annually, with a 60% growth rate.

	Number of Professionals and Educational Training Facilities	The Needs
Rehabilitation counselors	About 8,700 counselors were employed in 1969 in the Federal-State vocational rehabilitation program. By 1976 it is estimated that about 12,500 counselors will be employed in state agencies. Another large group of rehabilitation counselors serves veterans in the Veterans Administration and still others are employed in rehabilitation centers, sheltered workshops, and hospitals.	An additional 1,027 counselors trained in rehabilitation techniques, including adequately trained professional personnel to work with such disabled groups as the blind, deaf, mentally retarded, and other special groups, will be needed annually for several years in state vocational rehabilitation agencies. It is estimated that an additional 1,000 rehabilitation counselors will be needed for staffing private rehabilitation centers, sheltered workshops, and hospitals.
Speech and hearing therapists	In December 1972 the total membership of the American Speech and Hearing Association was approximately 15,756. Of this number, about 11,260 are certified in either speech or hearing. Although most speech and hearing therapists work with children in the public school system, the number of speech pathologists and audiologists working with adults in rehabilitation centers, speech and hearing centers, and hospitals has increased markedly.	An estimated 1,500 speech and hearing therapists should complete graduate training each year, as compared with about 1,000 now graduating each year.

*Medical and psychiatric social workers are reported together.

Physicians

There is an increasing recognition that rehabilitation is a part of total medical care. Many more refresher courses in modern rehabilitation methods are needed to reach a greater proportion of the 348,000 physicians in the United States.

Psychologists

The American Psychological Association reports that in fiscal year 1972 the association had a total membership of approximately 35,000. Of these, about 7,224 were employed as clinical psychologists and 2,750 in counseling and guidance, a number far short of the needs for mental hospitals, mental hygiene clinics, and rehabilitation.

Placement specialists

The state employment services employ placement specialists who devote most or all of their time to disabled clients. *The Vocational Rehabilitation and Education Program of the Veterans Administration* also includes placement specialists, as do the state vocational rehabilitation programs.

Special educators for handicapped children

Approximately 162,887 special educators now serve handicapped public school-age children. At least 16,587 of these persons are presently engaged in programs for speech impaired children.[8]

XIII. How Much Is the Social and Rehabilitation Service Spending for Research?

Federal grants are being made to public and voluntary agencies to *carry out research which holds promise of making a substantial contribution to the solution of vocational rehabilitation problems common to all or several states.*

From the beginning of the research and demonstration grants program in 1955 through June 30, 1969, 1,450 projects were activated, for which over $163 million of Federal funds were obligated. For the fiscal year 1972, the *appropriation for this program for new projects was $15 million.* Projects are funded for varying lengths of time, although the average is for three years. Geographically, projects have been approved in 50 states, the District of Columbia, Guam, Puerto Rico, and the Virgin Islands. The program includes studies on administrative and program problems, evaluation and counseling, rehabilitation workshops and centers, and international exchange of information, as well as projects covering a wide range of disabilities. (An annotated list of projects and a bibliography of published results are available from the SRS on request.)[5]

XIV. What Is Needed to Reduce the Problem of Disability and Its Effects?

1. *Additional funds* should be provided on all levels (Federal, state, local, public, and private) to assure *more adequate vocational rehabilitation programs to reach all who could benefit* from them, as well as for the *construction and staffing of rehabilitation research and training centers.*

2. *Funds are needed for research against the diseases that cause disability* so that fewer people will need rehabilitation in the future.

3. *More personnel trained in rehabilitation* are needed, particularly in the fields of rehabilitation medicine and nursing, psychiatry, physical therapy, occupational therapy, counseling, and social work. This will require more funds from public and private sources for undergraduate and graduate training, and for financial support to the training institutions required to produce the additional personnel needed.

4. Employers should be encouraged to establish *on-the-job training programs* so that disabled individuals can demonstrate to industrial personnel at all levels their ability to meet job demands.

5. *More facilities and workshops are needed,* including rehabilitation centers, for providing rehabilitation services of all types to the disabled.

6. *Public education in general preventive medical care,* including disease prevention programs.

Notes

1. Division of Monitoring and Program Analysis, Rehabilitation Services Administration, Social and Rehabilitation Service, U.S. Department of Health, Education, and Welfare, Washington, D.C.
2. Vital and Health Statistics. Series 10, No. 80. Data from National Health Survey. DHEW Publication no. (HSM) 73-1506. Public Health Service, Department of Health, Education, and Welfare, Washington, D.C.
3. *National Health Expenditures, 1929–73* by Barbara S. Cooper, Nancy L. Worthington, and Paula A. Piro. Social Security Bulletin, February 1974. U.S. Department of Health, Education, and Welfare, Washington, D.C. DHEW Publication No. (SSA) 74-11700.
4. Computation based on *Estimating the Cost of Illness*, Dorothy P. Rice, Health Economics Series 6. Publication of Division of Medical Care Administration, Public Health Service, Department of Health, Education, and Welfare, Washington, D.C., May 1966.
5. Office of Research, Demonstrations, and Training, Social and Rehabilitation Service, U.S. Department of Health, Education, and Welfare, Washington, D.C.
6. Division of Service Systems, Rehabilitation Services Administration, Social and Rehabilitation Service, U.S. Department of Health, Education, and Welfare.
7. Budget of the U.S. Government, fiscal year 1974, Appendix.
8. Bureau of Education for the Handicapped, Office of Education, U.S. Department of Health, Education, and Welfare.

NOTE: All other information obtained through the Rehabilitation Services Administration, Social and Rehabilitation Service, U.S. Department of Health, Education, and Welfare, Washington, D.C. 20201.

What Are the Facts About Tuberculosis?

I. How Many Deaths Are Caused by Tuberculosis Each Year?

1. In 1973, *3,870 Americans died from tuberculosis.*[1] Deaths from all causes in 1973 totaled an estimated 1,977,000.[1]
2. Of these deaths, 3,000 were caused by tuberculosis of the respiratory system.[1]
3. The greatest number of deaths occur in older age groups. About 71 percent of all tuberculosis deaths are among adults over 55.[1]
4. Almost 2½ times as many men died from tuberculosis as did women in 1971.[1]

II. How Has the Tuberculosis Death Rate Declined?

1. Between 1945 and 1973, the *death rate* from tuberculosis has *declined 95 percent.*[1]
2. *Between 1952 and 1973 alone,* tuberculosis *deaths* declined 89 percent.[1] The effectiveness of *streptomycin* against tuberculosis was announced in 1945 and it became generally available in 1947. The discovery of the usefulness of *isoniazid* was announced in 1952 and added dramatically to the decline in tuberculosis deaths.

COMPARISON OF TUBERCULOSIS DEATHS AND DEATH RATES IN THE UNITED STATES 1952-1973

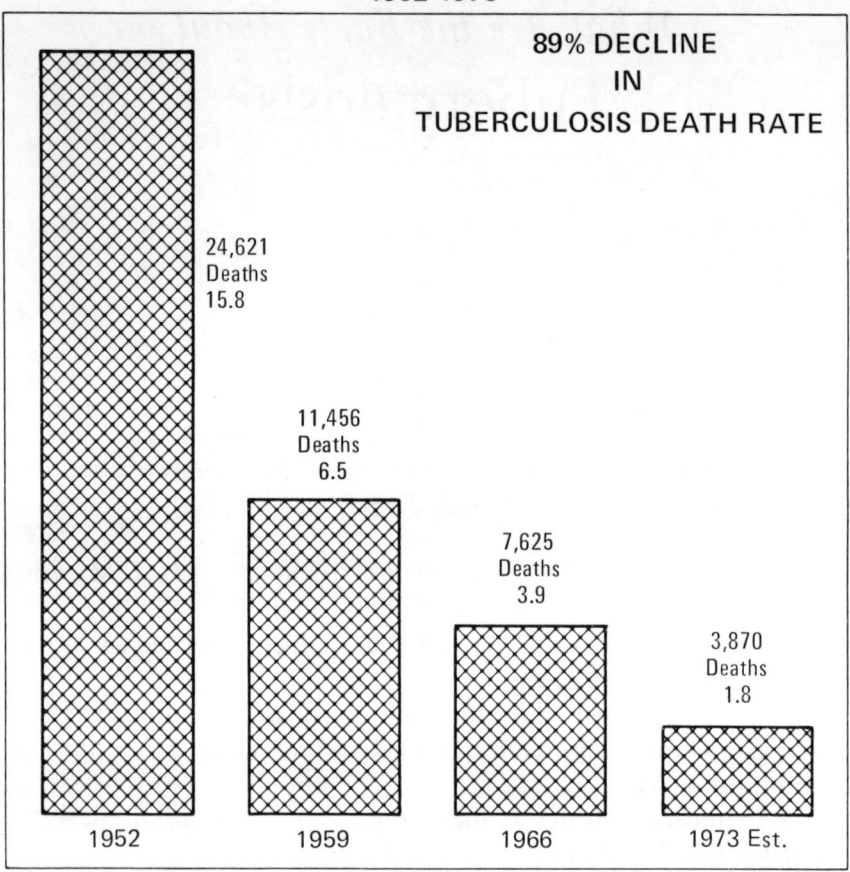

III. How Many New Cases of Tuberculosis Are Reported Each Year?

1. In 1973, *30,998 new active cases of tuberculosis were reported.*[4] *A 64 percent reduction from the 85,607 active cases reported in 1952,*[8] before isoniazid was generally used.
2. This is a case rate of 14.8 per 100,000 population.[4]
3. Thus, the goal of the U.S. Public Health Service and the National Tuberculosis Association for a new active case rate by 1970 of not more than 10 per 100,000 population[3] has not been realized.

COMPARISON OF NUMBER OF ACTIVE TUBERCULOSIS AND POLIO CASES REPORTED AND CASE RATES IN THE UNITED STATES

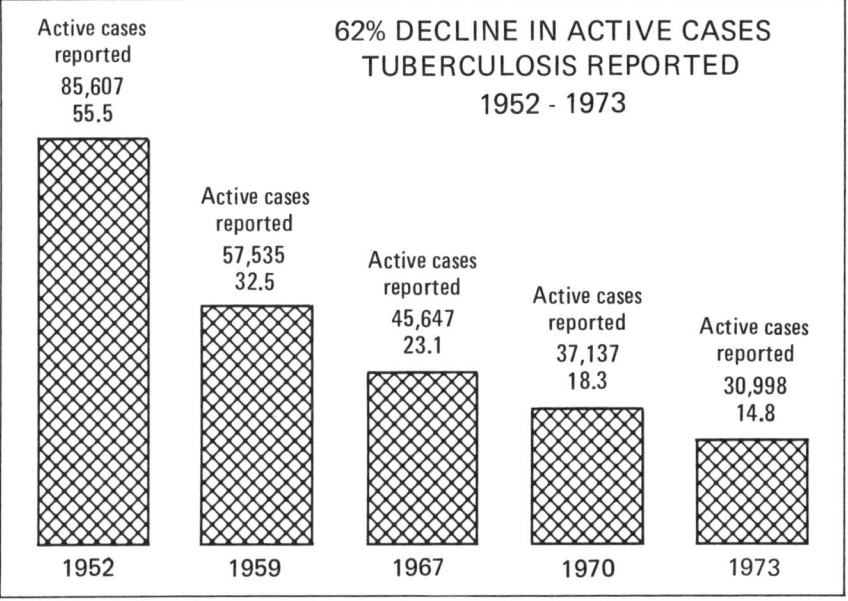

4. Nearly half of the tuberculosis cases are concentrated in cities with 100,000 or more population.[4]

5. In 1973, 58 cities with 250,000 or more population had a combined new active case rate of 25.7 compared to the average of 14.8 for the country. The cities with populations of 250,000 or more with the highest new active case rates in 1973 were:[4]

City	New Active Case Rate Per 100,000 Population
Newark	58.0
Honolulu	49.9
San Francisco	44.2
Washington, D.C.	41.2
Boston	38.9
Baltimore	38.5
Sacramento	37.5
Detroit	35.8
El Paso	35.3
Philadelphia	34.5

NEW ACTIVE TUBERCULOSIS CASES AND CASE RATES: STATES, 1973 AND 1972

State	New Active 1973	Cases 1972	Case 1973	Rate 1972	Rank According to Rate 1973	1972	Population July 1, 1973
United States	30,998	32,882	14.8	15.8	—	—	209,851,000
Alabama	790	918	22.3	26.2	5	2	3,539,000
Alaska	100	80	30.3	24.6	2	3	330,000
Arizona	416	396	20.2	20.4	8	11	2,058,000
Arkansas	460	434	22.6	21.9	4	6	2,037,000
California	3,210	3,326	15.6	16.2	18	21	20,601,000
Colorado	197	245	8.1	10.4	39	34	2,437,000
Connecticut	259	246	8.4	8.0	37	40	3,076,000
Delaware	74	103	12.8	18.2	24	15	576,000
District of Columbia	307	354	41.2	47.3	—	—	746,000
Florida	1,487	1,517	19.4	20.9	12	8	7,678,000
Georgia	1,010	897	21.1	19.0	7	13	4,786,000
Hawaii	303	315	36.4	38.9	1	1	832,000
Idaho	38	62	4.9	8.2	46	38	770,000
Illinois	1,520	1,940	13.5	17.2	21	18	11,236,000
Indiana	677	722	12.7	13.6	26	26	5,316,000
Iowa	125	117	4.3	4.1	50	50	2,904,000
Kansas	172	169	7.5	7.5	40	42	2,279,000
Kentucky	674	715	20.2	21.7	9	7	3,342,000
Louisiana	469	520	12.5	14.0	28	24	3,764,000
Maine	107	87	10.4	8.5	35	37	1,028,000
Maryland	719	838	17.7	20.7	15	10	4,070,000
Massachusetts	676	734	11.6	12.7	30	28	5,818,000
Michigan	1,121	1,261	12.4	13.9	29	25	9,044,000
Minnesota	183	202	4.7	5.2	48	47	3,897,000
Mississippi	445	400	19.5	17.7	11	17	2,281,000
Missouri	608	605	12.8	12.7	25	27	4,757,000

248

State							
Nevada	61	43	11.1	8.2	32	39	548,000
New Hampshire	52	38	6.6	4.9	44	48	791,000
New Jersey	1,075	1,208	14.6	16.4	19	20	7,361,000
New Mexico	221	194	20.0	18.2	10	16	1,106,000
New York	3,110	3,451	17.0	18.8	17	14	18,265,000
North Carolina	974	996	18.5	19.1	14	12	5,273,000
North Dakota	44	31	6.9	4.9	43	49	640,000
Ohio	1,218	1,252	11.4	11.6	31	30	10,731,000
Oklahoma	351	330	13.2	12.5	22	29	2,663,000
Oregon	239	234	10.7	10.7	33	32	2,225,000
Pennsylvania	1,689	1,772	14.2	14.9	20	22	11,902,000
Rhode Island	90	108	9.2	11.2	36	31	973,000
South Carolina	619	651	22.7	24.4	3	4	2,726,000
South Dakota	90	69	13.1	10.2	23	35	685,000
Tennessee	889	929	21.5	23.0	6	5	4,126,000
Texas	2,224	2,422	18.9	20.8	13	9	11,794,000
Utah	56	62	4.8	5.5	47	45	1,157,000
Vermont	32	36	6.9	7.8	42	41	464,000
Virginia	839	817	17.4	17.1	16	19	4,811,000
Washington	362	359	10.6	10.4	34	33	3,429,000
West Virginia	226	252	12.6	14.1	27	23	1,794,000
Wisconsin	238	240	5.2	5.3	45	46	4,569,000
Wyoming	25	20	7.1	5.8	41	44	353,000
Puerto Rico*	519	644	19.1	23.7	—	—	2,712,000

* Not included in totals.
District of Columbia is classed as a city, and is not ranked with the states.

June 12, 1974
Tuberculosis Control Division, BSS
Center for Disease Control
Atlanta, Georgia

In New York City, the new case rate was 26.6 in 1973.[4]

6. *High population densities, low living standards, and contact with tubercular persons* are considered to be among the major factors associated with a high incidence of the disease.[2]

7. One-fourth of active cases at home are not on chemotherapy, and only 37 percent of contacts are being treated, according to the 1970-1971 Annual Report of the National Tuberculosis and Respiratory Disease Association.

IV. How Many Cases of Tuberculosis Are There in the United States?

1. According to the National Health Survey, there were in the United States in 1970 *294,000 active and arrested cases of tuberculosis* reported in their Health Interview Surveys.[5]

157,000 active cases of tuberculosis, 57% of whom were under 45 years of age

137,000 cases of arrested tuberculosis, 66% of whom were over 45 years of age

2. Of these 294,000 people with active or arrested tuberculosis:

142,000 lived in the South
190,000 lived in metropolitan areas.[5]

3. Out of 23,237,000 persons in the United States reporting some activity limitation because of a chronic condition in 1970, *156,000 listed tuberculosis as the cause of their limitation.*[6]

V. How Can Tuberculosis Be Eliminated as a Public Health Menace?

1. In the United States—in addition to the traditional Public Health Service methods of TB control of case finding, tuberculin testing, X-ray screening and chemotherapy—BCG vaccination as a preventive against tuberculosis should also be

used in high incidence areas. *BCG vaccination is not being used routinely* in the United States today, as it is in other countries throughout the world.

The problem of tuberculosis in the slums and ghettos can be solved only by using all proven measures of prevention and control. These include BCG vaccination of children in the slums and ghettos in *high-incidence* areas of our American cities.

2. Two groups of people are referred to in any discussion of the tuberculosis problem:

    a. Those who are infected with the tubercle bacillus, even if they do not have active disease. These people remain at some risk of developing active disease as long as they live. The U.S. Public Health Service estimates that there are about *25 to 30 million such infected people* in the United States. *Seventy-five percent of new cases of active tuberculosis come from this group.*

    b. The second group consists of those who are *not* infected with the tubercle bacillus. Everyone is born "TB negative."[7]

The *"TB negative" can be protected by BCG vaccination* from becoming infected by the tubercle bacillus. *BCG has been found to be 80 percent effective* in the prevention of tuberculosis in this group.[9]

VI. How Many Special Tuberculosis Hospitals Are There in the United States?

1. In 1973, *64 special non-Federal tuberculosis hospitals* were listed in the United States with an *average daily census* of patients *of 4,840.*[4]

VII. What Is the Average Length of Stay of Patients in Special Tuberculosis Hospitals in the United States?

1. In 1973, the average length of stay in TB hospitals was *94 days, a 63 percent decline* from the average stay of 256 days in 1945.[4]

2. Between 1950 and 1970, the *admission rate* to these hospitals has *declined 71 percent*.[13]

VIII. What Other Hospital Facilities Are Available to Tuberculosis Patients?

1. As of June 30, 1973, there were 137 non-Federal hospitals (reporting 10 or more TB beds) with 11,721 beds available for tuberculosis—57.1 percent occupied by TB patients.[4]
2. The number of tuberculosis patients in non-Federal hospitals *had declined 78 percent* between 1965 and 1973—from an average per day of 30,798 to 6,687.[4]
3. Similarly, beds occupied by tuberculosis patients in Federal institutions *declined 75 percent* from 5,821 in 1965 to 1,469 in 1973.[4]

IX. How Much Is Tuberculosis Costing the Veterans Administration?

1. In fiscal 1972, hospital care costs plus compensation and pension benefits totaled an estimated *$154 million*.[11]

   a. There were 7,400 tuberculosis patients discharged from VA hospitals during fiscal year 1972. The average stay was 93.8 days. The average per diem cost in medical bed sections of VA hospitals was $57.83 during 1972. Thus, on the average, the hospitalization of these 7,400 patients cost the VA over $40 million in 1972.[11]

   b. 63,597 veterans were receiving compensation payments for service-connected disabilities due to tuberculosis. The average monthly value of these awards was $119 or *$90.8 million* for 1972. This does not include the costs of care of 1,581 veterans with tuberculosis who were discharged from non-VA hospitals during the same year.[11]

   c. 16,652 veterans were receiving pensions for non-service-connected disabilities due to tuberculosis, amounting to *$23.3 million* for the year (1972).[11]

2. As the number of veterans hospitalized for tuberculosis has declined, and the number of other types of pulmonary disease cases increased, the treatment of these patients has increasingly been placed under the supervision of the Medical Service under a Chief of the Pulmonary Disease Section. As of fiscal 1972, 9 VA hospitals which were still operating separate pulmonary disease services converted these services to sections under their Medical Service.[11] Since 1969, there have been no special tuberculosis hospitals in the VA system.

X. How Much Does TB Hospital Care Cost?

1. In 1973, the estimated expenses for non-Federal hospitals providing care for TB cases totaled *$155 million.*[4]

2. The per diem cost in non-Federal special tuberculosis hospitals in 1973 averaged $45. The per patient day expense for all types of hospitals caring for TB patients was $63.[4]

XI. How Much Is the U.S. Public Health Service Spending for Tuberculosis Control Programs?

1. Health department tuberculosis control programs are financed *mainly by state and local governments.* Supplementary money comes from the Federal Government through grant funding mechanism.[10]

2. *For fiscal year 1972,* the approximate amount reported to have been budgeted for *TB control programs* by state and, in a few instances, by local health departments totaled *$49,494,000,* as follows:[10]

State funds	$38,904,000—	79%
Federal funds	10,590,000—	21%
	$49,494,000—	100%

The above estimates do not include moneys expended for TB hospitalization.

XII. How Much Is the American Lung Association Spending to Support Its Programs to Aid Those Ill with Tuberculosis and Other Respiratory Diseases, Excluding Research?

For the year ended March 31, 1973, *$25,897,530* was spent by the American Lung Association (formerly the National Tuberculosis and Respiratory Disease Association and its affiliates).[14]

Community services	$13,327,939
Public education	7,148,506
Professional education and training	4,630,588
Patient services	790,497
	$25,897,530

Other support activities of the association include:

Fund raising	$10,914,025
Administrative and general expenses	3,983,956
Operating expenses (major property and equipment expenditures)	577,096
Total Expenditures	$41,372,607

Total income for the association and its affiliates for the period was $44,386,852.[14]

XIII. How Much Is Being Spent for Research Against Tuberculosis?

About *3.4 million* as follows:

1. *Veterans Administration* expenditures for research related to tuberculosis in fiscal 1974 totaled an estimated *$571,507*.[15]

Note: This total is undoubtedly understated since it does not include the dollar value of patient care in the clinical research conducted by the Veterans Administration, nor does it include the proportionate dollar value of full-time salaries

Tuberculosis

paid the investigators who are actually clinicians, and the related staffs, for research oriented activities.

2. The *American Lung Association* and its affiliate associations spent $1,654,000 for the year ended March 31, 1973, for research and fellowships in the area of tuberculosis as well as other respiratory diseases.[14]

3. The *National Institute of Allergy and Infectious Diseases* of the U.S. Public Health Service is spending about *$1.2 million* (fiscal 1974) for tuberculosis research.

4. In contrast to the $3.4 million currently being spent for research to find the answers to tuberculosis:

Tuberculosis cost the Veterans Administration in 1972 an estimated	$154 million
The costs of care in special tuberculosis hospitals alone in 1972 totaled	$155 million
	$309 million

XIV. How Has Medical Research Paid Off Against Tuberculosis?

1. Decline in the death rate from tuberculosis

Between 1945 and 1973, the *tuberculosis death rate has declined 95 percent*—due in major part to the medical research discovery of the effectiveness of streptomycin in 1945 and isoniazid in 1952. PAS has also been used in combination with these drugs.

2. Decline in number of cases

New active cases of tuberculosis reported *declined 64 percent* between 1952 (the year isoniazid was discovered) and 1973.

The Veterans Administration no longer operates any special TB hospitals because of the decline in the number of patients.

3. Decline in TB bed occupancy

The average daily census of patients in non-Federal TB hospitals has declined 78 percent between 1946 and 1970 (from 55,000 to 12,000).[12] Many patients whose disease is discovered soon enough do not have to go to the hospital at all. Hospitalization for other patients has been slashed from years to weeks.

a. Tuberculosis can now be controlled and prevented by the drug isoniazid. *A year* of pill taking is effective treatment. However, *one* BCG vaccination *prevents* the disease in 80 percent of people.

b. A new antituberculosis drug is now available called *Rifampin*. A number of recent studies have shown that Rifampin, used in combination with isoniazid, is one of the most promising new drugs in the primary treatment of tuberculosis. It is also effective in the treatment of drug-resistant TB.[16]

XV. *How Widely Used is BCG Vaccine in Other Countries?*

1. Between 15 and 20 million infectious cases of tuberculosis are in the world today. More than 80 percent of the world's tuberculosis sufferers are in the developing countries.[17]

BCG vaccination programs have been widely employed. BCG vaccination gives long lasting and substantial protection against tuberculosis under conditions prevailing in developing countries.[17]

2. Studies by the Medical Research Council of Great Britain established definitely, as a result of 10-year trials, that BCG is about 80 percent effective in the prevention of tuberculosis.[9] This preventive benefit lasts, among the vaccinated, from 10 to 15 years.

In other words, people who are given BCG vaccination are *5 times safer from tuberculosis infection* than those who have not been vaccinated.

3. BCG vaccination has been used for more than a quarter of a century in Japan, Norway, Sweden, Canada, Great Britain, India, and France, all of which have found BCG vaccination about 80 percent effective in preventing tuberculosis.

4. BCG vaccination programs are now in operation in most countries of the world, the majority of the programs being

assisted by the World Health Organization and usually by UNICEF also.

In 1972, some 12 million children were vaccinated in the Western Pacific Region, and in countries where vaccination is part of the national tuberculosis control program, the coverage of the susceptible population (generally speaking from preschool age to adolescence) was high enough to make an epidemiological impact in the years to come. High priority is also being given to BCG vaccination in countries of the African Region.

Many BCG vaccination programs are being combined with smallpox vaccination campaigns and have achieved high coverage of the susceptible population. Such combined campaigns have become possible since the adoption of the practice of direct BCG vaccination (without prior tuberculin testing), which can be carried out in one operation, since it has been shown that simultaneous BCG and smallpox vaccination is both harmless and effective.[17]

THE PARADOX OF BCG

(Editorial from the *New England Journal of Medicine*, September 1969)

The Great American Public accepts docilely, even enthusiastically, the recommendation of its pediatricians and public-health authorities, who propose routine immunization of children against three bacterial and five viral infections. Two of these five (mumps and rubella vaccines) are quite new, and one, smallpox vaccine (directed against a disease absent from this country for the past 20 years), is annually implicated in at least seven to 12 deaths. And yet a live, attenuated vaccine against tuberculosis, in use since 1922, holds little appeal in this country. One wonders exactly why.

Tuberculosis is still very much with us: over 40,000 new active cases of tuberculosis were reported in the United States last year. Granted that some 30,000 of these must, according to statistics, have developed in persons infected many years ago, another 10,000 or so developed in people infected only recently; at least some of those might have been prevented or minimized by the use of BCG.

The effectiveness of BCG has been proved past a shadow of a doubt in enormous, well controlled clinical trials, such as those of Aronson in American Indians, Frimodt-Moller in India and of the Medical Research Council in Great Britain. BCG vaccine presents practically no hazard: for safety, only polio vaccine is in the same league.

The objection that BCG vaccine produces hypersensitivity of a high enough order to render subsequent tuberculin tests useless for case finding is not borne out by the observations of many investigators, who have rather consistently shown marked waning of tuberculin reactivity within the year after inoculation with BCG, without, however, loss of the vaccine's protective power.

Even the proponents of BCG have never advocated its use in the United States for other than certain high-risk groups, such as hospital and laboratory workers, for military personnel and for children and adolescents perforce living in households or neighborhoods where they stand considerable chance of exposure to infectious tuberculosis. . . .

Despite its drawbacks, until a better vaccine has been developed and tested, BCG will no doubt continue to be one of the most widely used vaccines in the world. Sophisticated analysis by the biomathematicians of the WHO Tuberculosis Program show that, for great areas of the world, BCG is the only effective and economically feasible approach to tuberculosis control.

For countries such as ours, however, dedicated to elimination of tuberculosis rather than mere control, small, well designed BCG programs for individuals and groups at high risk should be used intensively to limit transmission of virulent tubercle bacilli to a potential new young reservoir of tuberculosis infection.

Notes

1. National Center for Health Statistics, U.S. Public Health Service, Department of Health, Education, and Welfare, Rockville, Md.
2. *Current Status of TB in the U.S.*, Statistical Bulletin, Metropolitan Life Insurance Company, New York, N. Y., January 1974.
3. *Goals and Standards for Eliminating Tuberculosis.* Statement of a committee appointed by the U.S. Public Health Service. Published by the National Tuberculosis and Respiratory Diseases Association, November 1960.
4. Information supplied by Tuberculosis Control Division, U.S. Public Health Service, Center for Disease Control, Atlanta, Ga.
5. *Prevalence of Selected Chronic Respiratory Conditions—United States —1970*, Series 10, no. 84. Data from the National Center for Health Statistics, U.S. Department of Health, Education, and Welfare, Rockville, Md., September 1973.
6. *Facts of Life and Death.* National Center for Health Statistics, Department of Health, Education, and Welfare, Rockville, Md.
7. Hearings before the U.S. Senate Appropriations Subcommittee for the Department of Health, Education, and Welfare, 91st Congress, 1st Session, fiscal year 1970, page 983.
8. Hearings before the U.S. House of Representatives Appropriations Subcommittee for the Department of Health, Education, and Welfare, 91st Congress, 2nd Session, fiscal year 1971, pt. 2, p. 849.
9. "BCG and Vole Bacillus Vaccines in the Prevention of Tuberculosis in Adolescence and Early Adult Life," Third Report to the Medical Research Council by their Tuberculosis Vaccines Clinical Trials Committee. Reprinted from the *British Medical Journal* 1:973–978 (April 13, 1963).
10. *Tuberculosis Programs 1972,* Tuberculosis Branch, Bureau of State Services, Center for Disease Control, U.S. Public Health Service, Atlanta, Ga. Published November 1973.
11. 1972 Annual Report of the Administrator of Veterans Affairs, Veterans Administration, Washington, D.C.
12. *Hospitals,* pt. 2, August 1971, Guide Issue, published by the American Hospital Association, Chicago, Ill.
13. *Statistical Abstract of the United States, 1972,* 93rd ed., U.S. Bureau of the Census, Washington, D.C.

14. 1973–74 Annual Report of the American Lung Association (formerly the National Tuberculosis and Respiratory Disease Association), New York, N. Y.
15. Information from Research Service, Department of Medicine and Surgery, Veterans Administration, Washington, D.C.
16. Irving Selikoff, M.D., Mount Sinai Medical School, New York, N.Y., personal communication, August 1974.
17. Information from the World Health Organization, United Nations, New York, N. Y.

Medical Research—
Does It Pay Off in Lives and Dollars?

I. How Has Medical Research Progress Aided in Reducing Deaths?

Medical research progress in the development and improvement of the antibiotics for the treatment of infectious diseases, the development of the antihypertensive drugs, as well as the development of vaccines and other improved methods of treatment, has achieved dramatic declines in the death rates from these diseases.

	1963–1973 *Percent Decline*
Polio (due to vaccines)	100%
Whooping cough (due to vaccine)	100%
Dysentery (due to use of antibiotics)	100%
Tuberculosis (due to use of antibiotics & other drugs)	62%
Maternal deaths (due to use of antibiotics)	58%
Hypertensive heart disease (with or without renal disease) (due to antihypertensive drugs)	57%
Appendicitis (due to use of antibiotics)	55%
Asthma (due to use of cortisone)	53%
Syphilis (due to use of antibiotics)	50%
Nephritis and nephrosis (due to use of antibiotics)	37%
Acute rheumatic fever and chronic rheumatic heart disease (due to use of antibiotics)	35%
Infant deaths (due to use of antibiotics)	30%
Meningitis (due to use of antibiotics)	27%
Pneumonia (due to use of antibiotics)	24%

II. How Many Years Have Been Added to the Average Life Expectancy of Americans?

Life expectancy for Americans *increased 8 years* between 1943 and 1973—from 63.3 years in 1943 to an estimated 71.3 years in 1973.

Since 1900, life expectancy has *increased 22 years.*

LIFE EXPECTANCY (IN YEARS)

Year	Total	White Male	White Female	Nonwhite Male	Nonwhite Female
1943	63.3	63.2	65.7	55.4	56.1
1953	68.8	66.8	72.9	59.7	64.4
1963	69.9	67.5	74.4	60.9	66.5
1971	71.1	68.3	75.8	61.6	69.7
1972	71.1	68.3	75.9	61.5	69.9
1973	71.3	68.4	76.1	61.9	70.0

SOURCE: Vital Statistics Division, National Center for Health Statistics, U.S. Public Health Service.

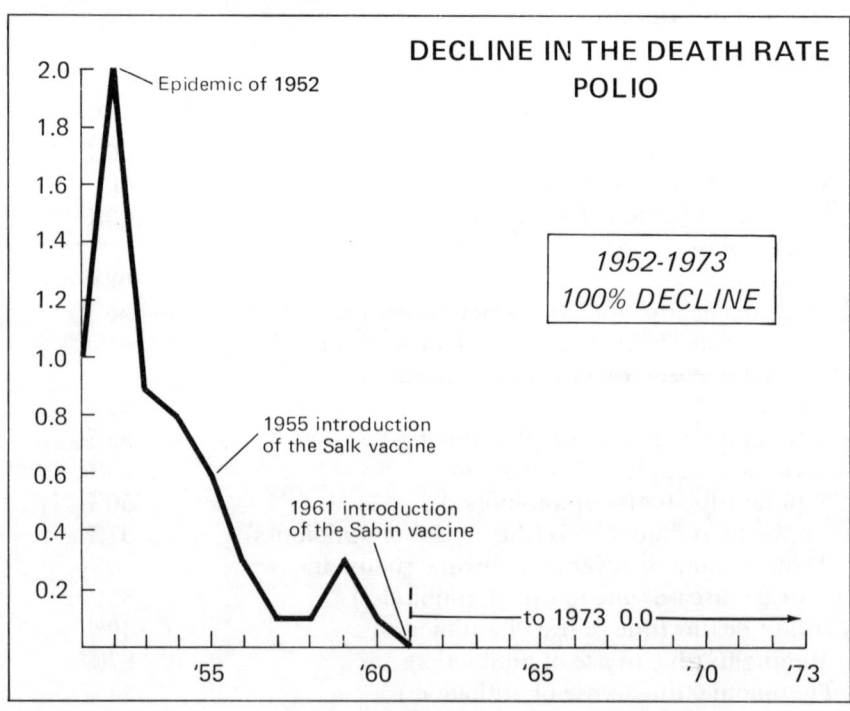

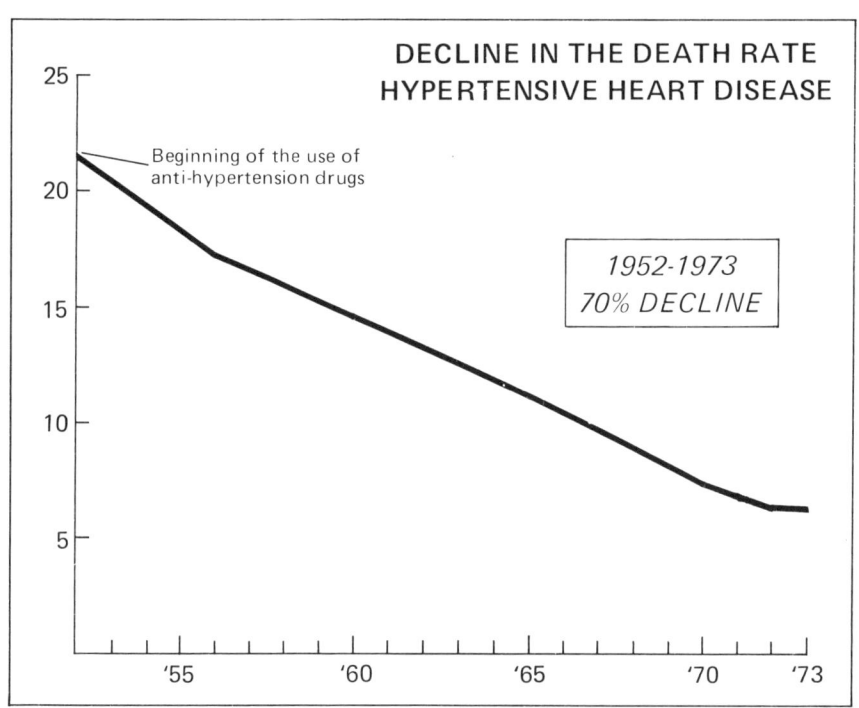

CRUDE DEATH RATE PER 100,000 POPULATION

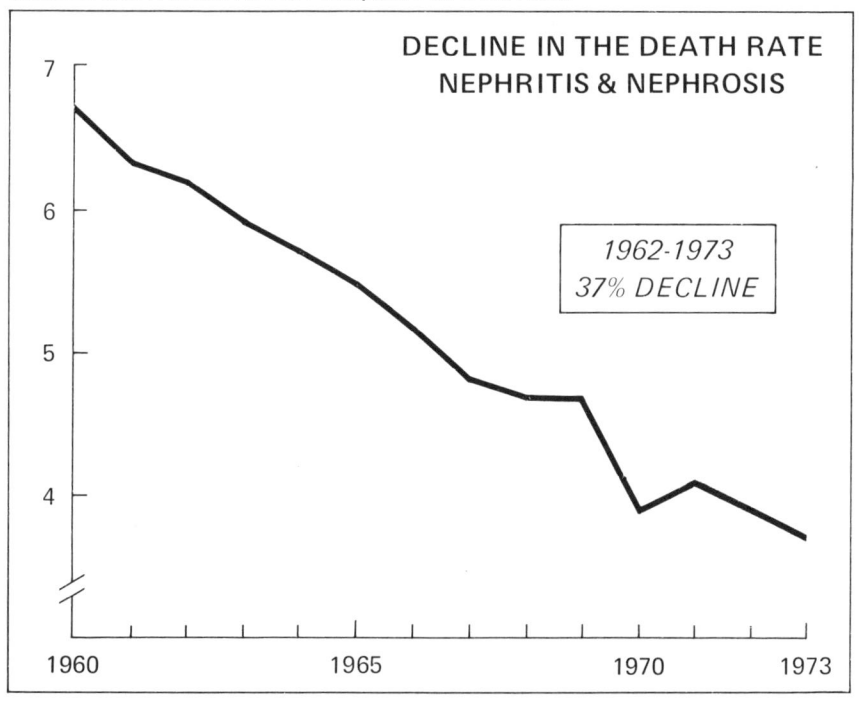

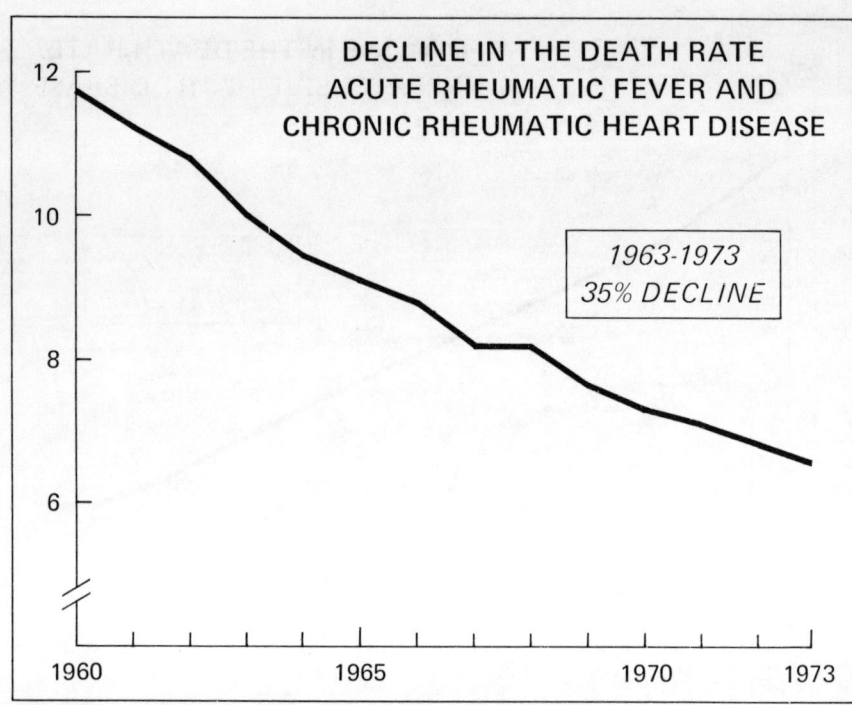

CRUDE DEATH RATE PER 100,000 POPULATION

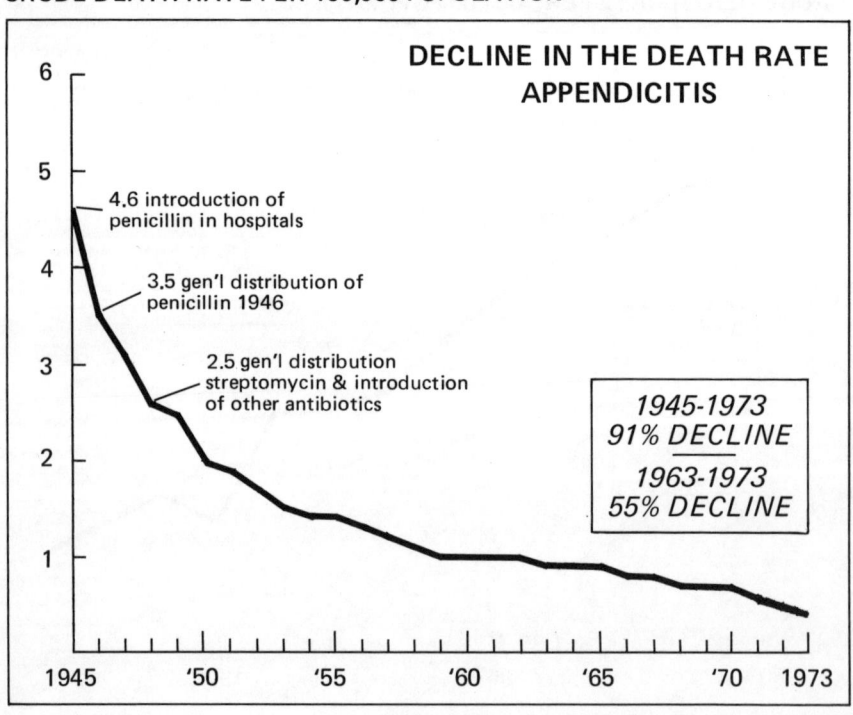

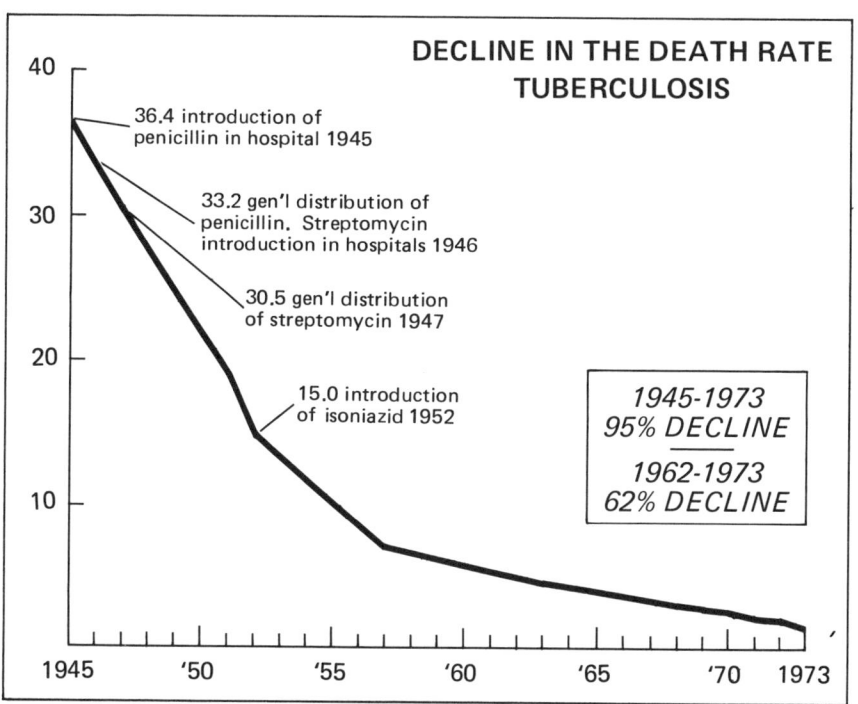

CRUDE DEATH RATE PER 100,000 POPULATION

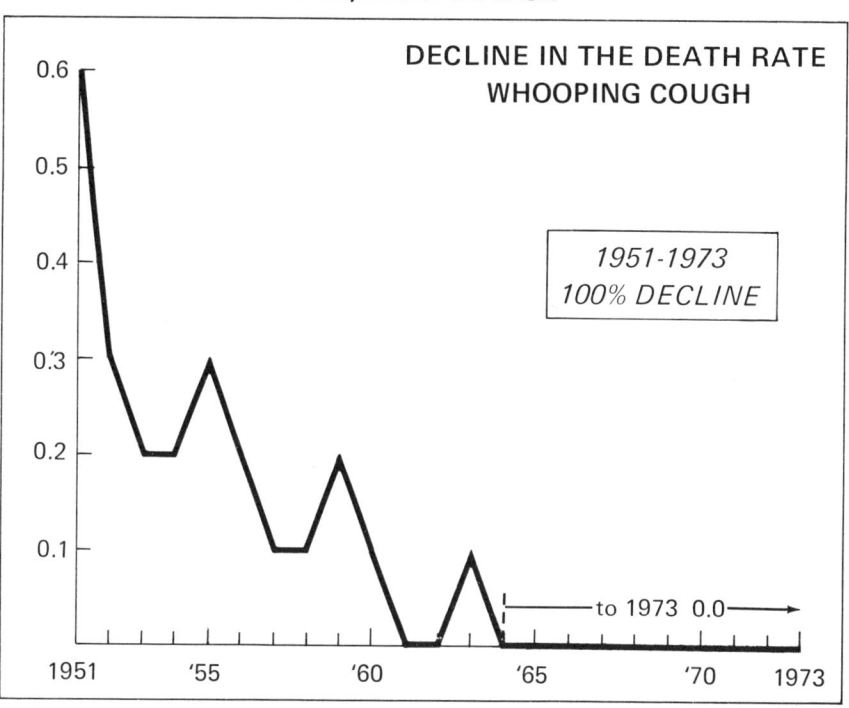

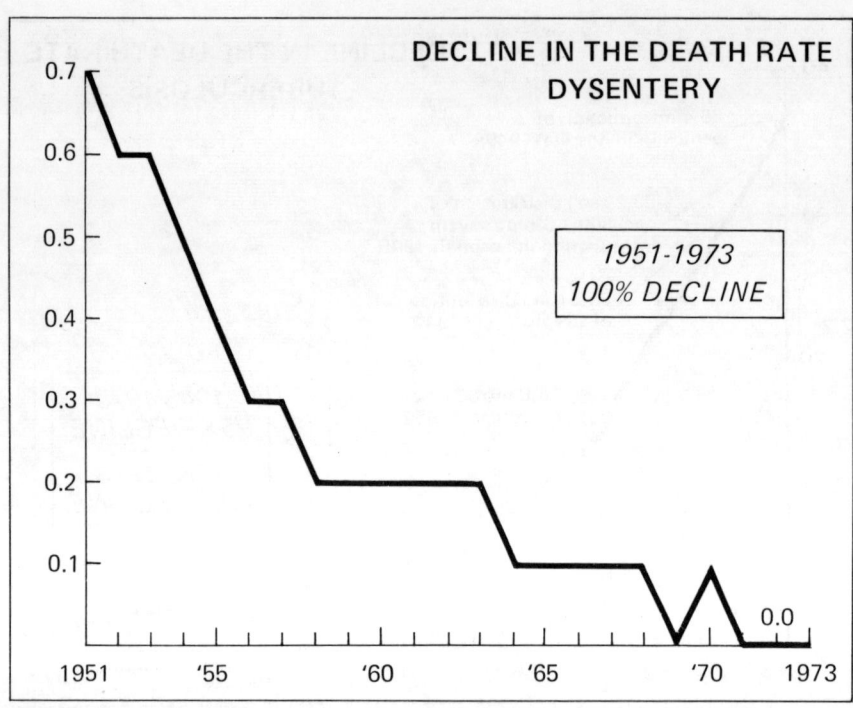

CRUDE DEATH RATE PER 100,000 POPULATION

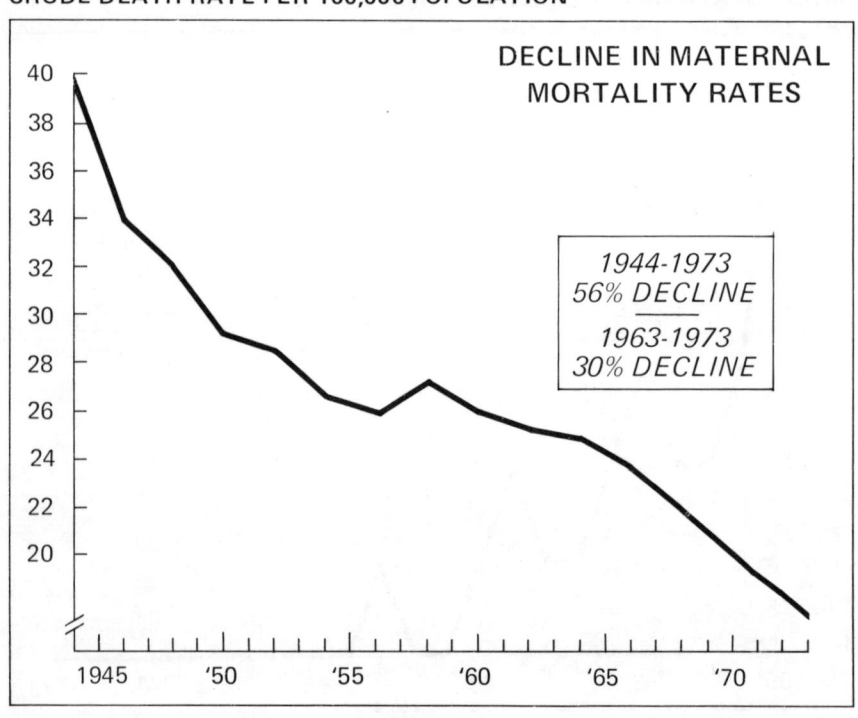

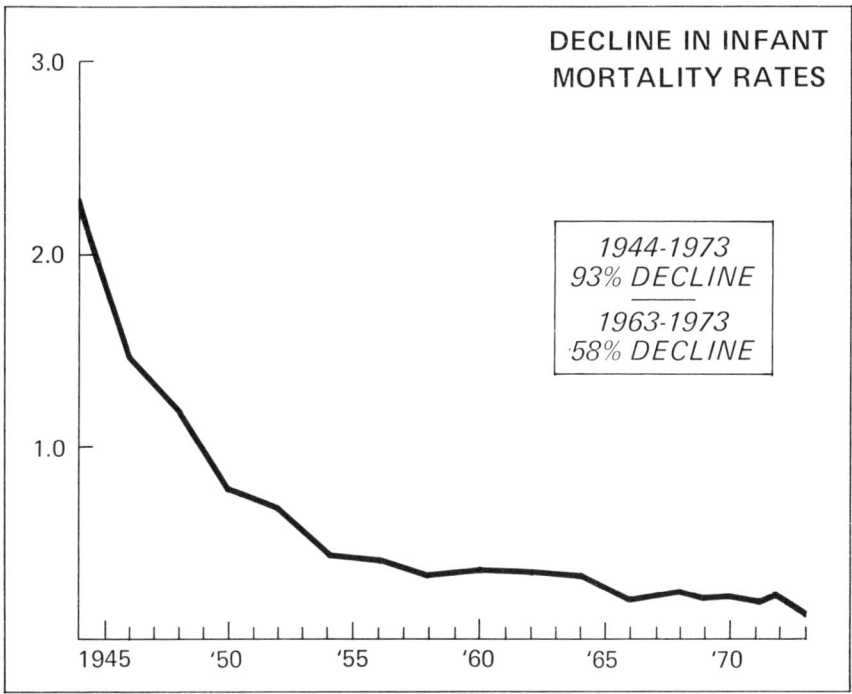

(Per 1000 Live Births)

The median age at death has increased 7.2 years from 63.4 years in 1943 to 70.6 years in 1971.

These added years of life, as well as the reduction in disabilities achieved through medical research advances, are certainly a major factor in the increase in our gross national product, which is almost 6 times greater than it was in 1945—from $211.9 billion in 1945 to $1,220.1 billion in 1972–73 (estimated).[18]

Medical advances are based on medical research breakthroughs supported by voluntary health agencies, the National Institutes of Health of the Department of Health, Education, and Welfare, and the pharmaceutical industry.

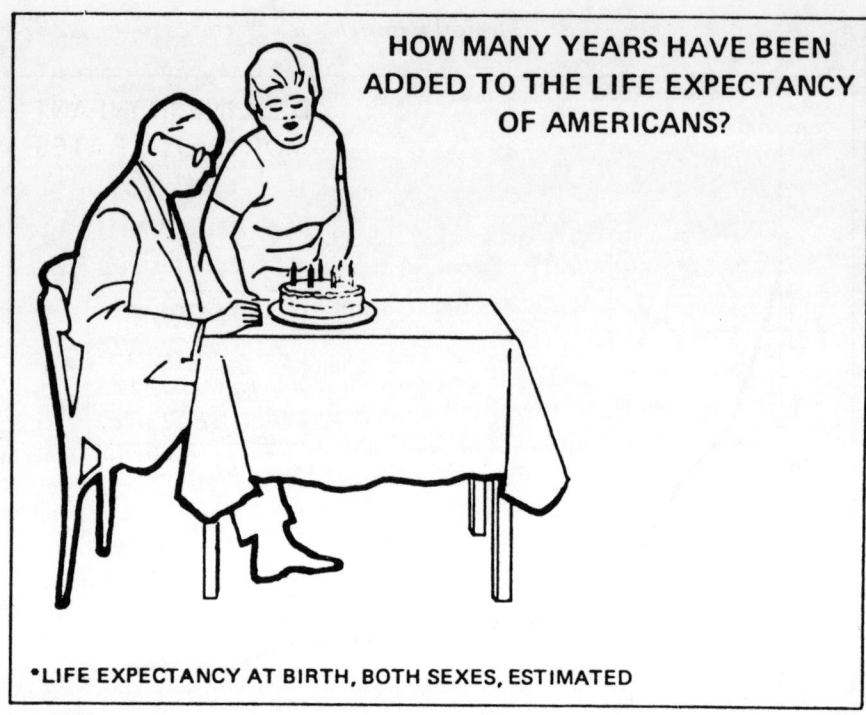
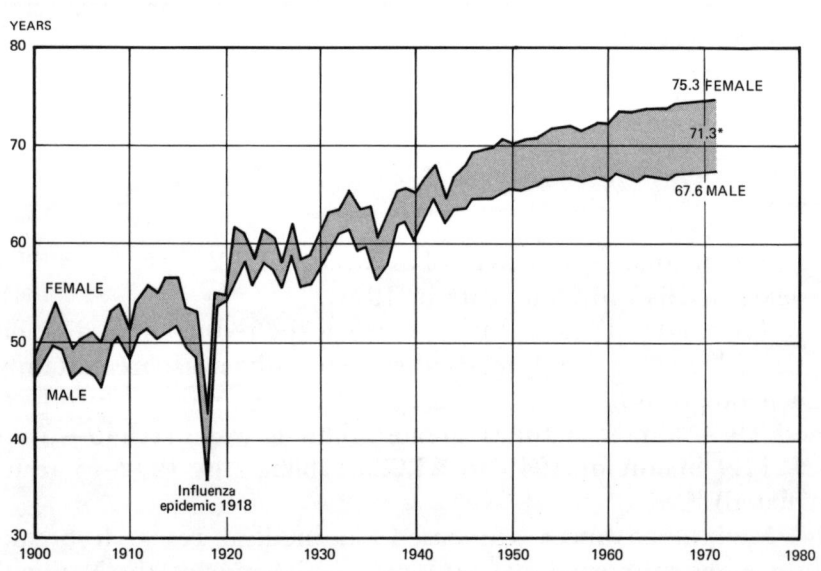
*Life expectancy at birth, both sexes, estimated.

III. How Has Medical Research Reduced Disabilities?

1. DECLINE IN STATE MENTAL HOSPITAL POPULATION

Following the advent of the psychiatric drugs in 1955, the number of patients confined to custodial institutions has been reduced 55 percent—from 558,000 in 1955 to 248,562 in 1973.[1]

Dollar Savings[2]

Between 1945 and 1955, the over-all rise in the number of patients in state mental hospitals averaged 13,000 a year.

If this average annual patient increase had continued through 1973, *234,000 more beds* would have been required at a unit cost of $20,000 and an *overall cost of $4.7 billion.*

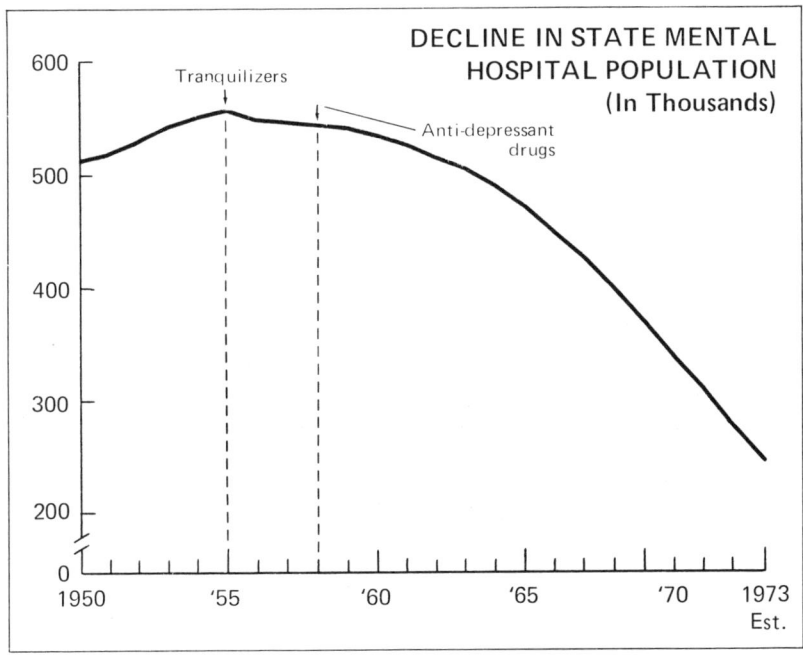

270 THE KILLERS AND CRIPPLERS

This $4.7 billion saving in bed construction costs does not include the additional reductions in patient care costs to the states which have been realized through the reduction of hospitalized mentally ill.

1. What is the outlook for patient population reductions by 1980?

A forecast made in 1963 to the effect that within 10 years there would be a 50 percent reduction in state mental hospital populations has now been achieved. It is now anticipated that by 1980, if the present rate of decline can be maintained, there will probably be a *two-thirds reduction* in the hospitalized

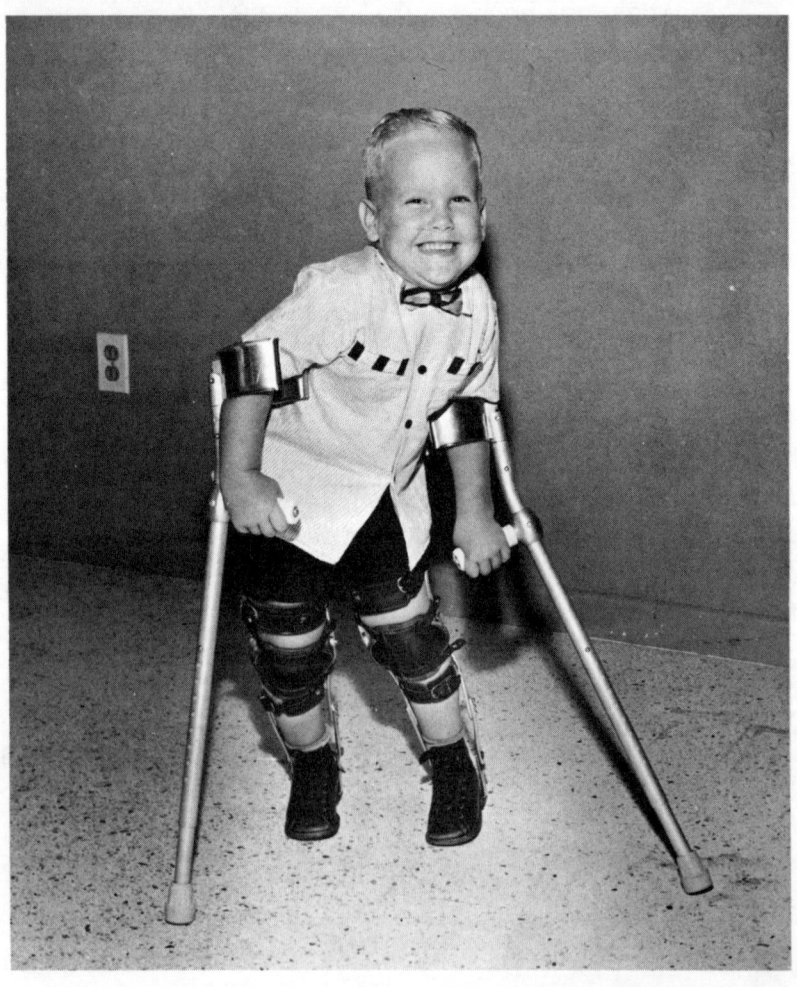

mentally ill. This means that the state mental hospital population will be reduced to 186,000 rather than 880,000, which would have been the projected population based on trends prior to 1955.[2]

Concomitant with the decline in state mental hospital populations is the increase in readmissions to outpatient clinics rather than to the mental hospitals, so that the patients remain with their families rather than going to distant mental hospitals.[2]

2. What has been the decline in the number of polio cases?

In 1952, 57,879 polio cases were reported; in 1970, only 33 cases of acute poliomyelitis were reported—*an almost 100 percent decline* from 1952.[3] This decline is due to the discovery and use of polio vaccines.

3. What has been the decline in the incidence of measles?

Until 1963, there was no vaccine available for measles, a common disease that once killed 500 children each year and left others with lasting handicaps, including hearing disorders and mental retardation.

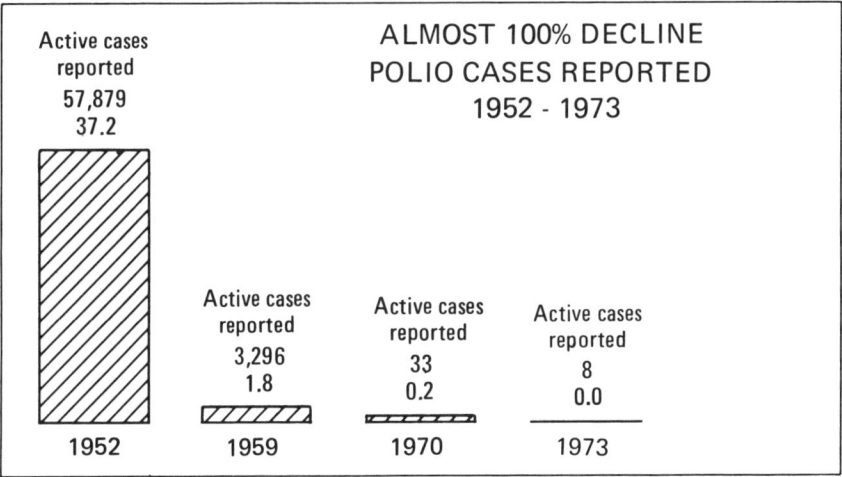

THE NUMBER OF CASES OF POLIO REPORTED DROPPED DRAMATICALLY FOLLOWING THE INTRODUCTION OF POLIO VACCINE IN 1952

The first measles vaccine became available in the spring of 1963. Since its introduction, the measles vaccine has *saved* an estimated *2,400 lives* (one in 10,000 cases), *prevented 8,000 cases* of *mental retardation* (one in 3,000 cases) and *averted 140,000 hospitalizations.*

If one considers that this represents 78 million schooldays saved and 12 million doctor visits averted, the monetary equivalent of these savings totals about *$1.3 billion.*[43]

4. What about the vaccine against German Measles (Rubella)?

Nearly 20,000 U.S. infants suffered congenital defects from the 1964 epidemic of German measles. An almost equal amount of fetal deaths were recorded. In 1969, a new vaccine was introduced and is being used on a national basis.[5]

The vaccine is strongly recommended for all boys and girls between the ages of 1 year and puberty, to reduce the possibility of exposure to German measles by pregnant women.

5. What has been the decline in the number of reported cases of tuberculosis?

In 1952, 85,607 active cases of tuberculosis were reported. In 1970, an estimated 37,137 active cases were reported—*a decline of 57 percent.*[3]

6. What is the decline in TB deaths?

Since the distribution of streptomycin, which began in 1946, the *TB death rate has declined 95 percent.* Following the discovery of the effectiveness of isoniazid (in combination with PAS) as a treatment for TB in 1952, the death rate declined (between 1952 and 1973) 89 percent.

7. What is the most important medical advance so far in recent years?

Without doubt, the discovery of the usefulness of a reliable contraceptive pill, such as Enovid and others, is the most practical medical advance in recent years. Since 1960, this breakthrough has made it possible for families to have children by

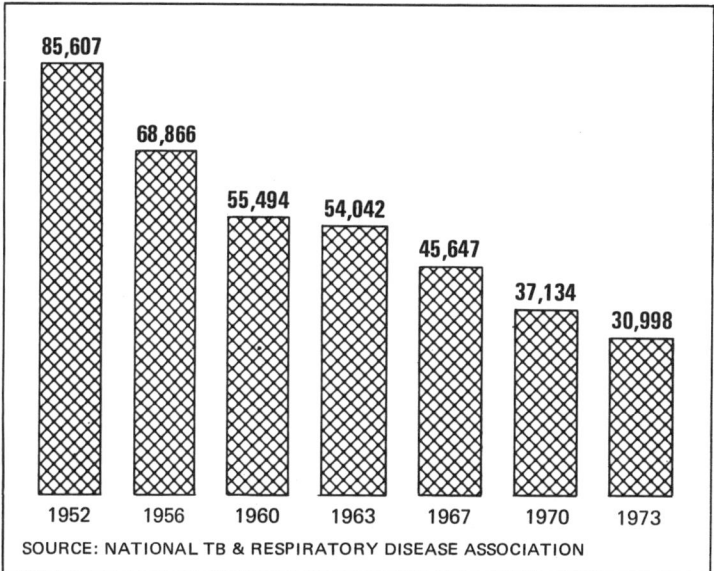

DECLINE IN NEW ACTIVE CASES OF TUBERCULOSIS

1952	1956	1960	1963	1967	1970	1973
85,607	68,866	55,494	54,042	45,647	37,134	30,998

SOURCE: NATIONAL TB & RESPIRATORY DISEASE ASSOCIATION

choice and not by chance, when they are physically and economically capable of caring for their children.

Although there are side effects to the pills, they are not commensurate with the tragic consequences of unwanted children for whom families cannot provide nor the grave risk frequently associated with pregnancy in women not physically capable of having or caring for additional children.

The birth rate in the United States (per 1,000 population) has declined over 36 percent—from 23.7 in 1960 to an estimated 15.0 in 1973.

IV. What Are the Major Research Payoffs and Developments?

1. In the treatment of arteriosclerosis of the heart (main cause of heart attack):

a. Approximately 50 percent of deaths from myocardial infarction occur before the patient reaches the hospital. Most of these sudden deaths are presumed to be due to *arrhythmias* (disturbances in heart rhythm).

If the patients can be reached by a specially equipped and staffed *intensive-care ambulance,* or if they have reached an *intensive-care unit in a hospital* (coronary care unit), *many of these arrhythmias can be controlled by medication, including Lidocaine and Procaine Amid, as well as digitalis and quinidine as indicated, or by D-C shock therapy.*[6]

Marked improvement in resuscitation after cardiac arrest has also been accomplished. All acute myocardial infarction cases should be monitored during the first 5 to 7 days in order to recognize the serious arrhythmias in time to provide effective treatment. Each of the above-mentioned life-saving refinements is the result of intensive research.[6]

Coronary-care units can effectively reduce in-hospital death from heart attack by about 30 percent. An estimated 50,000 lives could be saved annually if all heart attack victims received specialized coronary care promptly.[25]

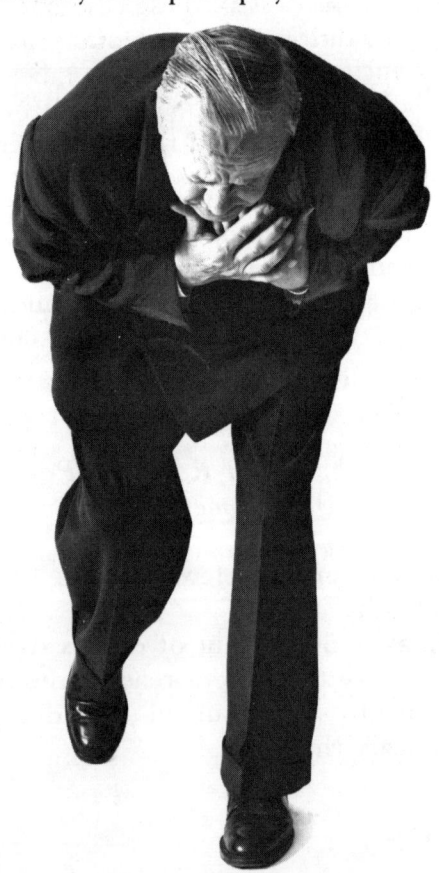

b. What Is the Present Status of Anticoagulants?

Anticoagulant therapy does not affect the development of these early serious arrhythmias. However, thromboembolic complications continue to occur during the acute phases of myocardial infarction and for the prevention of these, anticoagulant therapy is indicated.

Continued experience has served to emphasize the principle that *oral anticoagulant drugs are effective only if adequate dosage is administered. For patients who survive the first two days, the complications and the mortality rate are reduced by the administration of adequate anticoagulant dosage.*[32][33]

With the recent developments in the techniques of intensive care and the early ambulation for uncomplicated cases of myocardial infarction, the death rate has been lowered to the point where anticoagulant therapy does not further lower the death rate during the acute process in these cases. However, recent studies have confirmed that anticoagulant therapy does significantly reduce the incidence of venous thrombosis, pulmonary emboli, and embolic strokes, and is therefore warranted in most cases, especially those with a thromboembolic history as well as those who for whatever reason remain in bed five days or longer.[38][39]

c. What Research Progress Has Been Made in Cardiac Surgery?

Important advances have been made in the techniques and hardware now utilized in cardiac surgery.[19]

i. About 51,000 patients received *open heart surgery* in the United States in 1971. With new type valve replacements and anticoagulant therapy, a high percentage of these patients are enjoying a life which would otherwise be denied them.

ii. The introduction of the *coronary bypass procedure,* usually using a saphenous vein, has greatly broadened the potential application of cardiac surgery.

In 1971, approximately 22,500 procedures were done (44 percent of all open heart surgery) and it is probable that both this number and percentage were considerably higher in 1973.

iii. Since 1959 in the United States approximately 120,000

(or more) *pacemakers* have been implanted, and with these, 90,000 patients are still living. Since their average age was 70, this indicates significant progress in their outlook.

2. What are the payoffs in hypertension?

Since 1952, and the development of antihypertension drugs, the *death rate from hypertensive disease has declined more than 65 percent,*[7] but more strokes and heart failures could be prevented by intensive screening and treatment of high blood pressure in the adult population.

The results of the Framingham Study show that the *risk of every manifestation of coronary heart disease,* including angina, coronary insufficiency, myocardial infarction, and sudden death, *is distinctly and impressively related to the antecedent level of both systolic and diastolic blood pressure.*[37]

An earlier and more vigorous attack against this potent contributor to cardiovascular mortality and morbidity could have a major impact in reducing the incidence of clinical manifestations of arteriosclerosis, such as coronary heart disease.[37]

Dr. Theodore Cooper, formerly Director of the National Heart and Lung Institute and now Assistant Secretary for Health, Department of Health, Education, and Welfare, has estimated that a successful campaign in the public health sector for the detection and treatment of high blood pressure would result within 2 to 3 years in the *averting of about 200,000 deaths from stroke, heart attack, kidney failure, and heart failure per year.*

3. What are the payoffs in cancer?

a. Chemotherapy is now the key factor responsible for long-term survival in a number of types of widespread cancer occurring most frequently in children, adolescents, and young adults.[12]

Cancers Highly Responsive to Chemotherapy[12]
1. Choriocarcinoma
2. Retinoblastoma
3. Wilms' tumor (tumor of the kidney in children)
4. Hodgkin's disease
5. Acute lymphocytic leukemia

6. Lymphosarcoma
7. Mycosis fungoides
8. Embryonal testicular cancer
9. Ewing's sarcoma
10. Rhabdomyosarcoma
11. Burkitt's tumor

b. In many other cases, chemotherapy, while not yet curative in advanced metastatic disease, has delayed the progression of the disease and therefore prolonged survival.

This is true in *breast cancer* and *cancer of the prostate,* with the use of estrogen preparations in cancer of the prostate and the use of combinations of drugs and steroids in breast cancer, depending on the type of tumor and the age of the patient.

c. Forty-four drugs are now beginning to be used against 33 types of cancer.[8]

d. *Local chemotherapy* (5-FU in a salve, called Efudex) was recently introduced for the treatment of precancerous keratoses and *superficial skin cancers.* This form of therapy has been proven successful in thousands of patients. It is particularly valuable for the management of multiple extensive epithelio-

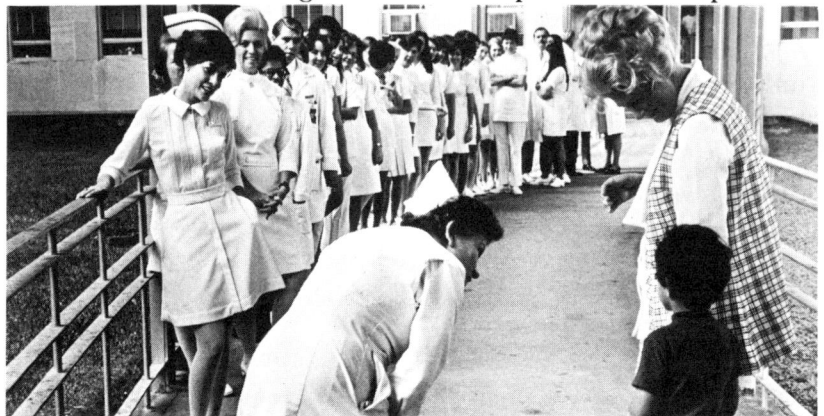

Doctors, nurses, technicians, and other staff members at Charity Hospital, New Orleans, are visited by young James Kole, who had spent his infancy in the hospital, a victim of a rare and generally fatal cancer in children. Fifteen-year-old Rhonda Kole, a volunteer at the hospital, captivated by the baby, had asked her parents' permission to bring the infant home for a weekend. The weekend never ended. The child was adopted by jazz pianist Ronnie Kole and his wife. Now in his sixth year, James is an active, normal boy. (COURTESY OF AMERICAN CANCER SOCIETY, INC., NEW YORK)

mas covering large portions of the body surface, which could not be adequately treated by other methods. Local chemotherapy is now being widely used as the first practical chemical treatment for the most common neoplasm in man.[14]

A cream containing an anticancer drug (5-FU) is applied to the area containing the lesions. The tumors undergo selective inflammatory reactions which result in their disappearance without serious side effects on the normal skin or other tissues. The selective effect on tumors permits healing with minimal and usually no scar formation.[14]

Lesions that are too small to be otherwise diagnosed react and undergo resolution. Early lesions are therefore cured before they become more serious clinical problems. Thus the subsequent incidence of tumors is reduced. Local chemotherapy therefore permits prevention, diagnosis, and cure of precancerous and malignant tumors.[14]

The results indicate that chemical agents can be selective for the destruction of malignant cells without causing serious effects on normal cells.[14]

e. Immunology

For the first time immunological methods have been used successfully for the treatment of precancerous and malignant tumors by inducing delayed hypersensitivity reactions in neoplasms of the skin.

Prevention, early diagnosis of clinically not diagnosed lesions, and cures lasting for more than 5 years have been accomplished by immunotherapy in more than 50 patients with extensive premalignant keratoses, superficial basal cell carcinomas, and squamous carcinomas in situ.

The immune response is induced by chemical agents that produce an allergy (delayed hypersensitivity) in the skin. This results in tumor destruction without adverse effect on the normal tissues. Immunotherapy has been shown to be associated with specific cell-mediated immunity predominantly due to hypersensitivity. The hypersensitivity reaction can be transferred from sensitized to nonsensitized patients by white blood cells.[14]

The selective curative effect of immunotherapy indicates

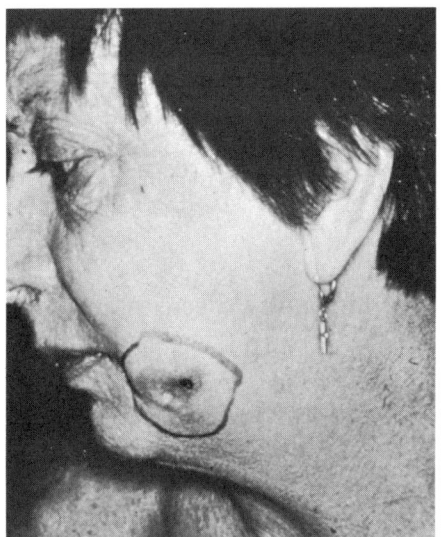 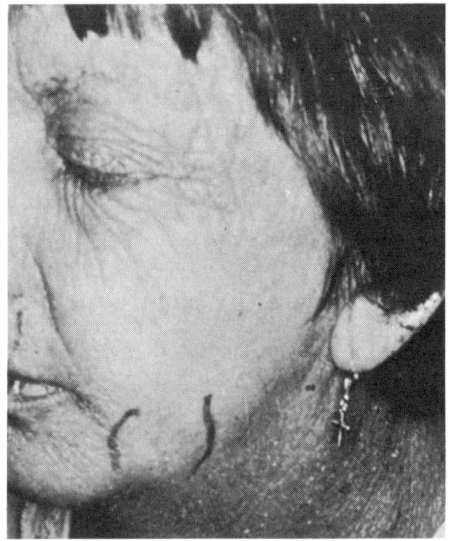

(Figure on left)
Lesion diagnosed as reticulum cell sarcoma in patient with mycosis fungoides. This cancerous lesion has resisted all known forms of treatment.

(Figure on right)
Same area as shown left, one month following administration of concentrated monocytes obtained from peripheral human blood. Lesion has disappeared and there has been no recurrence for observation period of two years.

(COURTESY EDMUND KLEIN, M.D., DEPARTMENT OF DERMATOLOGY, ROSWELL PARK MEMORIAL INSTITUTE, BUFFALO, NEW YORK)

that the body immune defense mechanisms can be induced to reject some cancers without adverse effects.[14]

f. *Leukemia and Hodgkin's Disease*

Chemotherapy (intensive treatment with drugs, often in combinations) of acute leukemia, Burkitt's tumor and Hodgkin's disease is producing a much higher percentage of long-term remissions and probable cures than conventional therapy with single agents or low-dose combination therapy.[9]

Drugs developed in recent years which have proved useful and life-saving include vincristine, methotrexate, daunomycin, cytoxan, mercaptopurine, adriamycin and cytosine arabinoside.[9]

The median survival time for children with acute leukemia has increased from just under four months prior to 1947 to approximately three years. Many patients have survived more than 5 years from the diagnosis of their disease—some show no evidence of disease 8 to 20 years after the first diagnosis.[9]

4. What are the payoffs in virus diseases?

Oral vaccines against adenovirus types 4 and 7—common causes of respiratory disease among military recruits—have been developed. Both vaccines appear to be 95 percent effective, thus saving millions of dollars in hospitalization costs and training time.[40]

5. What are the payoffs in arthritis, metabolic diseases and diabetes?

a. Arthritis

Among the newer treatments for rheumatoid arthritis developed in recent years are:[20]

    i. *Phenylbutazone*—an anti-inflammatory agent that alleviates pain in many types of arthritis, especially in spondylitis and gout. However, not all arthritics will benefit from it and a good many will experience undesirable side reactions.

    ii. *Antimalarial drugs*—certain compounds such as chloroquine, which have been developed against malaria, are used in the treatment of rheumatoid arthritis and systemic lupus erythematosus. Care must be taken in their use because of possible systemic toxic effects, including ocular involvement.

    iii. *Indomethacin (Indocin)*—a relatively new anti-inflammatory drug which may relieve certain symptoms associated with rheumatoid arthritis.

    iv. *Steroid hormones*—Cortisone and related steroid drugs are a special problem. They can bring about sensational reduction of pain and inflammation in a matter of hours, but they have been found to have serious side effects, sometimes worse than the rheumatoid disease. Also, they do not stop the disease process; they merely hide the fact that joint damage is still going on. So, although they are useful in special situations, they are being prescribed less and less often by arthritis specialists today in the routine treatment of rheumatoid arthritis.

v. An operation, developed by Dr. John Charnley of Lancaster, England, is now widely used by leading orthopedic surgeons in the United States. The operation involves *complete reconstruction of the hip joint* to relieve arthritis of the hip. This operation is successful in the majority of cases, and represents one of the greatest recent advances in arthritis treatment.

b. *What Has Research Discovered for Gout?*

The acute painful attacks of gout can be controlled quite well with several drugs now available, particularly colchicine, phenylbutazone, and indomethacin. Also, allopurinol, probenecid, and sulfinpyrazone now can be prescribed in long-term treatment to prevent the excessive accumulation of uric acid. Early treatment is important. If the gouty patient closely follows his treatment regimen, he can lead a virtually normal life free of the pain and complications of this form of arthritis.[20]

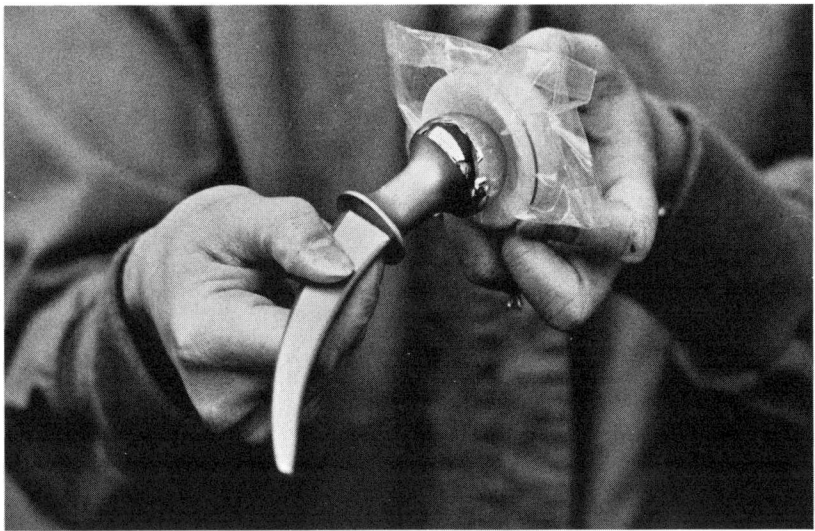

One of the greatest recent advances in arthritis treatment has been the development of new procedures for "total hip replacement." The artificial hip joint consists of a lower half—to be cemented into the femur—made of vitallium, with a polished ball-like top. The upper half is a cup made of polyethylene that functions as a socket and is cemented into the pelvic bone. (COURTESY OF THE ARTHRITIS FOUNDATION, NEW YORK)

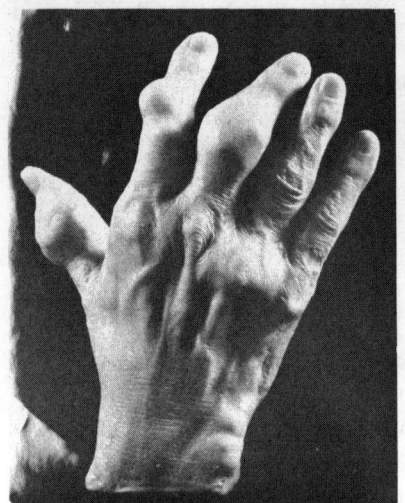 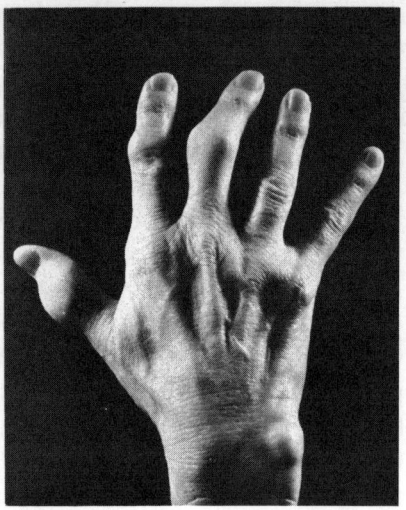

Left: *This is the hand of a person suffering from gout, one of the forms of arthritis. Lumps on fingers and knuckles are caused by excess of uric acid leading to formation of urate crystals around the joints.* Right: *The same hand after treatment with uricosuric agents. If left untreated, urate crystal accumulation would destroy the joint.* (COURTESY OF THE ARTHRITIS FOUNDATION, NEW YORK)

c. *What Improved Treatments for Other Rheumatic Diseases?*
Current synthetic derivatives of cortisone may be lifesaving in lupus erythematosus, dermatomyositis, acute rheumatic carditis with congestive heart failure.[15]

Steroids are also useful in the treatment of Addison's disease, and for patients who have undergone adrenalectomy or hypophysectomy. These steroids have revolutionized the treatment of certain diseases, such as thrombocytopenic purpura, severe chronic asthma, ulcerative colitis, polyarteritis nodosa and infections of the eyes.

d. *What Is the Status of Treatment for Diabetes?*
    i. Currently, investigators are placing emphasis upon studies of a *more fundamental nature* in the search for the precise mechanism of insulin secretion and action, which should yield information leading to a better understanding of the underlying cause of the disease.[15]

    ii. Other studies have concerned the question whether the small blood vessel disease characteristic of diabetes is an independent primary cause or an effect of long-term diabetes, and the possible role played by human growth hormone. In addition, there are a number of ongoing investigations of new approaches with a therapeutic potential, such as implantation of insulin-producing pancreatic beta cells, and various studies designed to understand better, and perhaps to forestall, development of the long-term complications of the disease.[15]

6. What are the payoffs in neurological diseases?[16]

a. *What About the New Drug for Parkinson's Disease?*

A major breakthrough in drug therapy for Parkinson's disease is the drug *L-DOPA*. About *75 percent of patients treated have benefited substantially.*[16]

One problem with L-DOPA has been that slow administration leading to the massive doses necessary for adequate penetration of the brain was sometimes not followed, causing intolerable side effects. A way around this problem has been found. *Enzyme inhibitors,* which slow the breakdown of L-DOPA in the body, allow much greater penetration and a subsequent reduction (up to 80 percent in dosage) permitting faster administration with reduction or elimination of peripheral side effects.[22]

b. *What Research Progress Has Been Made in Cerebral Palsy?*
    i. A method involving *multiple exchange blood transfusions* was discovered for preventing kernicterus, a leading cause of infant death (approximately 1,000 deaths annually) and of cerebral palsy.[34]

    Cerebral palsy from this cause has been *reduced from 15 percent to 1 percent.*[34]

    ii. The more recent introduction of *phototherapy* has further enabled successful treatment of these children in many instances without the need to resort to transfusion.[34]

    iii. The Rh-conflict type can be wiped out in the future through *preventive use of the Rh-O Immune globulin* within 72 hours of delivery or miscarriage of an Rh-positive baby by an Rh-negative mother.[34]

    iv. Some newly developed drugs have been helpful in the treatment or management of cerebral palsy patients:[34]

        The *tranquilizing* drugs have been helpful in ameliorating aberrant behavior in some cases and the amphetamines have been of special value in organic hyperactivity.

        L-DOPA has been useful in the athetoid type of cerebral palsy.

        Dantrolene has proven useful for the relief of spasticity in cerebral palsy.

Accurate monitoring of premature babies, especially as it relates to oxygen levels, blood acidity, and disturbances in blood chemistry along with appropriate remedial therapy, has greatly reduced the unusually high incidence of cerebral palsy in premature babies.[34]

  c. *What Research Progress Has Been Made in Epilepsy?*

In 1974, the Food and Drug Administration approved *carbamazepine (Tegretol) as an epilepsy drug.* This was the first time in 14 years that a drug for long-term treatment of epilepsy was approved. Scientists of the National Institute of Neurological Diseases and Stroke catalyzed the effort responsible for this advance.[44]

  d. *What Research Progress Has Been Made in Myasthenia Gravis?*

A new treatment for *myasthenia gravis* introduced by scientists in the medical neurology branch of the National Institute of Neurological Diseases and Stroke—a high, single dose, alternate day, oral prednisone regimen—has proven extremely beneficial over long periods in the majority of the patients studied.[4]

  e. *What Has Been the Medical Research Progress in Deafness?*

    i. The development of *microsurgery* (tympanoplasty) to restore hearing to those individuals suffering from middle-ear (conductive) deafness and mastoid infection.[41]

ii. Through the years improved techniques have been developed not only for the surgical but also for medical treatment of chronically infected mastoids and middle ears. *Acute mastoid disease* has been *dramatically reduced* and almost eliminated by the use of antibiotics.[41]
iii. The development of the *stapedectomy* operation for the removal of the stapes bone which is embedded in the otosclerotic proliferation in the middle ear and the substitution of a prosthesis to serve as a stapes. This operation gives a high return of the hearing function.[41]
iv. Recently advances have been made in the surgery for the correction of congenitally malformed external ear canals and middle ears in order to restore hearing and to remove tumors along the auditory nerve.[44]
v. An operation, devised by Dr. William House, for the congenitally deaf, involving an electronic device, gives promise that thousands born deaf will eventually be able to hear.

7. What are the major research payoffs and developments in eye disorders?[42]

1. *Cataract surgery is now safer* and its outcome more satisfactory because of advancements in suture techniques, improved instrumentation, operation under microscopic control, and other technical improvements.[42]

    a. An enzyme is now being used by some ophthalmic surgeons to weaken the ligaments holding the cataract in place. The cataract is then easily removed by grasping it with special forceps or a suction cup.[42]

    b. Another technique recently developed employs a very cold probe. In this technique, *cryoextraction,* the lens is frozen and the probe adheres to it. This produces a firm connection, and the cataract can be lifted easily from the eye.[42]

    c. *Ultrasound* is also being used for *cataract extraction.* In this method, called phacoemulsification, a hollow needle is attached to an ultrasound unit and inserted into the lens. The sound vibrations break up the cataract so it can be drawn out by suction through the hollow needle. This technique involves a smaller incision in the white of the eye than conventional cataract extraction. The period of hospitalization may be shorter.[42]

Clinical evaluation of these techniques is still under way.

2. Through research, *new and improved drugs* have been developed to control the high intraocular pressure associated with *glaucoma*. Glaucoma develops when the intraocular pressure is high enough to damage the optic nerve and cause visual loss. With the use of these drugs, most glaucoma patients can expect to retain useful vision throughout their lives.[42]

3. A few years ago it was found that some cases of *herpes simplex keratitis can be cured by idoxuridine (IDU)*, the first drug shown to be effective against this virus. The mechanisms by which antiviral drugs accomplish their task are now better understood, but research is continuing in an effort to broaden the use of antiviral drugs.[42]

4. The *hydrophilic or soft contact lens* is proving to be helpful for those people who have difficulty adjusting to the hard contact lens and is proving to be useful in treating corneal diseases. It has already been shown that the soft lenses may reduce the pain frequently associated with corneal disease. Studies are being conducted to determine whether the soft lens can also be effective in aiding the healing of certain corneal diseases.[42]

5. Progress has been achieved in treating *uveitis* through the use of antibiotics, antitumor drugs, steroids, electron microscopic studies, and other measures.[42]

6. The *Optacon,* a device which enables a blind person to read the same printed material any person with vision would use, has been developed. The user of the Optacon senses the outline of a regular letter conveyed through the raising and lowering of an array of tiny rods which fit onto a single finger. The entire system weighs only eight pounds and can be easily transported.[42]

7. A more complex vision substitution device uses the images captured by a television camera to activate a series of stimulators arranged on a grid and positioned over the skin of

the abdomen. *A sightless person, with training and practice, can learn to translate these impulses automatically into crude spatial images within his brain.* Both the Optacon and this system were developed with grant support from the National Eye Institute and other Federal agencies.[42]

8. A new diagnostic technique, *fluorescent angiography*, has made possible advancements in understanding retinal diseases. The technique involves the injection of a fluorescent dye into the arm. This dye circulates in the bloodstream and permits the direct viewing of the blood flow within the vessels of the retina and choroid, the tissue underlying the retina which is responsible for its nourishment. Fluorescent angiography improves the ability of doctors to distinguish among various kinds of diseases of the eye and to pinpoint the site of any leakage or blocking of blood flow in the retina or choroid. Research indicates that the technique will also improve the physician's ability to detect malignant melanoma, a cancer in the eye which causes severe visual loss and endangers life.[42]

9. *Cryosurgery,* a technique used for cataract extraction, is now being employed in the treatment of retinal detachment, a separation of the inner layer of the retina from its outer layer. The extreme cold produces adhesions between the two layers and can be used in those cases where photocoagulation (intense heat) cannot be used because it is difficult to see clearly the area to be treated. The two procedures complement each other.[42]

10. *Microsurgery* permits meticulous and precise placement of stitches during corneal transplantation so that a more nearly perfect placement of the graft in its recipient can be achieved. This minimizes the risk of scar tissue formation and subsequent growth of unwanted blood vessels. Microsurgery also allows the use of finer sutures which are less irritating to the eye.[42]

11. New methods of freezing and dehydrating corneas for long-range storage have also resulted in improved corneal transplants.[42]

12. Computer technology is being applied to the ERG (electroretinography), which is an electrical recording of the retina's response to light in an effort to increase its usefulness

in specific clinical diagnostic situations. Research is continuing in an effort to improve this technology and the range of its usefulness.[42]

13. Great advances have been made in the development of *optical devices for patients with low levels of visual acuity*. These devices include telescopic spectacles and a host of visual aids for the magnification of visual material both for direct observation and by projection.[42]

14. The cause of *retrolental fibroplasia,* formerly a major cause of blindness among infants, is now known and preventive measures have been developed. Research supported by the National Institutes of Health, the National Foundation for Eye Research, and the National Society for the Prevention of Blindness established the cause of RLF as the excessive exposure of premature babies to high oxygen concentration. As a result, the number of new cases of RLF per year has been substantially reduced.[42]

VI. How Many People Have Some Limitation of Activity Due to a Chronic Condition?

An estimated 25,868,000 persons, or 12.7 percent of the civilian, noninstitutionalized population, had some degree of activity limitation in 1972,[10] as a result of chronic disease or impairment.

Of these, 9.6 percent suffered with limitation of activity in their major activity (working, keeping house, school or preschool activities), or were unable to carry on their major activity.[10]

An estimated 66.7 million injuries occurred during July 1972–June 1973.[11]

The number of disability days per person resulting from acute conditions in 1973 were:[11]

16.5 days of restricted activity
6.4 days in bed
5.4 days lost from work per currently employed person
5.1 days lost from school per child aged 6 to 16 years

V. What Are the Main Causes of Death in the United States?

	Estimated 1973 Deaths	Percent of Total Deaths
1. Major cardiovascular diseases	1,037,460	52%
Diseases of the heart	754,460	
Active rheumatic fever and chronic rheumatic heart disease	13,580	
Hypertensive heart disease	7,810	
Hypertensive heart and renal disease	5,390	
Ischemic heart disease	682,910	
Chronic disease of endocardium and other myocardial insufficiency	4,870	
All other forms of heart disease	39,900	
Hypertension	8,010	
Cerebrovascular diseases	214,650	
Arteriosclerosis (general)	33,430	
Other diseases of arteries, arterioles, and capillaries	26,910	
2. Cancer	353,440	18%
3. Accidents	115,040	6%
4. Pneumonia and influenza (4,970 deaths)	61,160	3%
5. Diabetes mellitus	36,450	2%
6. Cirrhosis of liver	33,630	2%
7. Certain causes of mortality in early infancy (birth injuries, difficult labor, anoxic and hypoxic conditions)	31,030	2%
8. Bronchitis, emphysema, asthma	30,280	2%
9. Suicide	24,440	1.2%
10. Homicide	19,700	1%
11. Congenital anomalies	13,940	0.7%
12. Peptic ulcer	7,830	0.4%
13. Nephritis and nephrosis	7,740	0.4%
14. Hernia, intestinal obstruction	6,710	0.3%
15. Infections of kidney	6,100	0.3%
16. Benign neoplasms and neoplasms of unspecified nature	5,540	0.3%
17. Septicemia	4,290	0.2%
18. Tuberculosis	3,870	0.2%
	1,828,940	92%
Estimated deaths from all other causes	148,060	8%
Total estimated deaths, 1973	1,977,000	100%

Estimated death rate per 1,000 population in 1973—9.4

How Many Mothers and Infants Die Each Year in the United States?

Maternal deaths	470
Infant deaths (first years of life, not included above)	55,300
Estimated in 1973	55,770

The infant mortality rate was 12.9 per 1,000 live births for those infants under 28 days and 4.7 per 1,000 live births for those 28 days to 11 months.

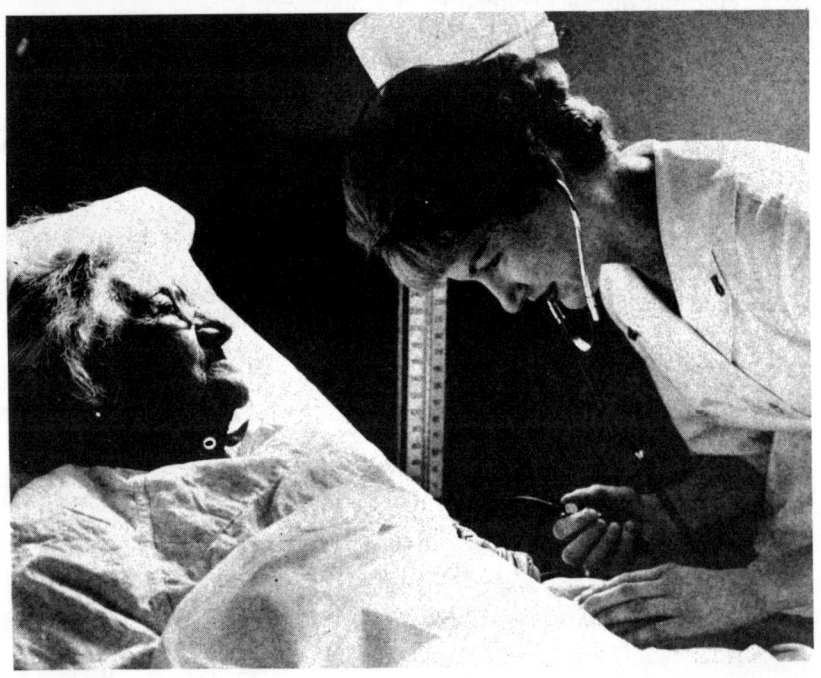

VII. What Are the Main Causes of Disability in the United States?

	Estimated Number of People Afflicted (in some degree)
1. Major cardiovascular diseases	
High blood pressure	23,000,000[7]
Coronary heart disease	4,040,000[25]
Rheumatic heart disease	1,670,000[25]
Cerebrovascular disease (strokes)	1,620,000[25]
	27,130,000*
2. Mental and emotional disorders (in some degree)	20,000,000[2]
3. Arthritis and rheumatic diseases	20,200,000[20]
4. Hearing impairments	11,500,000[16]
5. Mentally retarded	6,000,000[26]
6. Visual impairments	9,596,000[17]
Legally blind—475,000[35]	
7. Neurological disorders	
Epilepsy[16]	2,000,000 to 4,000,000[16]
Parkinsonism	1,000,000[16]
Cerebral palsy	750,000[13]
Multiple sclerosis and related disease	500,000[21]
Muscular dystrophy	200,000[23]
8. Diabetes mellitus	4,000,000[15]
9. Cancer—estimated under medical care now	1,025,000[24]

*The sum of the individual estimates exceeds 27,130,000 since many persons have more than one cardiovascular disorder.

VIII. What Does Illness Cost the United States?

1. *National health expenditures* in 1972–1973 totaled an estimated *$94 billion*. Of this amount:[18]

    $56.5 billion represented private expenditures
    $37.5 billion represented public expenditures

2. According to the National Health Survey, *over 301 million days were lost from work because of acute illness* by all persons 17 years and over during the year July 1972–June 1973.[11] Of these 301 million days lost from work:

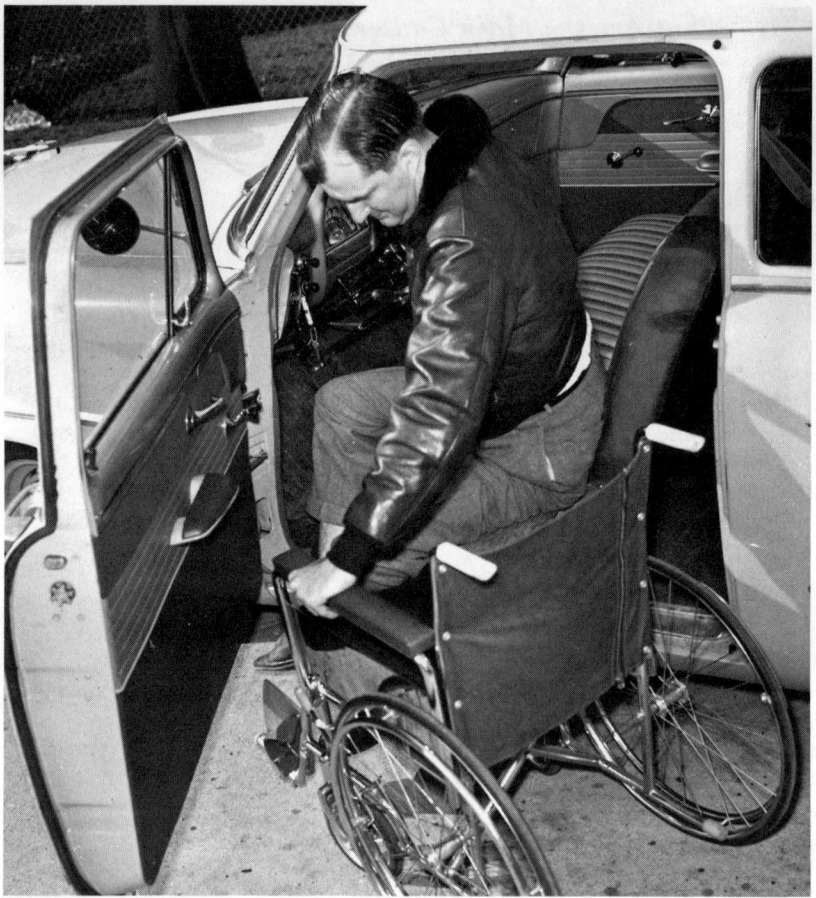

Days lost from work because of acute conditions:	Estimated wage loss*
132 million caused by respiratory conditions	$4,224,000,000
89 million caused by injuries	2,848,000,000
17 million caused by digestive diseases	544,000,000
20 million caused by infective and parasitic diseases	640,000,000
43 million caused by all other acute conditions	1,376,000,000
Total estimated wage loss from acute conditions	$9,632,000,000

*Based on estimated minimum daily wage of $32 (8 hours at $4.07 per hour). The average hourly earnings of production workers, manufacturing industries, 1973.[3]

While workers may not have actually lost this amount in wages, this nonetheless gives an indication of the loss in productivity.

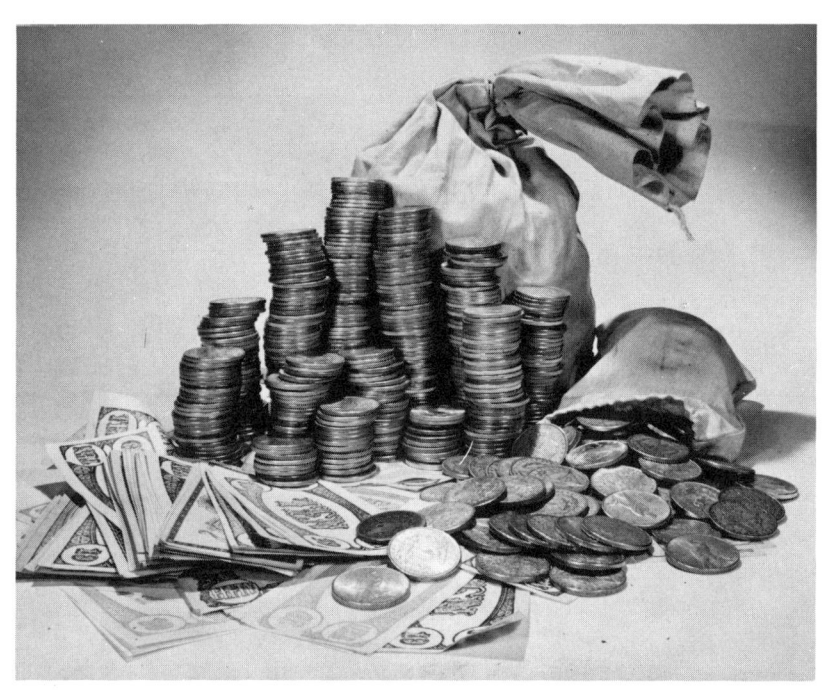

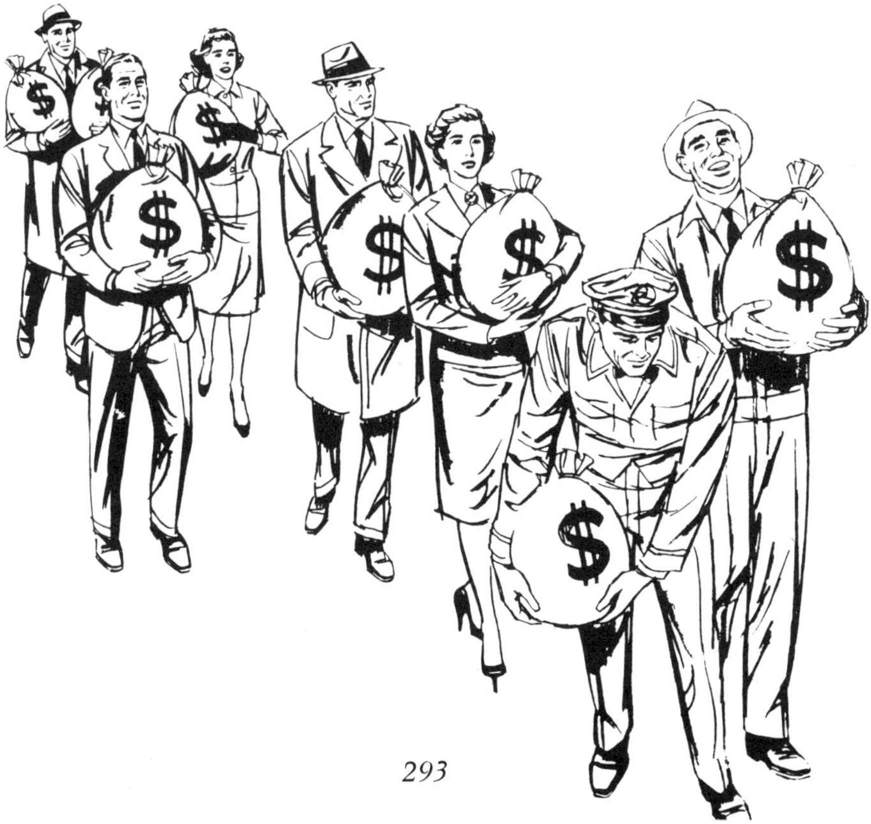

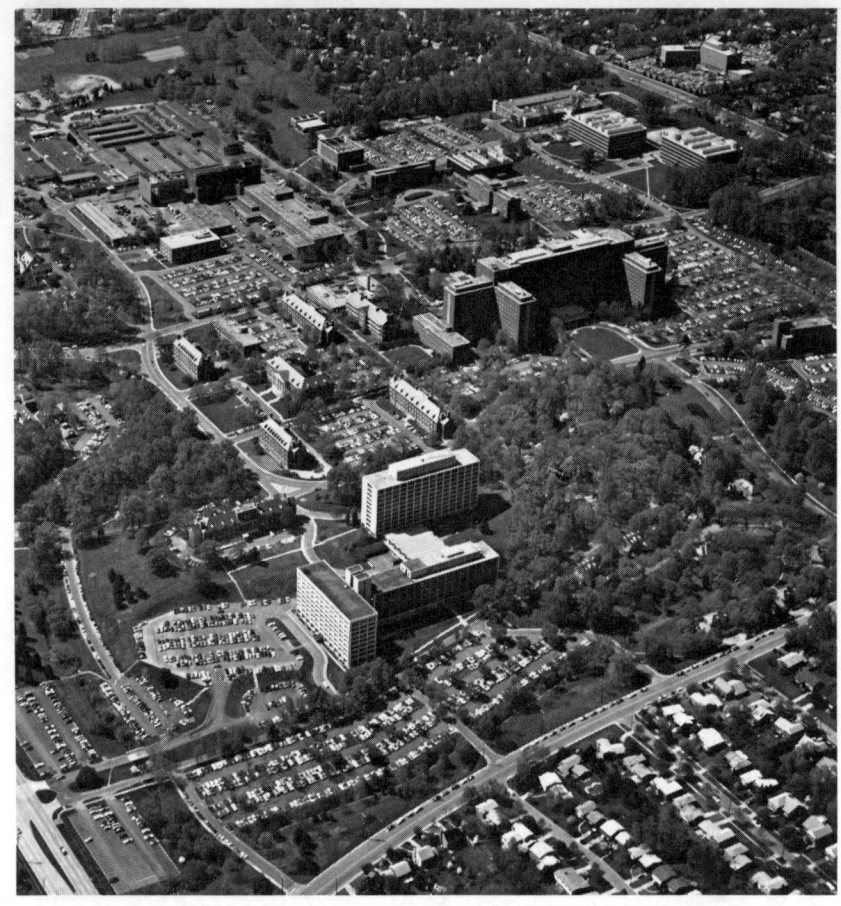
Aerial view of the National Institutes of Health, Bethesda, Maryland.

IX. What Does the Federal Government Spend Through Its Major Health Research Programs to Defend Us Against All the Diseases That Kill and Cripple Us?

Fiscal 1975 appropriations to the categorical National Institutes of Health, and to the Alcohol, Drug Abuse and Mental Health Administration totaled $2.9 billion, as follows:[30]

National Cancer Institute	$ 691,666,000
National Heart and Lung Institute	324,130,000

Medical Research

National Institute of Dental Research	49,864,000
National Institute of Arthritis, Metabolism and Digestive Diseases	173,121,000
National Institute of Neurological and Communicative Disorders and Stroke	142,498,000
National Institute of Allergy and Infectious Diseases	119,452,000
National Institute of General Medical Sciences	187,400,000
National Institute of Child Health and Human Development	141,966,000
National Eye Institute	44,133,000
National Institute of Environmental Health Sciences	34,949,000
Division of Research Resources	127,200,000
Fogarty International Center	5,589,000
	$2,041,968,000

Plus other programs under the National Institutes of Health:

National Library of Medicine	$28,450,000
Buildings and facilities	3,000,000
Office of the Director	17,000,000
Total, NIH	$2,090,418,000

Alcohol, Drug Abuse and Mental Health Administration:

National Institute of Mental Health	$405,989,000
National Institute of Drug Abuse	219,899,000
National Institute of Alcohol Abuse and Alcoholism	145,915,000
St. Elizabeth's Hospital	42,340,000
Program direction	9,555,000
	$823,698,000
Grand total	$2,914,116,000

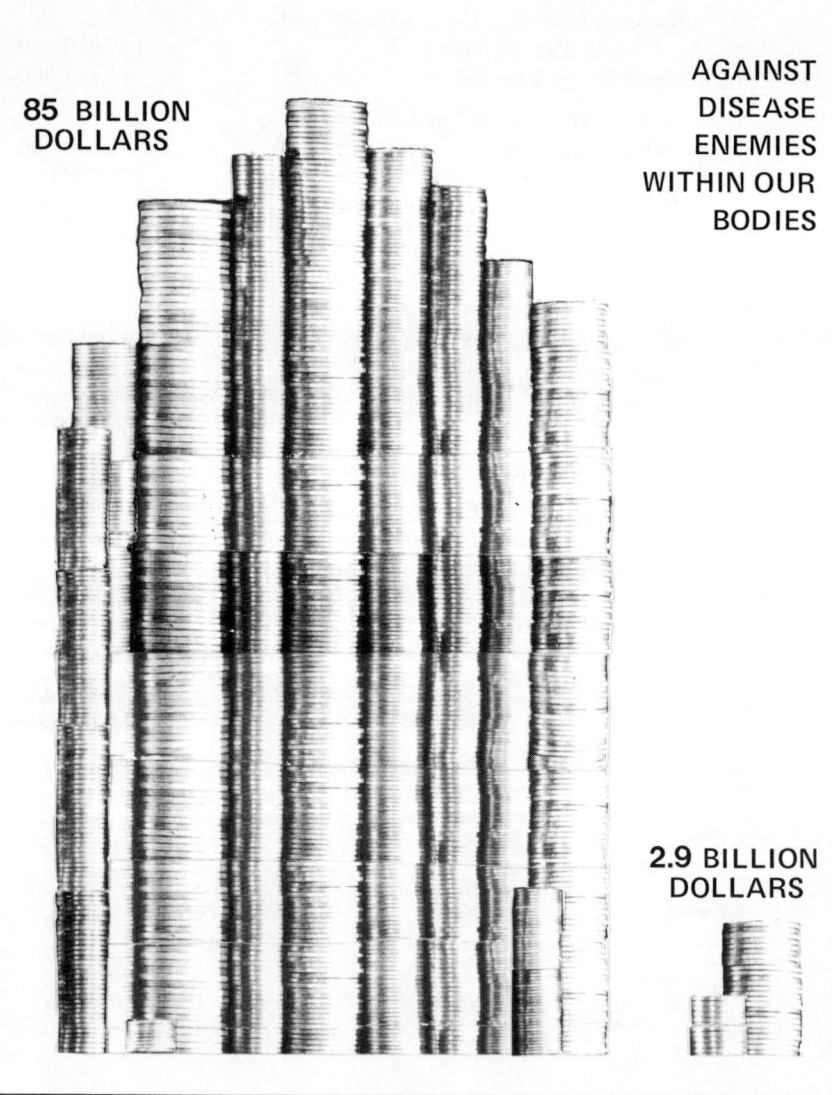

X. How Much Do the People Whose Lives Have Been Saved by Medical Research Repay the Federal Government?

The decline in the death rate between 1944 and 1970 has meant the *saving of 9,786,573 lives.*[27]

Of these, *8,985,056 are still alive and 3,292,326 are wage earners.* During these 26 years, these wage earners have *earned $156 billion in income.*[27]

Of this income, *they have paid $19.7 billion in income and excise taxes to the Federal Government.*[27]

Vast numbers of disabilities that would have been caused by polio, influenza, tuberculosis, syphilis, appendicitis, anemias, dysentery, acute rheumatic fever, hypertensive heart disease, acute nephritis, whooping cough, measles, and German measles *have been eliminated or reduced due to new drugs and vaccines.*

The above figures do not begin to take into account the billions of dollars in income added to the gross national product and the resulting tax revenues to the government which have been realized as well.

Fiscal 1975 appropriations to the *National Institutes of Health* totaled *$2 billion.* In addition, fiscal 1975 appropriations to the *Alcohol, Drug Abuse and Mental Health Administration* totaled *$823,698,000.*[30]

These fiscal 1975 appropriations have been repaid 10 times over to the Federal Government in income and excise taxes of wage earners whose lives were saved due to medical research successes in the 26 years 1944 to 1970, to say nothing of taxes paid by those who would otherwise have been disabled by diseases that are now curable or controllable through medical research advances.

In fact, in 1970 alone, the 3.3 million wage earners alive and working as a result of the decline in the death rate paid the Federal Government *$2.6 billion in income and excise taxes* on their earnings—*$600 million more than was appropriated to the National Institutes of Health in that year* (FY 1975).[27]

Income realized and tax revenue paid by people who would have been *disabled* had it not been for these medical research advances, but who received treatment with new drugs, vaccines, and other therapies in time to prevent long-term disability, are *incalculable and very much larger.*

The increase in production and gross national product in the United States due to the prevention of these deaths and disabilities *is so great that it cannot be accurately estimated.*

XI. What Have Been the Dollar Savings to State Governments in Construction Costs as a Result of Research in New Drugs for Mental Patients?

The 55 percent reduction in hospitalized patients in public mental hospitals since 1955 (following the advent of the psychiatric drugs) has meant *a saving of $4.7 billion to the states* in additional bed construction costs which would otherwise have been required, to say nothing of the reduction in patient care costs also realized through the decline in state mental hospital patient populations.

XII. How Much Did the Major Voluntary Health Agencies Raise and Allocate to Research in 1973 Against the Major Killers and Cripplers?

Agency	Public Support Funds Raised	Allocated To Research	% Allocated To Research
American Cancer Society	$93,013,644	$25,054,410	27%
The National Foundation	42,691,987	4,663,163	11%
American Heart Association	54,475,310	16,778,531	31%
United Cerebral Palsy	18.000,000 (est.)	864,928	5%
Nat'l Association for Mental Health	1,084,999*	186,139	17%
Muscular Dystrophy Association	17,815,893	4,364,209	24%
The Arthritis Foundation	10,718,000	1,359,005*	13%
Nat'l Multiple Sclerosis Society	12,125,366	2,406,645*	20%
Research to Prevent Blindness Committee	648,112	591,927	91%

Damon Runyon Memorial Fund for Cancer Research**	1,136,000	2,677,500	**
Nat'l Society for the Prevention of Blindness	2,668,528	148,513	6%
Fight for Sight (Nat'l Council to Combat Blindness)	296,728	316,769	80%
Deafness Research Foundation	488,610	303,722	62%
Nat'l Easter Seal Society for Crippled Children & Adults 1972	30,815,426	455,294	1.5%
American Lung Association	39,875,034	1,653,997	4%
	$325,953,637	$61,824,752	19%

*National Office expenditure only.
**All funds raised are used to support research.

NOTE: Many of the voluntary agencies devote the greater part of their funds to patient care, service and education.

XIII. How Much Does the National Heart and Lung Institute Spend to Defend Us Against Heart Disease, the Number 1 Killer?

In fiscal 1975, *$324 million* was appropriated to the National Heart and Lung Institute.[30]

Heart and circulatory diseases, largely due to arteriosclerosis and high blood pressure, are our *number 1 killer* in the United States today.

The incidence rate of clinical myocardial infarction (heart attack) is estimated at 1,000 to 1,500 cases per 100,000 middle-aged men per year, with 30 percent to 40 percent of first attacks fatal. For the survivors of an acute attack, a minimum of 20 percent are dead in 5 years, with as many as 40 percent of high-risk cases dead in 5 years.[29]

As Compared with the $3.2 Billion the Federal Government Wisely Spends for Our Space Exploration Program?

An estimated *$3.2 billion* was spent by the *National Aeronautics and Space Administration* in fiscal 1975 for the conduct of its research and development programs, including the exploration of space and its utilization for peaceful purposes, and to conduct and support advanced research and development related to space and aeronautics in support of civilian and mili-

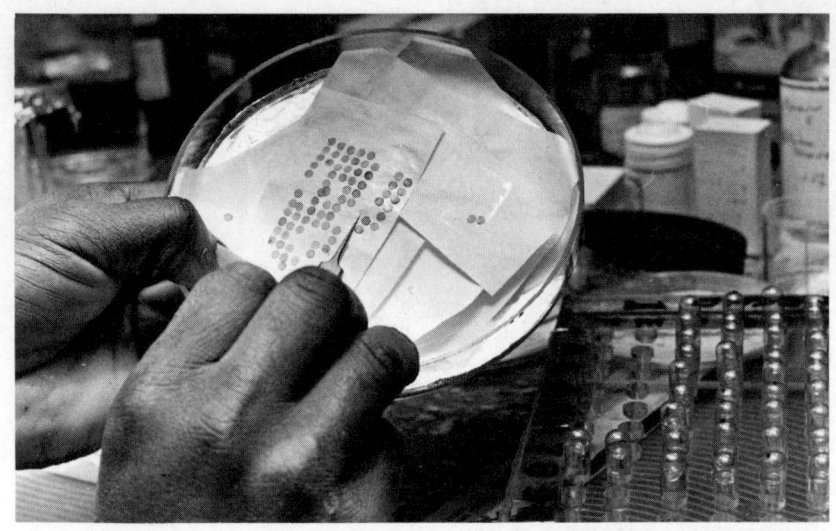
(COURTESY OF NATIONAL CANCER INSTITUTE, BETHESDA, MARYLAND)

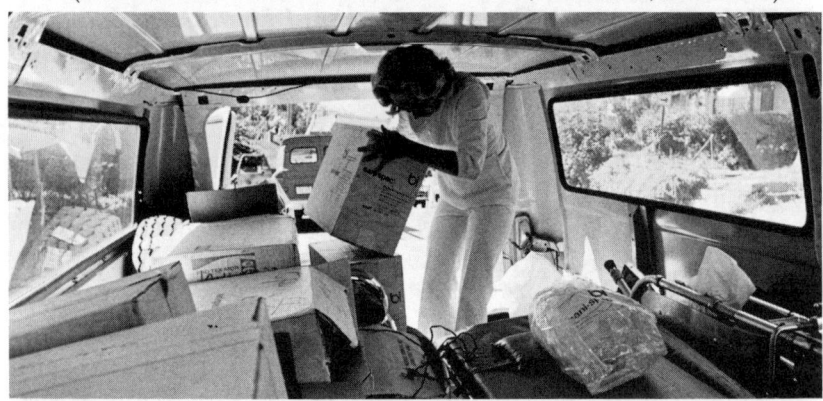
(COURTESY OF AMERICAN CANCER SOCIETY, INC., NEW YORK)

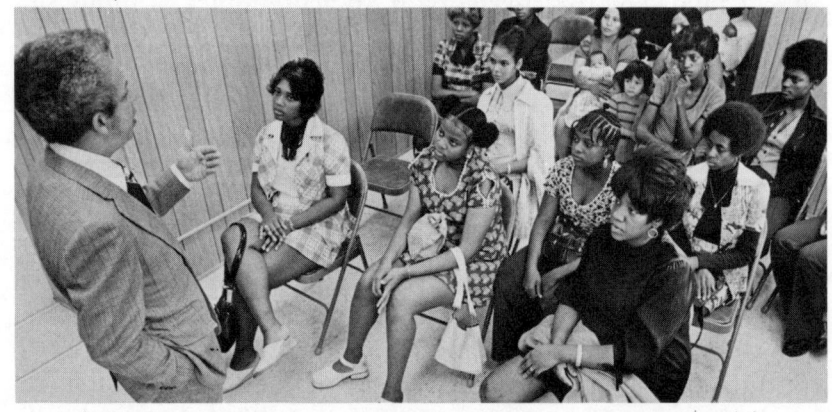
(COURTESY OF NATIONAL AERONAUTICS & SPACE ADMINISTRATION)

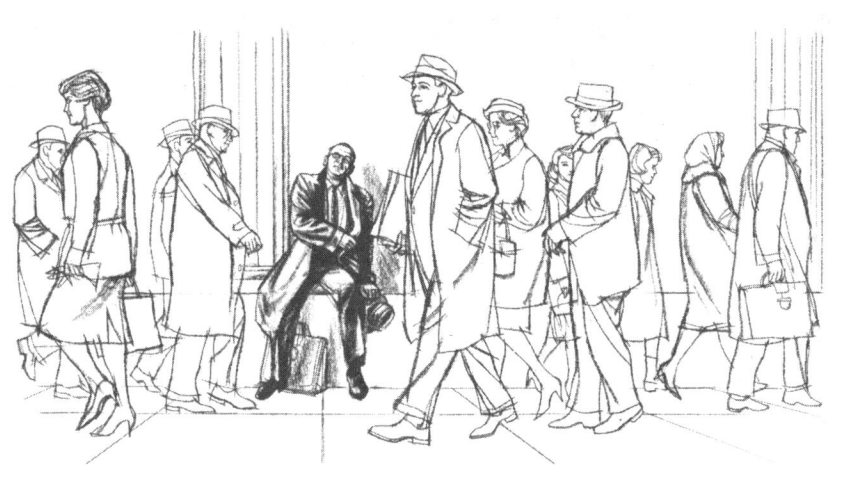

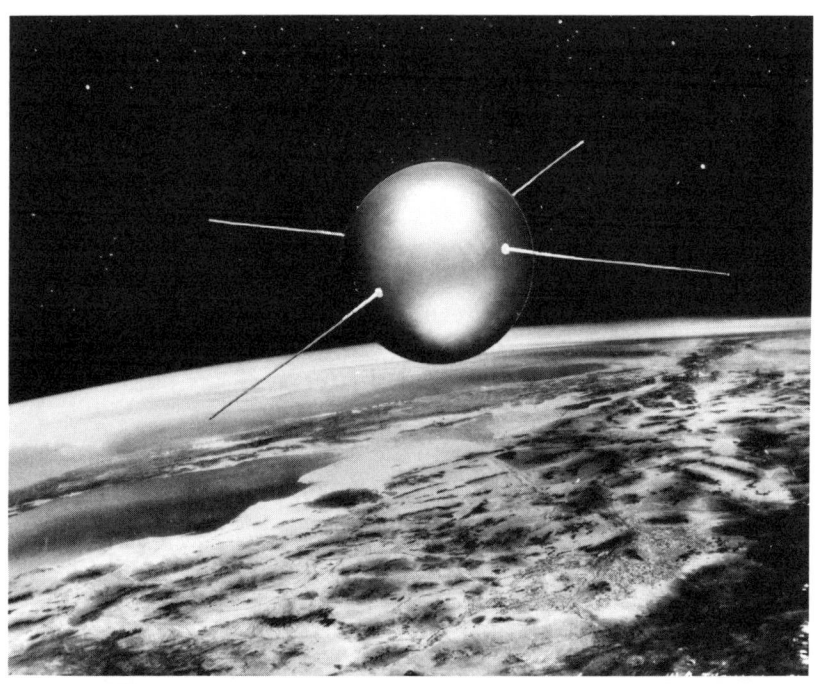

(COURTESY OF NATIONAL AERONAUTICS & SPACE ADMINISTRATION)

tary requirements,[30] *compared with $324 million* which the National Heart and Lung Institute spent for research against our number 1 killer.

XIV. How Much Does the National Cancer Institute Spend for Research to Defend Us Against Cancer?

In fiscal 1975, *$691 million* was appropriated to the National Cancer Institute.[30]

Cancer is our number 2 killer, causing 353,440 deaths in 1973. This means that almost 40 men, women, and children died from cancer every hour of every day during the year, or *one death every minute and a half.*

As Compared with the $2.1 Billion the Federal Government Necessarily Spends for the Development and Testing of Missiles and Related Equipment?

The *$2.1 billion* represents the fiscal 1975 estimated obligations of the Department of Defense for *research, development, testing, and evaluation* of missiles of all types and related equipment,[30] *compared with $691 million* which the National Cancer Institute spent for research against *our second leading cause of death.*

XV. How Much Does the Mental Health Administration Spend for Research, Training, and Clinics to Defend Us Against Mental Illnesses?

Fiscal 1975 appropriations to the Alcohol, Drug Abuse & Mental Health Administration totaled $824 million:[30]

Nat'l Institute of Mental Health	$405,989,000
Nat'l Institute of Drug Abuse	219,899,000
Nat'l Institute of Alcohol Abuse & Alcoholism	145,915,000
Program direction & other activities	51,895,000
	$823,698,000

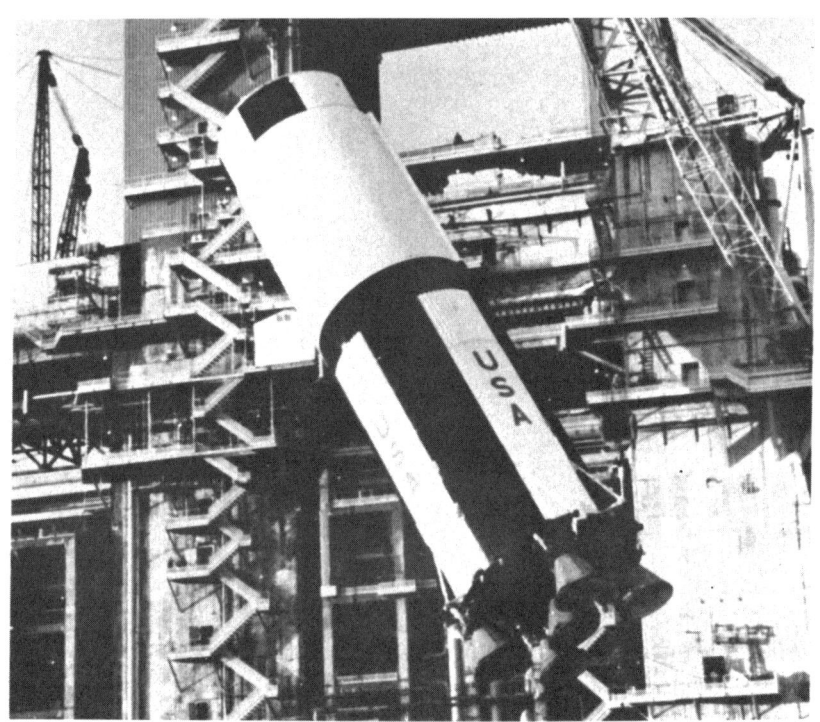

Saturn V booster being lifted onto test stand at Mississippi test facility operated for NASA by General Electric. (COURTESY OF GENERAL ELECTRIC COMPANY)

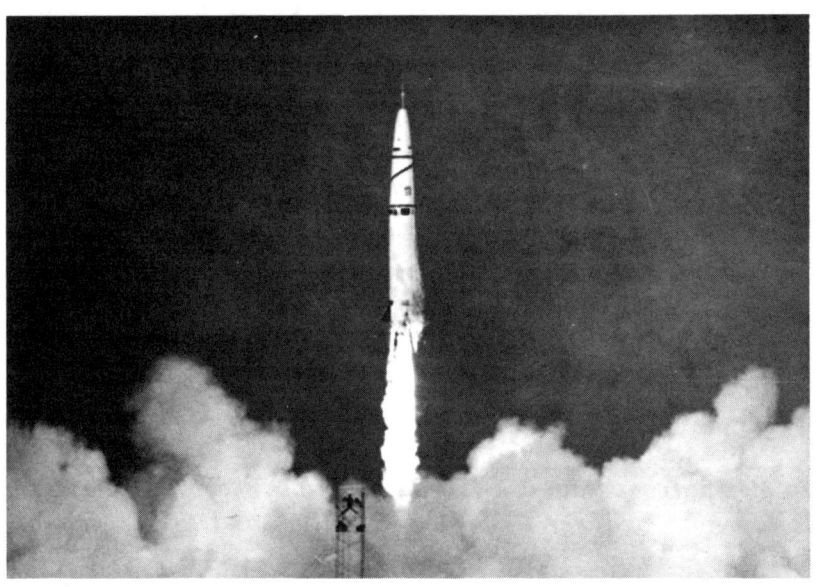

(COURTESY OF U.S. DEPARTMENT OF DEFENSE, WASHINGTON, D.C.)

Mental illnesses afflict an estimated 20 million Americans (in some degree), *and cost over $20 billion annually.*[2]

As Compared with $2.7 Billion the Commodity Credit Corporation of the Federal Government Wisely Spends for Its Price Support & Related Programs?

An estimated *$2.7 billion* was spent by the Commodity Credit Corporation of the Department of Agriculture in fiscal 1975 for its support, principally through loans and purchases, of agricultural commodities to producers of these commodities—and related programs—in order to stabilize prices at levels not in excess of those permissible by law,[30] compared with *$824 million* which the Alcohol, Drug Abuse and Mental Health Administration spent against all mental illnesses.

XVI. How Much Does the National Institute of Arthritis, Metabolism and Digestive Diseases Spend for Research to Defend Us Against These Diseases?

In fiscal 1975, *$173 million* was appropriated to the National Institute of Arthritis, Metabolism and Digestive Diseases.[30]

Arthritis and rheumatic diseases afflict (in varying degree) *20.2 million Americans;*[20] another *4 million people are victims of diabetes.*[15]

The estimated annual economic impact on the nation of arthritis and rheumatism is conservatively estimated at $9.2 billion.[20]

As Compared with the $428 Million the Federal Government Routinely Spends for Its Forest Protection and Utilization Programs?

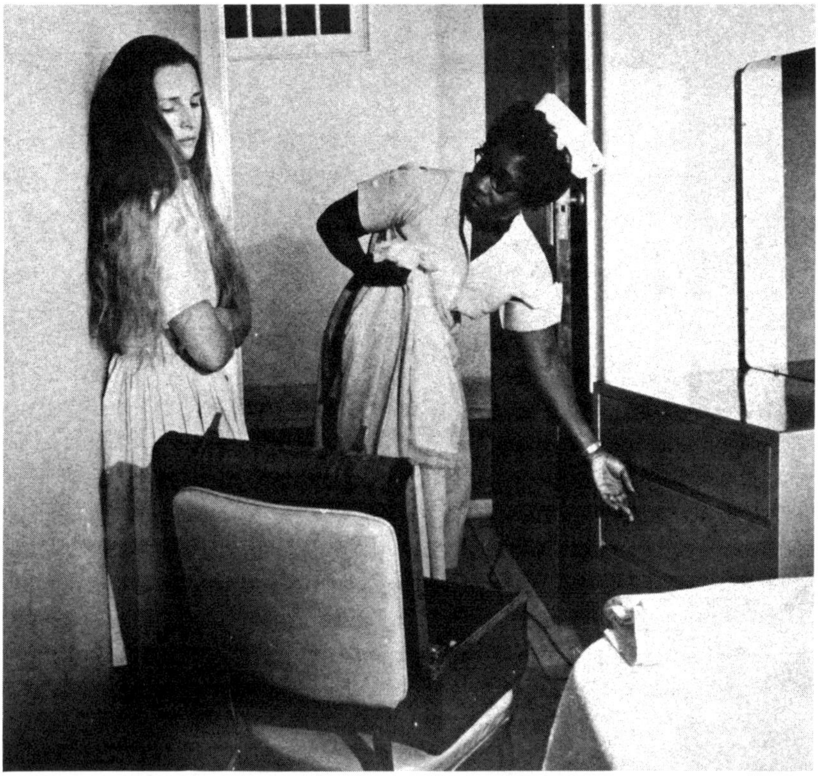

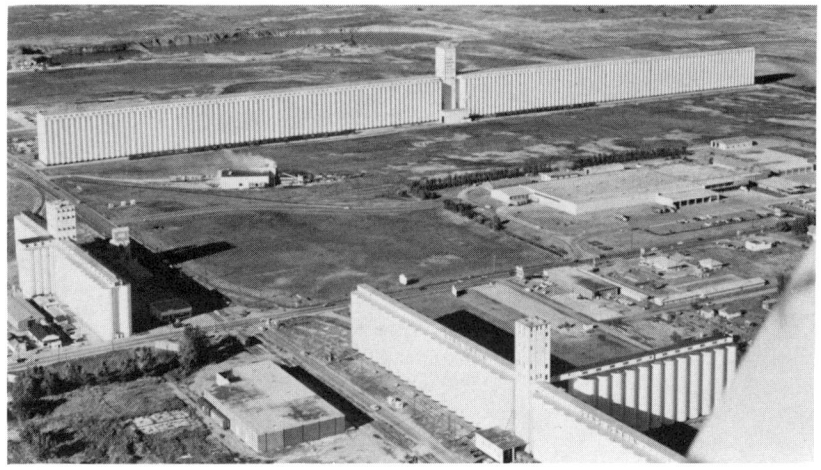

Nursing assistant at hospital helps patient to get settled in her room. (COURTESY OF NATIONAL INSTITUTE OF MENTAL HEALTH, ROCKVILLE, MARYLAND)

Storage grain elevators, Hutchinson, Kansas. (COURTESY U. S. DEPARTMENT OF AGRICULTURE, WASHINGTON, D.C.)

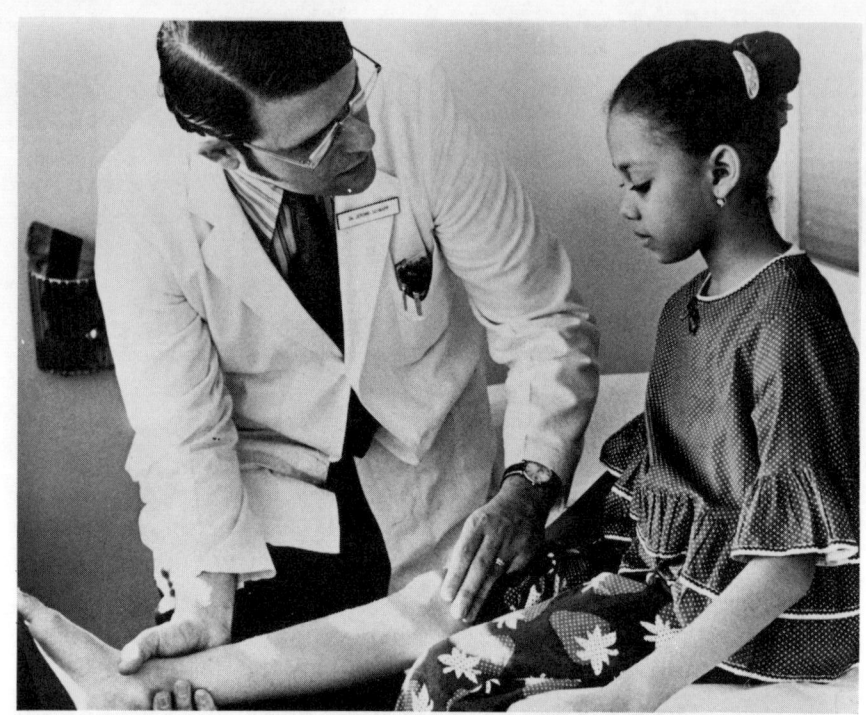

Young arthritis patient visits a special clinic at the Hospital for Special Surgery in New York City. (COURTESY OF THE ARTHRITIS FOUNDATION, NEW YORK)

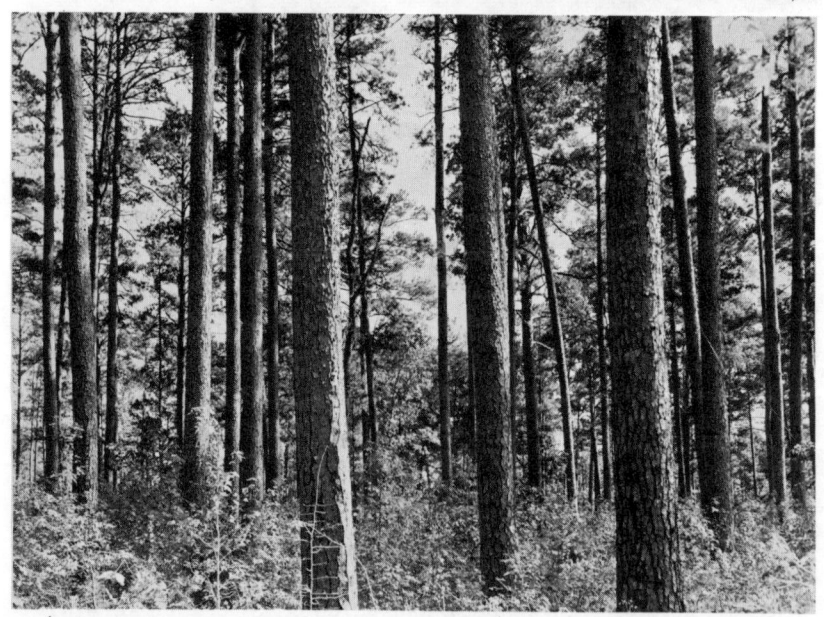

(COURTESY OF U.S. DEPARTMENT OF AGRICULTURE, WASHINGTON, D.C.)

Medical Research 307

It is estimated that *$428 million* was spent by the *Forest Service of the Department of Agriculture* in fiscal 1975 for forest protection and utilization programs,[30] *compared with $173 million,* which the National Institute of Arthritis, Metabolism and Digestive Diseases spent for research against such crippling and disabling diseases as arthritis, rheumatism, diabetes, and the digestive, nutritional, and metabolic disorders.

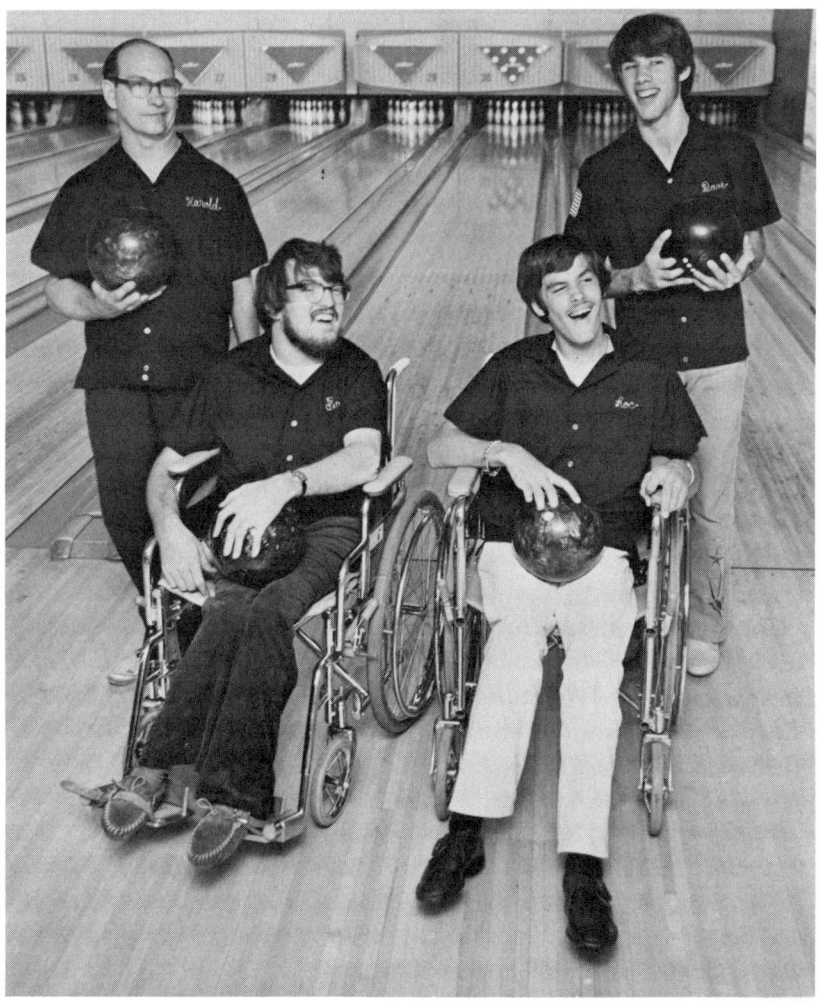

United Cerebral Palsy bowling team from San Mateo, California. (COURTESY OF UNITED CEREBRAL PALSY ASSOCIATIONS, NEW YORK)

308   THE KILLERS AND CRIPPLERS

XVII. How Much Does the National Institute of Neurological and Communicative Disorders and Stroke Spend for Research to Defend Us Against Neurological Diseases and Strokes?

In fiscal 1975, *$142 million* was appropriated to the National Institute of Neurological and Communicative Disorders and Stroke.[30]

Many millions of Americans are estimated to be disabled by such neurological disorders as epilepsy, cerebrovascular disease (stroke), cerebral palsy, Parkinsonism, multiple sclerosis, and other demyelinating diseases and muscular dystrophy.

There are *11,500,000 Americans who report hearing impairments,*[16] *9,596,000 who report visual impairments,*[17] *475,000 who are legally blind,*[35] *and an estimated 6 million who are mentally retarded.*[26]

As Compared with the $238 Million the Federal Government Constructively Spends for the Geological Survey Programs of the Department of the Interior?

An estimated *$238 million* was spent in fiscal 1975 by the Geological Survey programs of the Department of the Interior, which provides basic scientific data concerning water, land, and mineral resources, and supervises prospecting, development, and production of minerals and mineral fuels on leased Federal, Indian, and Outer Continental Shelf lands,[30] compared with *$142 million* spent by the National Institute of Neurological and Communicative Disorders and Stroke for research in these disease areas.

XVIII. How Much Does the Federal Government Spend for Research to Defend Us Against—

1. Allergies and infectious diseases?
$119 million through the National Institute of Allergy and Infectious Diseases, fiscal 1975.[30]

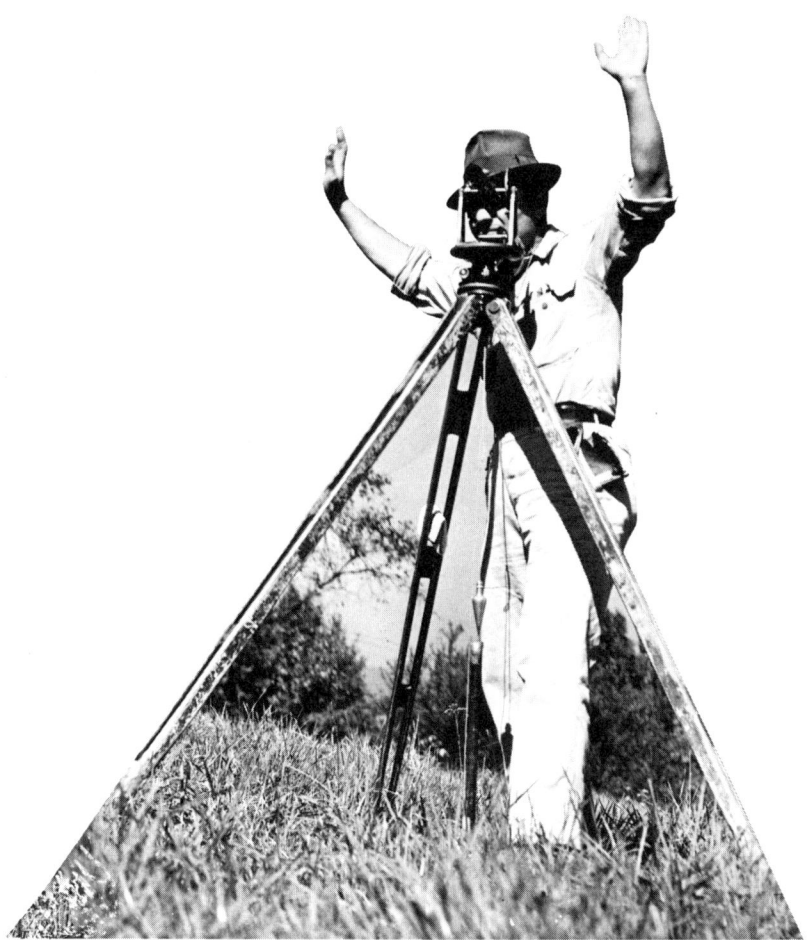

2. Child health and human development?

$142 million through the National Institute of Child Health and Human Development, fiscal 1975.[30]

3. Dental disorders?

$50 million through the National Institute of Dental Research, fiscal 1975.[30]

4. Eye disorders?

$44 million through the National Eye Institute, fiscal 1975.[30]

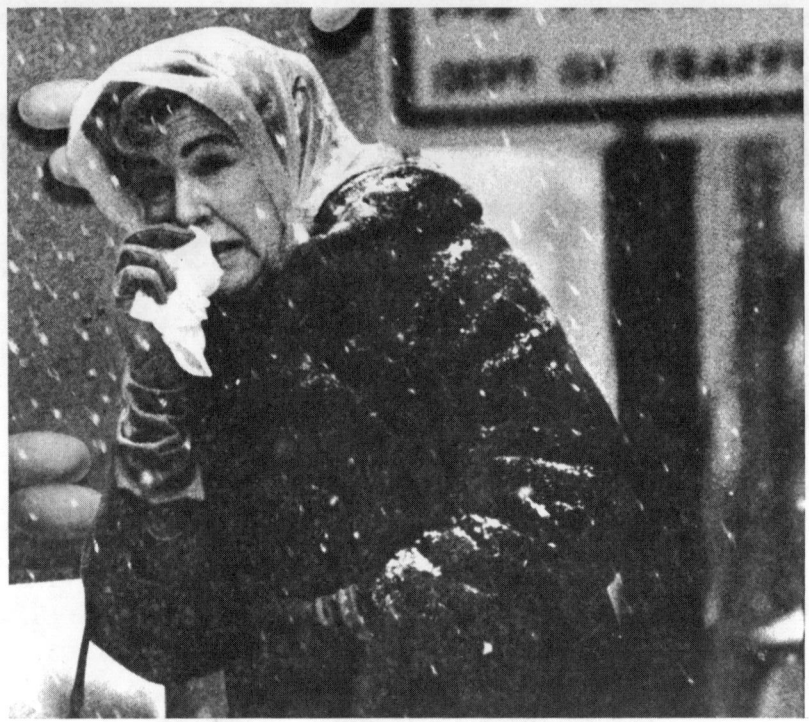
(COURTESY OF LEDERLE LABORATORIES)

5. Other disease areas?

$349.5 million through the National Institute of General Medical Sciences, the National Institute of Environmental Health Sciences and the Division of Research Resources appropriations, fiscal 1975.[30]

XIX. What Civilians Spent in 1972[31]

Alcoholic beverages	$17,076,600,000
Tobacco products and smokers' accessories	13,052,080,000
Photographic equipment and supplies	3,378,880,000
Greeting cards	1,290,130,000
Boxed candy	1,284,830,000
Cough and cold items	660,940,000
Aspirin and other internal analgesics	631,940,000
Chewing gum	496,090,000

WHAT AMERICANS ARE SPENDING — 1972

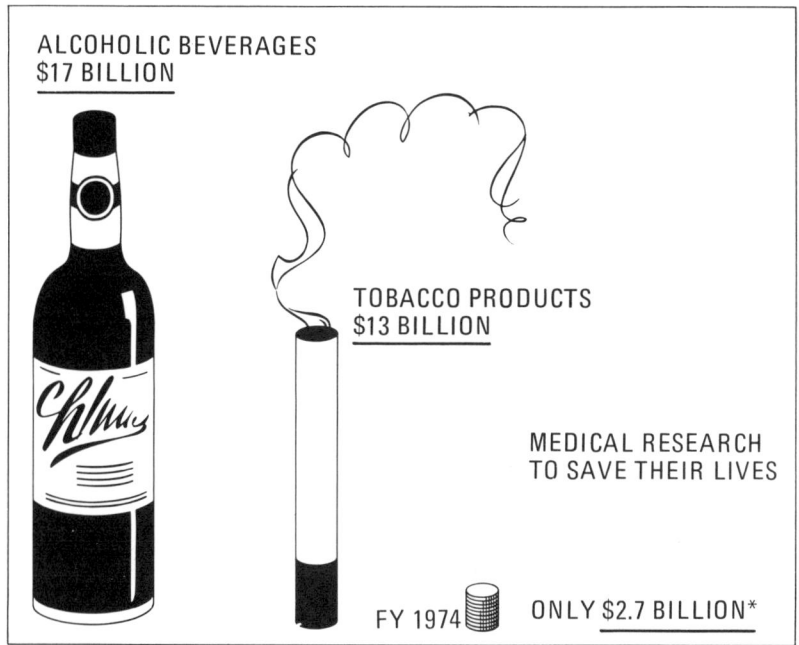

ALCOHOLIC BEVERAGES
$17 BILLION

TOBACCO PRODUCTS
$13 BILLION

MEDICAL RESEARCH
TO SAVE THEIR LIVES

FY 1974   ONLY $2.7 BILLION*

*THRU THE NAT'L INSTITUTES OF HEALTH & THE ALCOHOL, DRUG ABUSE & MENTAL HEALTH ADMINISTRATION.

Paperback books	475,740,000
External personal deodorants	465,950,000
Shampoos	441,560,000
Toilet water and cologne	302,870,000
Ballpoint pens and refills, porous point pens, felt tip markers	301,370,000
Lipsticks	300,230,000
Sunglasses (no corrective lenses)	280,840,000
Women's hair sprays	276,260,000
Hair coloring preparations	249,180,000
Mouth washes and gargles	245,390,000
After-shave lotions and men's cologne	223,700,000
Laxatives and cathartics	212,690,000
Eye makeup	194,100,000
Dieting aids	140,980,000
Stomach sweeteners (antacids)	116,680,000
Foot products	112,460,000
Men's hair dressings	99,910,000
Nail polish and enamel	91,160,000
Hand lotions and creams	81,180,000
Pressed cake face powder and blush makeup	76,340,000

Makeup bases	69,480,000
Suntan lotions and oils	64,880,000
Bath salts, tablets, oils, etc.	63,050,000
Elastic stockings	43,180,000
Playing cards	36,080,000

SOURCE: 1973 Marketing Guide, published by *Drug Topics,* Medical Economics Company, Oradell, N.J.

XX. What Does the Pharmaceutical Industry Spend for Research Against the Major Killing and Crippling Diseases?

The Pharmaceutical Manufacturers Association estimates the pharmaceutical industry spent *$728 million in 1972 for reearch and development of drugs for human and animal use.* The 1971 expenditures for these purposes totaled $684 million.[28]

These research and development expenditures have risen from $63 million in 1952 to $251 million in 1962 to the estimated $728 million in 1972.

XXI. What Are the Challenges That Remain in the Western World?

1. *Arteriosclerosis* and high blood pressure (main cause of heart attacks and strokes) and other heart diseases.
2. *Cancer,* the number 2 cause of death.
3. *Mental illnesses*—chronic schizophrenia, drug addiction, alcoholism, and others.
4. *Arthritis and rheumatic diseases, the metabolic diseases*—diabetes, cirrhosis and other liver diseases, obesity and nutritional diseases, diseases of the blood, aplastic anemia, disorders of bone metabolism, diseases of the endocrine glands, digestive diseases such as ulcers, colitis, ileitis, diverticulitis, kidney and gallstones, and other diseases of the kidneys.
5. *Neurological and sensory diseases,* including speech and hearing disorders, head and spinal cord injuries, epilepsy, Parkinsonism, multiple sclerosis, muscular dystrophy, cerebral palsy, and major eye diseases, such as glaucoma, cataracts, uveitis, diabetic retinopathy, detached retina, senile eye deterioration.
6. *Mental retardation,* which affects 3 percent of our entire

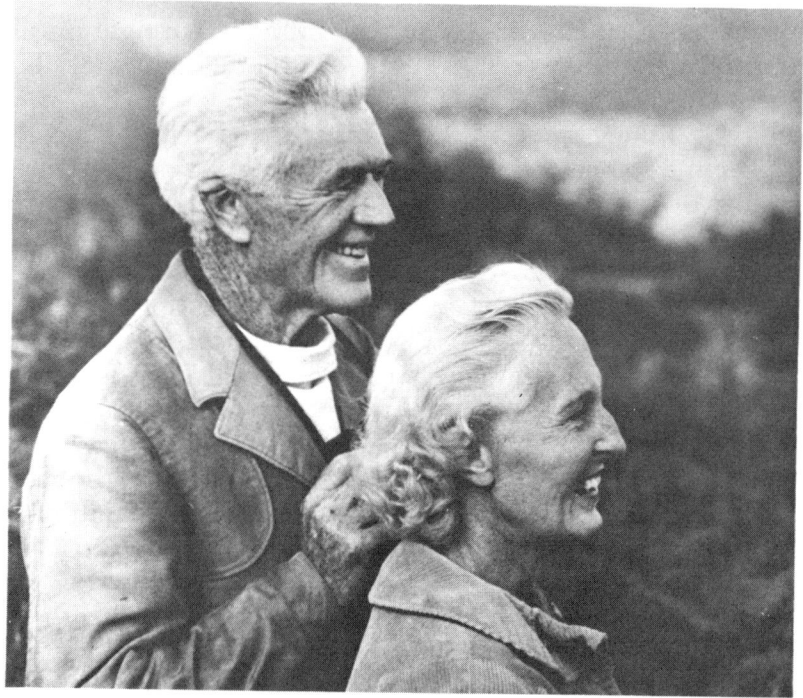

population (an estimated 6 million Americans are mentally retarded).

7. *Deaths associated with childbirth*—neonatal, fetal, and maternal deaths.

8. *Virus diseases*—hepatitis, new forms of influenza, the common cold, and others.

9. *Allergic diseases*—drug allergies, serum sickness, allergic skin disorders, and others.

10. *Genetic diseases.*

The prime of life has been prolonged 22 years from 49 years in 1900 to 71.3 in 1973. Let us prolong the *prime* of life even further and make the additional years happy and healthy ones.

REMEMBER:

... But what about someone who was born with a life expectancy of only 35 years and who can never forget that Death may visit him or his family at any time, and does, without even bothering to knock on the door? Most of mankind is surrounded by sickness and is helpless against disease. Whoever provides the tools to fight it will earn the gratitude and might win the allegiance of the multitude.

... Taking stock of the human capital at his disposal, Lenin discovered that Russia's death rate was nearly twice that of the West and that the average citizen had a life expectancy of only 40 years. Though there is no record that he was distressed from a humanitarian point of view, it is clear that the Soviet leader could translate these figures into national output. Financial capital for development of Russia, he knew, could come only from the production of workers and peasants. First, they had to be educated and trained. If, after that investment, they were weakened by disease and doomed to a short life, the rate of capital accumulation would be so slow that the Communists would never build a modern industrial state short of a hundred years.

... [Now] the Soviet Union ... had raised the health of its people up to the level of the West. It had slashed the crude mortality rate about 75% since before the Revolution and by 1956, at 7.7 per 1,000 population, it was comparable to ours. At the same time, it had lengthened average life expectancy from about 40 years at the beginning of World War I to a claimed 67 years in 1956. This was within reaching distance of longevity in the United States, which in the same year stood at 69.5.

... Because of our concentration on physical and financial capital, we are inclined to forget the importance of human capital, which is both the means and the end of industrialization. This concept of the relation between human capital and economic growth could turn out to be decisive as the Soviet sets forth to meet the rising expectations of Asia, Africa, the Middle East and even Latin America with a program of health, development and Communism.

Excerpts from an Address given by John T. Connor, November 6, 1958, at the American Management Association Conference on the Soviet Economic Offensive, in New York City. At the time, Mr. Connor was president of Merck & Co., Inc. He later served as Secretary of Commerce and is now president of Allied Chemical Corp.

Notes

All mortality and life expectancy data from the National Center for Health Statistics, U.S. Department of Health, Education, and Welfare, Washington, D.C.

1. *Statistical Note 106,* May 1974, Survey and Reports Section, National Institute of Mental Health, Chevy Chase, Md.
2. National Committee Against Mental Illness, Washington, D.C. Information from Mr. Mike Gorman, Executive Director, 1974.
3. The World Almanac & Book of Facts—1975. Published by Newspaper Enterprise Association, New York, Cleveland.
4. *Research Program Reports—1974—Summary of Research at the National Institute of Neurological Diseases and Stroke.* DHEW Publication No. (NIH) 74-697. U.S. Department of Health, Education, and Welfare, Public Health Service, National Institutes of Health, 1974.
5. *New England Journal of Medicine,* August 8, 1968.
6. Irving S. Wright, M.D., and associates, Cornell University Medical College, New York. Information confirmed October 1973.
7. Robert L. Ringler, M.D., Acting Director, National Heart and Lung Institute, National Institutes of Health, Bethesda, Md. Personal communication August 22, 1974.
8. *Drugs Against Cancer, April 1973,* National Cancer Institute, National Institutes of Health, Bethesda, Md.
9. James F. Holland, M.D., Roswell Park Memorial Institute, Buffalo, N.Y. Personal communication, August 30, 1974.
10. *Limitation of Activity and Mobility Due to Chronic Conditions, U.S., 1972 and 1970,* Series 10, no. 96. Data from the National Center for Health Statistics, U.S. Department of Health, Education, and Welfare, Rockville, Md., November 1974.
11. *Acute Conditions, U.S., July 1972-June 1973,* Series 10, no. 98. Data from National Center for Health Statistics, U.S. Department of Health, Education, and Welfare, Rockville, Md., January 1975.
12. *Ca—A Cancer Journal for Clinicians,* published by the American Cancer Society, New York, N.Y., July-August 1973.
13. Mrs. Sara W. Kelley, Director of Public Relations, United Cerebral Palsy Associations, Inc., New York, N.Y. Personal communication, March 8, 1973.
14. Edmund Klein, M.D., Chief, Department of Dermatology, Roswell Park Memorial Institute, Buffalo, N.Y., 1970.

15. Information supplied in 1973 and 1974 by Victor Wartofsky, Office of Public Information, National Institute of Arthritis, Metabolism and Digestive Diseases, National Institutes of Health, Bethesda, Md.
16. Information supplied by Ms. Margaret Suter, Information Office, National Institute of Neurological Diseases and Stroke, National Institutes of Health, Bethesda, Md., June 1973.
17. National Center for Health Statistics, unpublished data based on household interviews of the 1971 civilian, non-institutional population of 202,360,000, 1971.
18. National Health Expenditures, 1929-73, by Barbara S. Cooper, Nancy L. Worthington, and Paula A. Piro. Social Security Bulletin, February 1974. Department of Health, Education and Welfare, Washington, D.C.
19. "Optimal Resources for Cardiac Surgery." Reports of Inter-Society Commission for Heart Disease Resources, *Circulation* 44:A22 (September 1971), and *Circulation* 46:A325 (October 1972).
20. Charles C. Bennett, Director, Public and Professional Education. The Arthritis Foundation, New York, N.Y., October 1973.
21. Douglas McAlpine, Charles E. Lumsden, and E.D. Acheson, National Multiple Sclerosis Society, New York, N. Y., *Multiple Sclerosis—A Reappraisal, 2nd ed.* (Edinburgh and London: Churchill Livingstone, 1972).
22. George C. Cotzias, M.D., Brookhaven National Laboratory, Upton, L.I., N.Y., in personal communication dated July 30, 1974.
23. Ms. Helene Lindow, Public Relations Officer, Muscular Dystrophy Associations of America, Inc., New York, N.Y. Personal communication, November 1973.
24. *1973 Cancer Facts and Figures,* American Cancer Society, New York, N.Y.
25. *1973 Heart Facts,* American Heart Association, New York, N.Y.
26. Testimony of Dr. Philip A. Corfman, Acting Director, National Institute of Child Health and Human Development, before House of Representatives Subcommittee on Appropriations for the Department of Health, Education, and Welfare for 1975, March 28, 1974.
27. Based on computation prepared December 1969, by Owen McCrory, Consultant in Medical Economics, Ann Arbor, Mich.
28. Annual Survey Report 1971-72, Pharmaceutical Manufacturers Association, Washington, D.C.
29. Jeremiah Stamler, M.D., Director, Heart Disease Control Pro-

gram, Chronic Disease Control Division, Chicago Board of Health, "Breakthrough Against Hypertensive and Atherosclerotic Diseases?" *Geriatrics,* January 1962.
30. Budget of the U.S. Government, 1976.
31. *1973 Marketing Guide,* published by *Drug Topics,* Medical Economics Company, Oradell, N.J.
32. I.S. Wright, "Recent Developments in Antithrombotic Therapy," *Annals of Internal Medicine* 71:823 (October 1969).
33. I.S. Wright, "Anticoagulant Therapy—Practical Management," *American Heart Journal* 77:280 (1969).
34. William Berenberg, M.D., Professor of Pediatrics, Harvard Medical School, Boston. Personal communication dated July 26, 1974.
35. Elizabeth Macfarlane Hatfield, M.P.H., "Estimates of Blindness in the U.S.," *The Sight-Saving Review* 32, no. 2 (Summer 1973).
36. *Acute Conditions, Incidence and Associated Disability, U.S., July 1971-72,* Vital and Health Statistics, Series 10, no. 88, National Center for Health Statistics, Department of Health, Education, and Welfare, Rockville, Md.
37. William B. Kannel, M.D., Melvin J. Schwartz, M.D., and Patricia M. McNamara, "Blood Pressure and Risk of Coronary Heart Disease: The Framingham Study," *Diseases of the Chest* 56, no. 1 (July 1969).
38. "Anticoagulants in Acute Myocardial Infarction—Results of a Cooperative Clinical Trial (Veterans Administration)," *Journal of the American Medical Association* 4:225-724 (1973).
39. R. Wray, B. Maurer, and J. Shillingford, "Prophylactic Anticoagulant Therapy in the Prevention of Calf Vein Thrombosis After Myocardial Infarction," *New England Journal of Medicine* 228:815 (April 19, 1973).
40. Robert L. Schreiber, Information Officer, National Institute of Allergy and Infectious Diseases, Bethesda, Md. Information supplied 1973.
41. Harry Rosenwasser, M.D., Division of Medical Affairs, Deafness Research Foundation, New York, N.Y., August 1973.
42. Ms. Bonnie A. Friedman, Information Office, National Eye Institute, Bethesda, Md., May 1973.
43. *New England Journal of Medicine,* article by Dr. Herbert A. Schreier, Children's Hospital Medical Center, Boston, Mass., April 4, 1974, p. 8040.

Vital Statistics and Other Tables

Personal Consumption Expenditures by Type of Product, 1970

Food, alcoholic beverages, and tobacco	$142,900,000,000
Food—$114,000,000,000	
Alcoholic beverages—$17,000,000,000	
Tobacco—$11,200,000,000	
Housing	91,200,000,000
Household operation	85,600,000,000
Transportation	77,900,000,000
Clothing, accessories, and jewelry	62,300,000,000
Medical care expenses	47,300,000,000
Recreation	39,000,000,000
Personal business	35,500,000,000
Private education and research	10,400,000,000
Personal care (other than medical)	10,100,000,000
Religious and welfare activities	8,800,000,000
Foreign travel and remittances, net	4,800,000,000
Total personal consumption expenditures, 1970	$615,800,000,000

SOURCE: *Statistical Abstract of the United States, 1972*, 93rd. ed., U.S. Bureau of the Census, Washington, D.C., 1972.

Total Deaths and Death Rates, Deaths Under 60 Years of Age, Median Age at Death and Life Expectancy by Race and Sex: Death-Registration States, 1930–1972[1]

(Exclusive of fetal deaths. Rates per 1,000 population enumerated as of April 1 for 1940 and 1950 and estimated as of July 1 for other years)

Year	Total Deaths Number	Rate	Deaths under 60 years of age	Median Age at Death (in Years) White Total	Male	Female	Nonwhite Male	Female	Life Expectancy (in Years) White Total	Male	Female	Nonwhite Male	Female
1930	1,327,240	11.3	743,645	55.5	57.2	59.6	41.3	38.8	59.7	59.7	63.5	47.3	49.2
1931	1,307,273	11.1	721,871	56.2	57.8	60.2	41.3	39.1	61.1	60.8	64.7	49.5	51.5
1932	1,293,269	10.9	682,305	58.0	59.4	61.7	42.8	40.9	62.1	62.0	64.5	52.8	54.6
1933	1,342,106	10.7	704,060	58.2	59.6	61.8	43.0	41.4	63.3	62.7	66.3	53.5	56.0
1934	1,396,903	11.1	730,885	58.3	59.7	62.1	43.1	41.3	61.1	60.5	64.6	50.2	53.7
1935	1,392,752	10.9	716,419	59.0	60.1	62.7	43.9	42.3	61.7	61.0	65.0	51.3	55.2
1936	1,479,228	11.6	742,739	59.8	60.7	63.7	44.8	43.0	58.5	58.0	61.9	47.0	51.4
1937	1,450,427	11.3	721,648	60.1	60.9	64.0	45.4	43.2	60.0	59.3	63.8	48.3	52.5
1938	1,381,391	10.6	667,903	60.9	61.7	64.8	46.0	44.1	63.5	63.2	66.8	51.7	54.3
1939	1,387,897	10.6	644,786	62.0	62.5	65.8	47.3	45.7	63.7	63.3	66.6	53.2	56.0
1940	1,417,269	10.8	641,436	62.6	63.0	66.4	48.6	46.7	62.9	62.1	66.6	51.5	54.9
1941	1,397,642	10.5	635,047	62.5	62.9	65.4	48.2	46.3	64.8	64.4	68.5	52.5	55.3
1942	1,385,187	10.3	621,504	62.8	62.9	66.7	48.8	47.3	66.2	65.9	69.4	55.4	58.2
1943	1,459,544	10.9	639,065	63.4	63.4	67.2	50.0	48.6	63.3	63.2	65.7	55.4	56.1
1944	1,411,338	10.6	610,621	63.6	63.6	67.4	50.6	48.5	65.2	64.5	68.4	55.8	57.7
1945	1,401,719	10.6	596,369	63.9	63.8	67.7	51.0	49.3	65.9	64.4	69.5	56.1	59.6
1946	1,395,617	10.0	586,847	64.2	63.9	68.1	51.2	50.0	66.7	65.1	70.3	57.5	61.0
1947	1,445,370	10.1	590,058	64.8	64.4	68.7	52.2	51.1	66.8	65.2	70.5	57.9	61.9
1948	1,444,337	9.9	575,414	65.2	64.8	69.2	52.8	51.9	67.2	65.5	71.0	58.1	62.5

Year										
1949	1,443,607	9.7	560,777	65.6	65.2	69.6	53.1	52.6	68.0	66.2	71.9	58.9	62.7
1950	1,452,454	9.6	545,405	66.2	65.7	70.2	54.2	53.5	68.2	66.5	72.2	59.1	62.9
1951	1,482,099	9.7	551,387	66.4	65.9	70.4	54.3	54.0	68.4	66.5	72.4	59.1	63.3
1952	1,496,838	9.6	553,123	66.5	65.9	70.6	54.4	54.0	68.6	66.6	72.7	59.1	63.7
1953	1,517,541	9.6	542,670	67.0	66.3	71.0	55.1	54.9	68.8	66.8	72.9	59.7	64.4
1954	1,481,091	9.2	519,600	67.3	66.6	71.3	55.2	55.0	69.6	67.4	73.6	61.0	65.8
1955	1,528,717	9.3	519,734	67.8	67.0	71.9	55.9	56.1	69.5	67.3	73.6	61.2	65.9
1956	1,564,476	9.4	523,868	68.0	67.2	72.2	56.3	56.7	69.6	67.3	73.7	61.1	65.9
1957	1,633,128	9.6	541,380	68.2	67.4	72.2	56.3	57.1	69.3	67.1	73.5	60.3	65.2
1958	1,647,886	9.5	538,948	68.5	67.6	72.7	57.0	57.4	69.4	67.2	73.7	60.6	65.5
1959	1,656,814	9.4	539,646	68.7	67.6	72.9	56.9	57.6	69.9	67.6	74.2	61.4	66.5
1960	1,711,982	9.5	547,771	68.9	67.9	73.1	57.8	58.6	69.7	67.4	74.1	61.1	66.3
1961	1,701,522	9.3	538,320	69.2	68.1	73.4	58.1	59.5	70.2	67.8	74.5	61.9	67.0
1962	1,757,000	9.5	546,329	69.5	68.3	73.7	58.6	60.2	70.0	67.6	74.4	61.5	66.8
1963	1,813,549	9.6	557,938	69.7	68.5	74.0	59.1	60.5	69.9	67.5	74.4	60.9	66.5
1964	1,798,051	9.4	557,593	69.6	68.4	74.0	58.3	60.4	70.2	67.7	74.6	61.1	67.2
1965	1,828,136	9.4	556,150	69.9	68.6	74.3	58.8	60.9	70.2	67.6	74.7	61.1	67.4
1966	1,863,149	9.5	559,590	70.1	68.6	74.6	59.0	61.6	70.1	67.6	74.7	60.7	67.4
1967	1,851,323	9.4	551,936	70.7	68.7	74.7	59.0	61.8	70.5	67.8	75.1	61.1	68.2
1968	1,930,082	9.7	567,483	70.3	68.8	75.0	59.3	62.7	70.2	67.5	74.9	60.1	67.5
1969	1,921,990	9.5	575,340	70.3	68.7	75.1	58.9	62.7	70.4	67.8	75.1	60.5	68.4
1970*	1,921,000	9.4	564,070	70.3	68.6	75.1	58.7	63.3	70.8	68.1	75.4	60.5	68.9
1971*	1,921,000	9.3	548,730	70.6	68.9	75.5	59.8	63.4	71.1	68.3	75.7	61.3	69.4
1972*	1,962,000	9.4	N.A.	N.A.	N.A.	N.A.	N.A.	N.A.	N.A.	N.A.	N.A.	N.A.	N.A.

NOTE: Figures exclude deaths among armed forces overseas. Rates based on population excluding armed forces overseas. All figures from Vital Statistics Division, National Center for Health Statistics, U.S. Public Health Service, Washington, D.C.

1. The death-registration states increased in number from 43 states and the District of Columbia in 1927 to the entire continental United States in 1933. All medians are based on deaths by 5-year age groups except for 1961.

*Figures are estimated.

N.A.—figures not presently available.

Maternal Mortality Rates and Infant Mortality Rates: Birth-Registration States,[1] 1930–1972

(Maternal mortality rates and infant mortality rates per 1,000 live births)

Year	Maternal mortality rates[2]	Infant Mortality Rates[3]		
		Under 1 year	Under 1 month	1-11 months
1930	6.73	64.6	35.7	28.9
1931	6.60	61.6	34.6	27.0
1932	6.33	57.6	33.5	24.1
1933	6.19	58.1	34.0	24.1
1934	5.93	60.1	34.1	26.0
1935	5.82	55.7	32.4	23.3
1936	5.68	57.1	32.6	24.6
1937	4.89	54.4	31.3	23.2
1938	4.35	51.0	29.6	21.4
1939	4.04	48.0	29.3	18.7
1940	3.41	47.0	28.8	18.3
1941	2.88	45.3	27.7	17.7
1942	2.35	40.4	25.7	14.7
1943	2.23	40.4	24.7	15.6
1944	2.28	39.8	24.7	15.1
1945	2.07	38.3	24.3	13.9
1946	1.57	33.8	24.0	9.7
1947	1.35	32.2	22.8	9.4
1948	1.17	32.0	22.2	9.8
1949	0.90	31.3	21.4[4]	9.9[5]
1950	0.83	29.2	20.5[4]	8.7[5]
1951	0.75	28.4	20.0[4]	8.4[5]
1952	0.68	28.4	19.8[4]	8.6[5]
1953	0.61	27.8	19.6[4]	8.2[5]
1954	0.52	26.6	19.1[4]	7.5[5]
1955	0.47	26.4	19.1[4]	7.3[5]
1956	0.41	26.0	18.9[4]	7.1[5]
1957	0.41	26.3	19.1[4]	7.3[5]
1958	0.38	27.1	19.5[4]	7.6[5]
1959	0.37	26.4	19.0[4]	7.4[5]
1960	0.37	26.0	18.7[4]	7.3[5]
1961	0.37	25.3	18.4[4]	6.9[5]
1962	0.35	25.3	18.3[4]	7.0[5]
1963	0.36	25.2	18.2[4]	7.0[5]
1964	0.33	24.8	17.9[4]	6.9[5]
1965	0.32	24.7	17.7[4]	7.0[5]
1966	0.29	23.7	17.2[4]	6.5[5]
1967	0.28	22.4	16.5[4]	5.9[5]

1968	0.25	21.8	16.1[4]	5.7[5]
1969*	0.27	20.7	15.4[4]	5.4[5]
1970*	0.25	19.8	14.9[4]	4.9[5]
1971*	0.21	19.2	14.3[4]	4.9[5]
1972*	0.24	18.5	13.7[4]	4.8[5]

1. The birth-registration states increased in number from 40 states and the District of Columbia in 1927 to the entire continental United States in 1933.
2. The rates are based on deaths classified by the International List of Causes of Deaths.
3. Exclusive of fetal deaths.
4. Under 28 days.
5. From 28 days to 11 months.

All figures from the Vital Statistics Division, National Center for Health Statistics, U.S. Public Health Service, Washington, D.C.

National Health Expenditures

Expenditures for medical care reached *$71 billion in 1970; preliminary estimates for 1971 put the figure at more than $75 billion.* Medical care outlays have grown at a rapid pace, faster than that of the economy in general. In 1929, they represented 3.5 percent of the gross national product; by 1970, the share of GNP for this purpose had reached 7.3 percent.

Deaths for Selected Causes: United States, 1968-1973

(For 1972 and 1973, based on a 10-percent sample of deaths; for all other years, based on final data)

Cause of death		Number					
		1973	1972	1971	1970	1969	1968
All causes		1,977,000	1,962,000	1,927,542	1,921,031	1,921,990	1,930,082
Bacillary dysentery and amebiasis	004,006	90	70	84	89	94	111
Enteritis and other diarrheal diseases	008,009	2,370	2,180	2,466	2,567	2,612	2,940
Tuberculosis, all forms	010-019	3,870	4,550	4,501	5,217	5,567	6,292
Tuberculosis of respiratory system	010-012	3,000	3,580	3,590	4,162	4,492	5,009
Tuberculosis, other forms	013-019	870	970	911	1,055	1,075	1,283
Whooping cough	033	10	—	18	12	13	36
Streptococcal sore throat and scarlet fever	034	20	—	23	29	41	28
Meningococcal infections	036	290	420	509	550	744	741
Septicemia	038	4,290	4,180	3,907	3,535	3,009	2,991
Acute poliomyelitis	040-043	20	20	18	7	13	24
Measles	055	10	—	90	89	41	24
Infectious hepatitis	070	700	700	906	1,014	1,011	877
Syphilis and its sequelae	090-097	410	320	375	461	543	586
Other infective and parasitic diseases	Remainder of 000-136	3,350	3,360	3,130	3,079	3,103	3,126
Malignant neoplasms, including neoplasms of lymphatic and hematopoietic tissues	140-209	353,440	346,930	337,398	330,730	323,092	318,547
Malignant neoplasms of buccal cavity and pharynx	140-149	8,350	7,520	7,725	7,612	7,553	7,294
Malignant neoplasms of digestive organs and peritoneum	150-159	97,610	97,180	94,914	94,703	93,986	93,563
Malignant neoplasms of respiratory system	160-163	78,330	76,860	72,898	69,517	66,038	63,485
Malignant neoplasms of breast	174	31,980	31,070	30,277	29,917	29,083	29,081
Malignant neoplasms of genital organs	180-187	42,460	42,470	42,017	41,190	41,008	40,936
Malignant neoplasms of urinary organs	188,189	16,810	15,520	15,288	15,514	14,897	14,792
Malignant neoplasms of all other and unspecified sites	170-173,190-199	43,020	41,870	40,685	39,068	37,825	37,247
Leukemia	204-207	15,050	14,630	14,469	14,492	14,450	14,375
Other neoplasms of lymphatic and hematopoietic tissues	200-203,208,209	19,830	19,810	19,125	18,717	18,252	17,774

Benign neoplasms and neoplasms of unspecified nature	210-239	5,540	5,870	4,958	4,828	4,677	4,948
Diabetes mellitus	250	36,450	39,070	38,256	38,324	38,541	38,352
Avitaminoses and other nutritional deficiencies	260-269	2,360	2,400	2,537	2,470	2,534	2,543
Anemias	280-285	3,250	3,060	3,449	3,427	3,318	3,494
Meningitis	320	1,600	1,350	1,553	1,701	1,719	1,707
Major cardiovascular diseases	390-448	1,037,460	1,028,560	1,017,145	1,007,984	1,013,015	1,023,399
Diseases of heart	390-398,402,404,410-429	754,460	752,450	743,368	735,542	739,265	744,658
Active rheumatic fever and chronic rheumatic heart disease	390-398	13,580	14,090	14,644	14,889	15,432	16,358
Hypertensive heart disease	402	7,810	7,570	7,860	8,413	8,976	9,811
Hypertensive heart and renal disease	404	5,390	5,550	6,190	6,578	7,310	7,887
Ischemic heart disease	410-413	682,910	688,100	674,292	666,665	669,829	674,747
Acute myocardial infarction	410	348,010	357,590	357,714	357,241	361,583	369,610
Other acute and subacute forms of ischemic heart disease	411	4,330	4,400	4,027	4,246	4,677	4,691
Chronic ischemic heart disease	412	330,440	320,950	312,351	304,962	303,362	300,216
Angina pectoris	413	130	160	200	216	207	230
Chronic disease of endocardium and other myocardial insufficiency	424,428	4,870	5,330	6,132	6,705	7,475	7,836
All other forms of heart disease	420-423,425-427,429	39,900	36,810	34,250	32,292	30,243	28,019
Hypertension	400,401,403	8,010	7,680	7,837	8,273	8,426	9,063
Cerebrovascular diseases	430-438	214,650	210,050	209,092	207,166	207,179	211,390
Cerebral hemorrhage	431	34,270	36,580	38,563	41,379	43,303	47,002
Cerebral thrombosis	433	56,260	56,460	57,229	57,845	58,748	60,331
Cerebral embolism	434	940	890	954	884	1,005	1,136
All other cerebrovascular diseases	430,432,435-438	123,180	116,120	112,346	107,058	104,123	102,921
Arteriosclerosis	440	33,430	32,820	31,521	31,682	33,063	33,568
Other diseases of arteries, arterioles, and capillaries	441-448	26,910	25,560	25,327	25,321	25,082	24,720
Acute bronchitis and bronchiolitis	466	810	1,080	1,154	1,310	1,286	1,432
Influenza and pneumonia	470-474,480-486	61,160	61,160	57,194	62,739	68,365	73,492
Influenza	470-474	4,970	5,010	1,504	3,707	5,971	7,062
Pneumonia	480-486	56,190	56,150	55,690	59,032	62,394	66,430
Bronchitis, emphysema, and asthma	490-493	30,280	28,760	30,284	30,889	31,144	33,078
Chronic and unqualified bronchitis	490,491	5,810	5,360	5,591	5,846	5,843	6,205
Emphysema	492	22,540	21,310	22,539	22,721	22,939	24,185
Asthma	493	1,930	2,090	2,154	2,322	2,362	2,688

Cause of death		1973	1972	1971	1970	1969	1968
Peptic ulcer	531-533	7,830	7,660	8,120	8,607	9,312	9,460
Appendicitis	540-543	940	1,130	1,295	1,397	1,407	1,485
Hernia and intestinal obstruction	550-553,560	6,710	6,280	6,989	7,235	7,500	7,758
Cirrhosis of liver	571	33,630	32,760	31,808	31,399	29,866	29,183
Cholelithiasis, cholecystitis and cholangitis	574,575	3,280	3,630	3,735	3,973	4,262	4,385
Nephritis and nephrosis	580-584	7,740	8,190	8,443	8,877	9,417	9,311
Acute nephritis and nephrotic syndrome	580,581	1,380	1,550	1,373	1,354	1,392	1,294
Chronic and unqualified nephritis and renal sclerosis	582-584	6,360	6,640	7,070	7,523	8,025	8,017
Infections of kidney	590	6,100	7,010	7,558	8,190	8,750	9,395
Hyperplasia of prostate	600	1,700	1,900	1,918	2,168	2,499	2,647
Complications of pregnancy, childbirth, and the puerperium	630-678	470	780	668	803	801	859
Abortions	640-645	10	140	99	128	132	133
Other complications of pregnancy, childbirth, and the puerperium	630-639,650-678	460	640	569	675	669	726
Congenital anomalies	740-759	13,940	15,050	15,957	16,824	17,008	16,793
Certain causes of mortality in early infancy	760-769.2,769.4-772,774-778	31,030	34,240	38,494	43,205	43,171	43,840
Birth injury, difficult labor, and other anoxic and hypoxic conditions	764-768,772,776	17,790	18,940	20,992	22,801	21,939	22,132
Other causes of mortality in early infancy	Remainder of 760-778	13,240	15,300	17,502	20,404	21,232	21,708
Symptoms and ill-defined conditions	780-796	38,310	36,170	26,534	25,781	26,160	23,656
All other diseases	Residual	112,700	110,910	104,680	101,128	97,982	97,305
Accidents	E800-E949	115,040	113,670	113,439	114,638	116,385	114,864
Motor vehicle accidents	E810-E823	55,690	56,590	54,381	54,633	55,791	54,862
All other accidents	E800-E807,E825-E949	59,350	57,080	59,058	60,005	60,594	60,002
Suicide	E950-E959	24,440	24,280	24,092	23,480	22,364	21,372
Homicide	E960-E978	19,700	18,880	18,787	16,848	15,477	14,686
Other external causes	E980-E999	5,370	5,690	5,070	5,427	5,147	4,315

SOURCE: National Center for Health Statistics, U.S. Public Health Service, Rockville, Maryland.

Aggregate National Health Expenditures, by Type of Expenditure, Selected Years, 1950–1970
(In Millions)

Type of service	1950	1955	1960	1965	1968	1969	1970
Total	$12,867	$18,036	$26,973	$40,591	$57,103	$63,989	$71,161
Health services and supplies	11,910	17,099	25,263	37,210	53,078	59,114	65,797
Hospital care	3,845	5,929	9,044	13,520	20,751	24,223	27,961
Short-term	2,234	3,640	6,032	9,545	15,418	—	—
Long-term	1,611	2,289	3,012	3,975	5,333	—	—
Physicians' services	2,755	3,680	5,684	8,745	11,562	12,378	13,600
Dentists' services	975	1,525	1,977	2,808	3,612	4,047	4,440
Other professional services	395	559	862	1,038	1,342	1,343	1,431
Drugs and drug sundries	1,730	2,385	3,657	4,850	6,149	6,731	7,211
Eyeglasses and appliances	490	597	776	1,230	1,718	1,818	1,884
Nursing-home care	142	222	526	1,328	2,282	2,650	3,100
Expenses for prepayment and administration	300	614	863	1,297	1,847	2,109	2,097
Government public health activities	361	377	412	696	969	1,227	1,439
Other health services	917	1,211	1,462	1,698	2,846	2,588	2,634
Research and medical-facilities construction	957	937	1,710	3,381	4,025	4,875	5,364
Research	117	216	662	1,469	1,765	1,819	1,934
Construction	840	721	1,048	1,912	2,260	3,056	3,430

Source: Barbara S. Cooper, Nancy L. Worthington, and Mary F. McGee, *Compendium of National Health Expenditures, 1929-70*, Office of Research and Statistics, Social Security Administration, U.S. Department of Health, Education, and Welfare, Washington, D.C.

Cause of death		1973	1972	1971	Number 1970	1969	1968
All causes		942.1	942.2	932.2	945.3	951.9	965.7
Bacillary dysentery and amebiasis	004,006	0.0	0.0	0.0	0.0	0.0	0.1
Enteritis and other diarrheal diseases	008,009	1.1	1.0	1.2	1.3	1.3	1.5
Tuberculosis, all forms	010-019	1.8	2.2	2.2	2.6	2.8	3.1
Tuberculosis of respiratory system	010-012	1.4	1.7	1.7	2.0	2.2	2.5
Tuberculosis, other forms	013-019	0.4	0.5	0.4	0.5	0.5	0.6
Whooping cough	033	0.0	—	0.0	0.0	0.0	0.0
Streptococcal sore throat and scarlet fever	034	0.0	—	0.0	0.0	0.0	0.0
Meningococcal infections	036	0.1	0.2	0.2	0.3	0.4	0.4
Septicemia	038	2.0	2.0	1.9	1.7	1.5	1.5
Acute poliomyelitis	040-043	0.0	0.0	0.0	0.0	0.0	0.0
Measles	055	0.0	—	0.0	0.0	0.0	0.0
Infectious hepatitis	070	0.3	0.3	0.4	0.5	0.5	0.4
Syphilis and its sequelae	090-097	0.2	0.2	0.2	0.2	0.3	0.3
Other infective and parasitic diseases	Remainder of 000-136	1.6	1.6	1.5	1.5	1.5	1.6
Malignant neoplasms, including neoplasms of lymphatic and hematopoietic tissues	140-209	168.4	166.6	163.2	162.8	160.0	159.4
Malignant neoplasms of buccal cavity and pharynx	140-149	4.0	3.6	3.7	3.7	3.7	3.6
Malignant neoplasms of digestive organs and peritoneum	150-159	46.5	46.7	45.9	46.6	46.5	46.8
Malignant neoplasms of respiratory system	160-163	37.3	36.9	35.3	34.2	32.7	31.8
Malignant neoplasms of breast	174	15.2	14.9	14.6	14.7	14.4	14.6
Malignant neoplasms of genital organs	180-187	20.2	20.4	20.3	20.3	20.3	20.5
Malignant neoplasms of urinary organs	188,189	8.0	7.5	7.4	7.6	7.4	7.4
Malignant neoplasms of all other and unspecified sites	170-173,190-199	20.5	20.1	19.7	19.2	18.7	18.6
Leukemia	204-207	7.2	7.0	7.0	7.1	7.2	7.2
Other neoplasms of lymphatic and hematopoietic tissues	200-203,208,209	9.4	9.5	9.2	9.2	9.0	8.9
Benign neoplasms and neoplasms of unspecified nature	210-239	2.6	2.8	2.4	2.4	2.3	2.5
Diabetes mellitus	250	17.4	18.8	18.5	18.9	19.1	19.2
Avitaminoses and other nutritional deficiencies	260-269	1.1	1.2	1.2	1.2	1.3	1.3

Anemias	280-285	1.5	1.5	1.7	1.7	1.6	1.7	
Meningitis	320	0.8	0.6	0.8	0.8	0.9	0.9	
Major cardiovascular diseases	390-448	494.4	493.9	491.9	496.0	501.7	512.1	
Diseases of heart	390-398,402,404,410-429	359.5	361.3	359.5	362.0	366.1	372.6	
Active rheumatic fever and chronic rheumatic heart disease	390-398	6.5	6.8	7.1	7.3	7.6	8.2	
Hypertensive heart disease	402	3.7	3.6	3.8	4.1	4.4	4.9	
Hypertensive heart and renal disease	404	2.6	2.7	3.0	3.2	3.6	3.9	
Ischemic heart disease	410-413	325.4	328.0	326.1	328.1	331.7	337.6	
Acute myocardial infarction	410	165.8	171.7	173.0	175.8	179.1	184.9	
Other acute and subacute forms of ischemic heart disease	411	2.1	2.1	1.9	2.1	2.3	2.3	
Chronic ischemic heart disease	412	157.5	154.1	151.1	150.1	150.2	150.2	
Angina pectoris	413	0.1	0.1	0.1	0.1	0.1	0.1	
Chronic disease of endocardium and other myocardial insufficiency	424,428	2.3	2.6	3.0	3.3	3.7	3.9	
All other forms of heart disease	420-423,425-427,429	19.0	17.7	16.6	15.9	15.0	14.0	
Hypertension	400,401,403	3.8	3.7	3.8	4.1	4.2	4.5	
Cerebrovascular diseases	430-438	102.3	100.9	101.1	101.9	102.6	105.8	
Cerebral hemorrhage	431	16.3	17.6	18.6	20.4	21.4	23.5	
Cerebral thrombosis	433	26.8	27.1	27.7	28.5	29.1	30.2	
Cerebral embolism	434	0.4	0.4	0.5	0.4	0.5	0.6	
All other cerebrovascular diseases	430,432,435-438	58.7	55.8	54.3	52.7	51.6	51.5	
Arteriosclerosis	440	15.9	15.8	15.2	15.6	16.4	16.8	
Other diseases of arteries, arterioles, and capillaries	441-448	12.8	12.3	12.2	12.5	12.4	12.4	
Acute bronchitis and bronchiolitis	466	0.4	0.5	0.6	0.6	0.6	0.7	
Influenza and pneumonia	470-474,480-486	29.1	29.4	27.7	30.9	33.9	36.8	
Influenza	470-474	2.4	2.4	0.7	1.8	3.0	3.5	
Pneumonia	480-486	26.8	27.0	26.9	29.0	30.9	33.2	
Bronchitis, emphysema, and asthma	490-493	14.4	13.8	14.6	15.2	15.4	16.6	
Chronic and unqualified bronchitis	490,491	2.8	2.6	2.7	2.9	2.9	3.1	
Emphysema	492	10.7	10.2	10.9	11.2	11.4	12.1	
Asthma	493	0.9	1.0	1.0	1.1	1.2	1.3	
Peptic ulcer	531-533	3.7	3.7	3.9	4.2	4.6	4.7	
Appendicitis	540-543	0.4	0.5	0.6	0.7	0.7	0.7	
Hernia and intestinal obstruction	550-553,560	3.2	3.0	3.4	3.6	3.7	3.9	

Cause of death		1973	1972	1971	1970	1969	1968
Cirrhosis of liver	571	16.0	15.7	15.4	15.5	14.8	14.6
Cholelithiasis, cholecystitis and cholangitis	574,575	1.6	1.7	1.8	2.0	2.1	2.2
Nephritis and nephrosis	580-584	3.7	3.9	4.1	4.4	4.7	4.7
Acute nephritis and nephrotic syndrome	580,581	0.7	0.7	0.7	0.7	0.7	0.6
Chronic and unqualified nephritis and renal sclerosis	582-584	3.0	3.2	3.4	3.7	4.0	4.0
Infections of kidney	590	2.9	3.4	3.7	4.0	4.3	4.7
Hyperplasia of prostate	600	0.8	0.9	0.9	1.1	1.2	1.3
Complications of pregnancy, childbirth, and the puerperium	630-678	0.2	0.4	0.3	0.4	0.4	0.4
Abortions	640-645	0.0	0.1	0.0	0.1	0.1	0.1
Other complications of pregnancy, childbirth, and the puerperium	630-639,650-678	0.2	0.3	0.3	0.3	0.3	0.4
Congenital anomalies	740-759	6.6	7.2	7.7	8.3	8.4	8.4
Certain causes of mortality in early infancy	760-769.2,769.4-772,774-778	14.8	16.4	18.6	21.3	21.4	21.9
Birth injury, difficult labor, and other anoxic and hypoxic conditions	764-768,772,776	8.5	9.1	10.2	11.2	10.9	11.1
Other causes of mortality in early infancy	Remainder of 760-778	6.3	7.3	8.5	10.0	10.5	10.9
Symptoms and ill-defined conditions	780-796	18.3	17.4	12.8	12.7	13.0	11.8
All other diseases	Residual	53.7	53.3	50.6	49.8	48.5	48.7
Accidents	E800-E949	54.8	54.6	54.9	56.4	57.6	57.5
Motor vehicle accidents	E810-E823	26.5	27.2	26.3	26.9	27.6	27.5
All other accidents	E800-E807,E825-E949	28.3	27.4	28.6	29.5	30.0	30.0
Suicide	E950-E959	11.6	11.7	11.7	11.6	11.1	10.7
Homicide	E960-E978	9.4	9.1	9.1	8.3	7.7	7.3
Other external causes	E980-E999	2.6	2.7	2.5	2.7	2.5	2.2

SOURCE: National Center for Health Statistics, U.S. Public Health Service, Rockville, Maryland.

DISTRIBUTION OF FAMILIES BY TOTAL MONEY INCOME—1972—UNITED STATES

Money Income	No. of Families	Percentage
Under $4,000		
Under $1,000	683,000	1.3%
$1,000 to $1,999	1,183,000	2.2%
$2,000 to $2,999	2,018,000	3.7%
$3,000 to $3,999	2,494,000	4.6%
Total	6,378,000	11.8%
$4,000 to $6,000		
$4,000 to $4,999	2,670,000	4.9%
$5,000 to $5,999	2,735,000	5.0%
Total	5,405,000	9.9%
$6,000 and over		
$6,000 to $6,999	2,828,000	5.2%
$7,000 to $7,999	3,030,000	5.6%
$8,000 to $9,999	6,063,000	11.1%
$10,000 to $14,999	14,192,000	26.1%
$15,000 and over	16,478,000	30.3%
Total	42,591,000	78.3%
Grand total	54,374,000	100.0%
Median income	$11,116	

SOURCE: Current Population Reports, Series P-60 No. 90, December 1973. Consumer Income, Bureau of the Census, U.S. Department of Commerce, Washington, D.C.